To Susan,

With grateful thanks!

Love,

John.

Medical Embryology

John C. McLachlan

3rd March, 1994.

Medical Embryology

JOHN McLACHLAN

University of St Andrews

 Addison-Wesley Publishing Company

Wokingham, England • Reading, Massachusetts • Menlo Park, California • New York
Don Mills, Ontario • Amsterdam • Bonn • Sydney • Singapore
Tokyo • Madrid • San Juan • Milan • Paris • Mexico City • Seoul • Taipei

ACQUISITIONS EDITOR: Jane Hogg
PRODUCTION EDITOR: Susan Keany
PRODUCTION CONTROLLER: Jim Allman
PRODUCTION MANAGER: Stephen Bishop
COPYEDITORS: Jane Bryant and Helen Juden
PROOFREADERS: Judith Ockenden and Helen MacDonald
INDEXER: Liza Weinkove
COVER DESIGNERS: Designers & Partners incorporating a photograph by
    James Stevenson/Science Photo Library
ILLUSTRATIONS: Angela Christie
TEXT DESIGN: Valerie O'Donnell
TYPESETTER: VAP Group Ltd
Printed in Singapore

First printed 1994

ISBN 0-201-54420-2

British Library Cataloguing in Publication Data
A catalogue record for this book is available from the British Library.

Library of Congress Cataloging in Publication Data applied for.

Acknowledgements
The publishers wish to thank the following for permission to use photographs in this book:
Dr David Edgar; Dr Martin Milner; Dr G. B. Shellswell; Ninewells Hospital, Dundee; and the Anatomy Museum, University of St Andrews.

Preface

Embryology has always been of value to medical students in understanding anatomy. In addition, abnormalities arising during development are important both to the individual and to society. But until recently little could be done about such abnormalities before birth, so their study was of theoretical rather than practical interest. Now that methods of diagnosis exist for the prenatal detection of many abnormalities, termination of pregnancy is exerting a significant effect on the incidence of such conditions at birth. Intervention is possible at many stages and difficult calculations of relative risk arise, along with complex ethical dilemmas. The ability to manipulate human fertility also requires a new level of understanding of the early stages of development. Also, embryology, or more accurately the wider field of developmental biology, has increasing importance in understanding cancer and other developmental diseases.

These advances must be reflected in textbooks of human development aimed at medical students. However, a new style is desirable for such a textbook in addition to new content. Developmental biology is an experimental subject: the inferences it draws are conditional and liable to alteration. It is essential that students appreciate this, for the sake of the subject itself and to promote their understanding of the scientific process as a whole. The experimental bases for at least some of the current beliefs about development are therefore indicated in this book. This inevitably requires reference to animal models: however, the dramatic discoveries of the last 5 years have confirmed the unity of developmental mechanisms throughout the animal kingdom and validated the applicability of these models.

All this cannot be done merely by adding new material to the magisterial canon of descriptive embryology: the medical curriculum is already overloaded to the point that students lose sight of general principles in the morass of detail. The material appropriate for teaching must be reconsidered and reduced where possible. In addition, some curious myths have grown up about human development and have been passed from textbook to textbook over a period of decades. Revision of these requires a return to original source material; however, it is unrealistic to expect students to pursue topics through extensive reading lists and brief references are given more as a guide to teachers than to students.

Developmental biology is also part of the grand unification of cellular and molecular biology currently taking place. While this is outside the scope of this book I have tried to indicate links between classical embryology and modern cell biology where possible. I would regard the book as a success if students came to realize through it that a description is not the same as an explanation.

I believe that an appreciation of the evolutionary background to the appearance of certain structures is the key to understanding their morphogenesis during development, and so brief notes on evolution are included where appropriate.

Development can be approached either chronologically or by region; most embryology textbooks use both methods. In this book, Part I deals mainly with events in the pre-embryonic period. Part II considers the major tissue types on a systematic basis and Part III describes regional development during the embryonic period. Regional structures are considered in craniocaudal sequence, as far as possible. Part IV deals with the succession of generations. This plan means that there is occasional overlap with the systematic section, but I believe that this is justifiable in the interests of clarity.

I wish to acknowledge with gratitude the friends and colleagues, too many to name, who reviewed sections of the manuscript or helped me with particular questions. Particular thanks, however, are due to Dr Susan Whiten, who read the complete manuscript and made many valuable suggestions and Dr David Sinclair who helped me with clinical questions. I also wish to thank Jane Hogg and Susan Keany of Addison-Wesley for all their help and encouragement. Finally, thanks to my undergraduate students who have made the teaching of human development so interesting and stimulating and whose curiosity contributed greatly to the book as it now stands.

John McLachlan
Balmullo, Scotland
December 1993

Contents

27 The menstrual cycle and pregnancy   376

Timing and orientation

A necessary preliminary to understanding human development is that we learn how to describe when and where various events take place.

Timing

The various stages of human life before birth have specific names which are also, unfortunately, in common non-specific use. It is therefore necessary to provide definitions of these right at the beginning.

The time from fertilization to birth can be divided into three main phases, each of which has unique properties.

During the first 3 weeks after fertilization a number of subphases exist which, in recent times, have been grouped together as the **pre-embryonic period**. The **embryonic period** runs from the beginning of the fourth week after fertilization to the end of the eighth week. The third phase runs from the beginning of the ninth week until birth, and is known as the **fetal period**. The terms **pre-embryo**, **embryo** and **fetus** should used only when referring to these periods.

A useful distinction can be drawn between the tissues that will contribute to the baby that is born, and those, the **extraembryonic membranes**, which contribute to life support mechanisms but will not be part of the baby itself. Thus the terms **embryo** and **fetus** are sometimes used to refer to the tissues giving rise to the baby only. The products of fertilization as a whole – the embryo and its extraembryonic membranes, for instance – can conveniently be described as the **conceptus**.

Of course, in vivo, the moment of fertilization cannot be easily distinguished. The first time at which pregnancy is usually detected by the mother is when the next menstrual period fails to occur. The imprecision of the menstrual cycle means that failure of manstruation often cannot be dated exactly, so the convention is that the duration of pregnancy is calculated from the date of the last menstrual period. This is referred to as weeks or months of **gestation**.

Ironically, this means that for the first 2 weeks of gestation, the mother was not yet pregnant! Unless otherwise specified, times in this book refer to time after fertilization.

The pre-embryonic period

The pre-embryonic period is divided into a number of named subphases (see also Chapter 2). The newly fertilized egg is known as the **zygote**. During the first few days after fertilization, the zygote divides several times to form a ball of cells called the **morula**. At about day 4 the morula begins to develop an internal space and is thereafter described as the **blastocyst**. This will implant in the wall of the uterus at about day 6. Towards the end of the second week after fertilization the main body axis begins to become apparent, though at first in rather subtle ways. This process is called **gastrulation**, and this stage is therefore referred to as the **gastrula**. Next, the existence of the main body axis is confirmed by the development of the neural tube (corresponding to the brain and spinal cord in the adult). This process is known as **neurulation**: hence this stage is known as the **neurula**. By the time neurulation is completed, the embryonic period is about to begin.

During the pre-embryonic period, rapid cell division occurs. The main axis of the embryo, and the progenitors of all the body tissues, are established by the end of this phase. However, this time is marked by strongly regulative behaviour. Damage to any part of the conceptus has a good chance of being repaired completely: many cells are not committed to a particular fate, and can change their nature to compensate for any deficiencies. As a result the pre-embryo can be exposed to quite severe environmental insults, and still the resulting embryo may develop unscathed: however, so many cells may be damaged that the conceptus is no longer viable.

The embryonic period

During the embryonic period, development is much more sensitive to disturbance. During this time all the main body organs are laid down, and by the end of the embryonic period the embryo is recognizably human in appearance, although it is still tiny: only 3 cm from head to tail. The complexity of tissue interactions during organ formation offers a likely explanation as to why the embryo is so susceptible to environmental damage and, as a result, this period is sometimes known as the **critical period** of development.

The fetal period

From 9 weeks to birth the fetus, as it can now be called, grows in size and maturity. All its organs have been laid down, at least in rudimentary form, during the embryonic period, but their tissues still have to mature towards their functional state, and overt sexual differentiation has only just begun. Two kinds of tissue in particular undergo major changes: bone is laid down largely during the fetal period, and the delicate interconnections in the central nervous system are made. Environmental insults during this time are particularly likely to affect growth, the skeleton, and mental functioning.

How to interpret the diagrams in this book

For most of the illustrations in this book the time after fertilization is indicated by means of a notepad. Approximate size is indicated by a scale bar. Be alert for the varying units of measurement in notepads and bars!

A consistent colour code is adopted throughout. Ectoderm and derivatives are shown in red tints, mesoderm and derivatives in blue tints, and endoderm and derivatives in yellow tints. Occasionally, it will be necessary to depart briefly from this convention – for example when comparing arteries and veins, use of red and blue is too well established to resist – but at these times solid colours will be used, and such departures will be clearly indicated.

Orientation

At first the embryo is a flat two-dimensional structure, but it then begins to fold into a three-dimensional shape. The main body axis also becomes strongly concave during the embryonic period, so that the head is close to the tail. The fetus remains in a curled position, due to the constraint of the extraembryonic membranes, and further changes after birth are required before it begins to adopt the erect anatomical position. These changes make it difficult to describe orientation consistently and simply. The following convention is therefore adopted throughout this book (Figure I.1). The neural tube provides a constant frame of reference. A section which cuts the neural axis at 90° is described as **transverse** to the neural tube; **sagittal** sections are parallel to the axis of symmetry of the neural tube; a **frontal** section is at mutual right angles to both of these, though in practice this will rarely be used. Where necessary, section orientations will be shown on a reduced-scale embryo.

In a transverse section, the neural tube is in contact with, or in close proximity to, the dorsal surface of the embryo. This is used to define movements and positions as **dorsal** (literally, 'towards the back'). The opposite direction is **ventral** ('towards the belly'). Similarly, in a sagittal section, we can describe movements and positions as **cranial** ('towards the head') or **caudal** ('towards the tail'), even though this may sound a little odd at times – in describing one part of the brain as 'cranial' to another, for instance – but it brings advantages in terms of simplicity and consistency.

The neural tube occupies the midline. Structures on either side can be described as lying **laterally** to this, which defines the **lateral** direction. The opposite direction, towards the midline, is **medial**. Wherever possible, diagrams in this book will be presented with the **dorsal** direction facing *up* the page.

A number of reference stages (particularly in the early embryonic period) have been selected and, where possible, diagrams refer to these reference stages to promote familiarity with the changing three-dimensional nature of development.

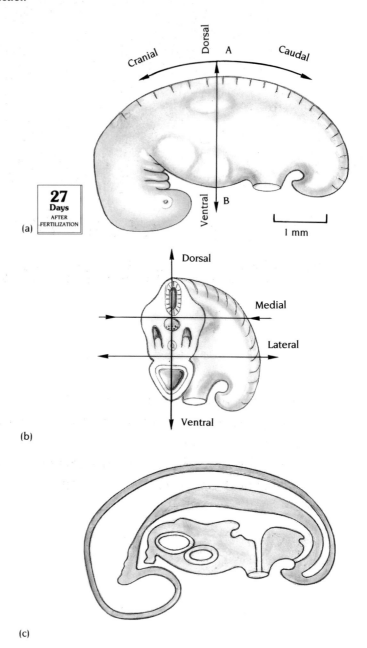

FIGURE I.1 (a) Side view of 27-day human embryo (based on an embryo in the University of St Andrews collection) showing time, scale, and orientation conventions employed in this book; (b) transverse section through this embryo along the line marked AB in (a). The embryo is shown in three-dimensional style, with the tail to the left; (c) sagittal section through the same embryo.

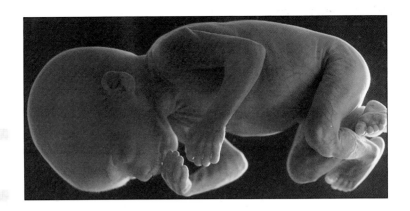

PART I

The pre-embryo from fertilization to neurulation

1

The genesis of organization

Introduction: the central enigma

There is a central riddle at the heart of development that, although profound, can be illustrated in a simple manner. The newly fertilized human egg is a small and apparently simple structure (Figure 1.1). It is less than 0.1 mm in diameter and, apart from the pronuclei, has no obvious internal organization. Yet this fertilized egg, under the right conditions, will develop into a human baby, which is dramatically different in its nature: it is very much larger than the egg, and is composed of billions of cells. These cells are of many different kinds (there are muscle cells, nerve cells, bone cells, and so on, each divided into further subtypes) and the cells are arranged in complex relative positions in space. This is the mystery of development – the central enigma of how complex order can arise from apparently simple structures. This enigma remained intractable until very recently, and only now are profound answers beginning to emerge.

Three underlying processes are involved: cell division, cell differentiation and positioning of cells in space. Of these, cell division is perhaps the simplest concept to understand. In the early stages of development it is regulated inside the cell by a complex internal oscillating system, located in the cytoplasm but interacting with the nucleus so that the DNA replication cycle is coupled to that of the cell. Later, it is regulated outside the cell, both by the availability of nutrients and by **growth factors** (extracellular polypeptide molecules that bind to receptors on the cell surface and modulate cell division both positively and

3

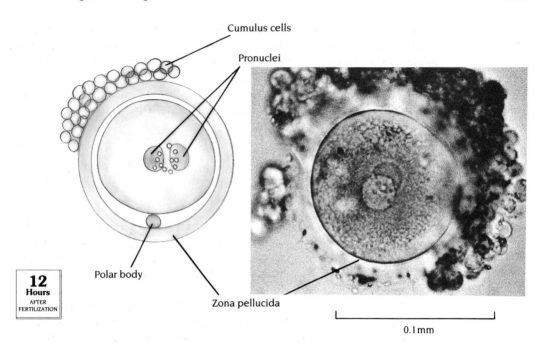

FIGURE 1.1 Fertilized human egg. (Photograph courtesy of Dr David Edgar, Ninewells Hospital, Dundee.)

negatively). Expression of these factors can lead to local growth of structures relative to the rest of the body. The limbs, for example, grow out from the flanks in this manner; similar changes in relative size occur continuously throughout development and long after birth. Cell division is of vital importance in terms of both development and pathology. Embryos grow faster than the fastest tumours, and it is likely that cancer in many ways represents a reversion to this embryonic state. (This idea is further explored in Special Topic 10, pp. 384–5.) Details of the fine control of cell division are, however, outside the scope of this book.

Cell differentiation leads to the formation of about 200 major categories of cell in the mammalian body. Some of these are terminally differentiated and will no longer divide: erythrocytes and nerve cells fall into this category. Others remain as stem cells, and retain the ability to replace missing or damaged cells as required. There is an inverse relationship between cell division and differentiation; in many cases the more differentiated a cell is the more slowly it divides (this too has implications for cancer studies). Growth factors are often involved in regulating differentiation. Differentiation arises from the expression within the cell of a particular subset of its genes, which is a result of interaction of special signal molecules with the DNA within the nucleus. This concept is explored further in Special Topic 6, pp. 174–7.

Finally, cells are deployed in different relative positions in space. The leg, for example, consists of exactly the same cell types as the arm, but their arrangement in space is recognizably different. Similarly, a pig has essentially the same cell types as a human, but they are deployed in a different way. This is perhaps the most subtle of the developmental processes to understand but rapid advances have recently been made, for which the development of the limbs will be used as a paradigm (see Chapter 18).

In this chapter we will examine how cells initially become different from each other. First, it is necessary to consider the role of DNA in this process.

DNA in early development

It might be thought that development is merely the unfolding of the genetic programme. However, although the genetic material is of vital importance in development – after all, cell differentiation results from the differential expression of genes – it does not provide the initial mechanism of differentiation itself. This is demonstrated by four observations.

The first is that essentially the same DNA is present in all cells of an organism. This can be shown in amphibia by transferring nuclei from differentiated cells to eggs from which the normal nuclei have been removed. These hybrid eggs then give rise to the complete range of tissue types, and in a few cases to normal tadpoles. This demonstrates that the nuclei from differentiated cells, and hence their DNA, have not become irrevocably specialized during development. Molecular biology techniques confirm that, while a limited subset of genes is expressed in particular differentiated cells, all the other genes are present though silent, and that, with a few exceptions, those genes that are being expressed are present in a single copy only. (Lymphocytes are one important exception to this general principle. New genes can be created in these cells by rearrangement of their genome, to aid in generating the enormous diversity required in the immune system. This is a special case, however, and in general cells do not become different from each other by inheriting different regions of DNA.)

Second, in a number of animals (generally where the egg is large), the fertilized egg can divide and undergo the early stages of development without expressing its DNA at all. In the toad *Xenopus*, transcription does not get under way until the 12th cleavage division, when about 4000 cells are present. Genes are actively transcribed during formation of the egg, but transcription then ceases and may not recommence until the early stages of development have already taken place. Indeed, in some cases the nucleus can be completely removed from a fertilized egg and development will proceed as normal through the early stages. This is not the case for human embryos, which commence transcription early in development (between the four- and eight-cell stages), but this is probably only because the eggs are so small.

Third, the cells produced by cleavage of the fertilized egg are often **totipotent** – capable of producing a complete individual. This is particularly true of mammalian embryos. If the component cells of a four-cell sheep embryo are

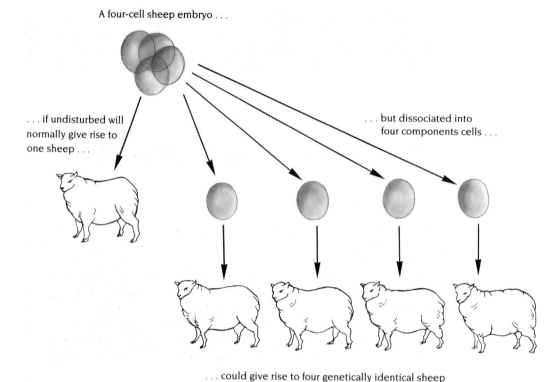

A four-cell sheep embryo . . .

. . . if undisturbed will normally give rise to one sheep . . .

. . . but dissociated into four components cells . . .

. . . could give rise to four genetically identical sheep

FIGURE 1.2   Multipotency of early blastomeres.

separated, each of them can go on to form a complete, normal-sized, sheep (Figure 1.2); yet if the embryo had been left alone it would have developed into only one sheep rather than four. Thus, the component cells are able to change their behaviour markedly in response to such a manipulation, even though the manipulation did not in itself alter their DNA content. Something else must be influencing their behaviour.

Fourth, in a number of cases, aspects of development can be inherited in a non-mendelian way (see Box 1.1). This is generally because the egg inherits information from the mother that influences its own development. Its own genome may be silent during this time. The form of the embryo therefore reflects the genetic make-up of its mother. However, in time, the genome of the embryo will influence the form of its own offspring, and so on. DNA is the controlling element in development in such cases but it is the DNA of the mother, rather than that of the embryo, which is important. Such maternal influences explain how early development can occur in the absence of DNA. Recently, it has also been learned that complex patterns of gene activation may result from passage through the parental male or female germline – a phenomenon known as **genetic imprinting** (see Box 1.1).

Box 1.1 Unusual modes of inheritance • 7

Generally we may suggest that the embryo's DNA does not initiate major changes during initial development: rather, it will in time respond to other influences by switching on particular genes. Of course, the gene products may act during subsequent development to induce differentiation in other cells, for

Box 1.1 Unusual modes of inheritance

Maternal effect mutants

Some gene defects are evident in an unusual way. A simple point mutation in the Mexican axolotl serves as a good example of how this phenomenon operates. Each individual has, as usual, two copies of the relevant gene. The gene can be present in the normal wild-type (+) form or the mutant (o) form. The mutation brings about developmental arrest, but in the *next* generation, and only through the maternal line, as illustrated below.

If a normal **homozygous** female (both copies of the relevant gene are normal) is mated with a homozygous male mutant (both copies abnormal) then all of the offspring are **heterozygous**. In such a mating combination, all the offspring survive.

$$\begin{array}{cc} ♀ & ♂ \end{array}$$

Parents: +/+ ×   o/o
Offspring: +/o   +/o   +/o   +/o

However, if the homozygous mutant is female, and the male is the homozygous normal individual, the outcome is very different. All the offspring arrest during development, despite the fact that they are all heterozygous, as before.

$$\begin{array}{cc} ♀ & ♂ \end{array}$$

Parents: o/o ×   +/+
Offspring: +/o   +/o   +/o   +/o

That is, the fate of the offspring is not controlled by their own genome. In fact, they arrest because their *mother* carried two mutant copies of the gene. If the mother carries even one normal copy, then they will be normal.

$$\begin{array}{cc} ♀ & ♂ \end{array}$$

Parents: +/o ×   +/o
Offspring: +/+   +/o   +/o   o/o

This explains how an individual can survive when it is homozygous for the defect.

This kind of inheritance is non-mendelian in character.

All this reveals that the embryos behave in a way that corresponds to the genotype of their mother, irrespective of their own genome. It is possible to show that eggs from o/o mothers can be rescued by cytoplasm from eggs with normal or heterozygous mothers. This rescue effect can be removed by heat and trypsin treatment. This in turn suggests that the wild-type gene produces a protein that is required during development.

A homozygous mutant mother cannot pass the product of the gene on to her offspring, because she lacks the gene altogether. However, some genes can behave differently depending on whether they pass through the male or the female germ line. This phenomenon is known as **genetic imprinting** (also discussed in Special Topic 9, pp. 369–74).

An example of the possible complexity of inheritance is found in the human fragile X syndrome, perhaps the most common genetic cause of mental retardation, with an incidence of approximately 1 per 2000 live births. Males are affected more often than females. Here, part of the X chromosome is attached only by a thread and can detach easily (hence the name). However, the associated expression of mental retardation is curiously related to the mode of inheritance. Unexpectedly, some males show the fragile X appearance without showing mental retardation, despite the fact that they have only one X chromosome. Their daughters are also asymptomatic. This might be expected because daughters have two X chromosomes, and the normal X from the mother might compensate for the abnormal X from the father. But the daughters' daughters may express the symptoms. Plainly, the mode of inheritance can have effects on the expression of the syndrome which are not yet fully understood.

Non-nuclear inheritance

A different kind of non-DNA inheritance is found in unicellular ciliates such as *Paramecium* and *Tetrahymena*. These have organized rows of cilia on their surface, which are asymmetric (Figure 1). Manipulations can disturb the pattern of these rows: for example, a region can be produced in which the rows run at right angles to normal. Although this disruption was produced by a manipulation that did not affect DNA, this new pattern is inherited stably through succeeding generations.

At first glance, ciliates might not seem very relevant to human development. However, the unity of developmental processes is such that this view would be mistaken. For instance, it is currently suspected that the causative agent of the sheep disease scrapie, and its analogues in cattle and humans (bovine spongiform encephalopathy and Creutzfeldt–Jakob disease respectively), is a protein-like material that can copy itself in a non-DNA manner. Perhaps in this case, and in that of *Paramecium*, membrane structures act as a template for copying information directly to the next generation without the intervention of DNA.

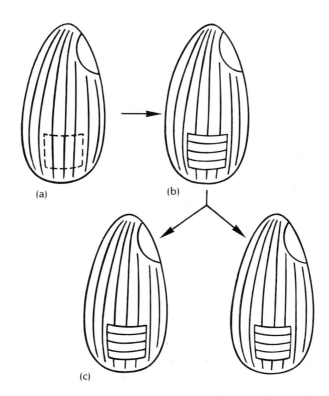

FIGURE 1   An individual *Paramecium* shows distinct rows of cilia on its surface (a). If a patch is experimentally rotated (b), this is transmitted to subsequent generations (c).

example by binding to specific regions of their DNA, and cascades of differentiation can result from these changes. But something must first initiate the expression of these factors.

Organization inherent in the egg

It might be that the structure of the egg initially influences differentiation. The egg could possess different regions, established perhaps in the ovary, that as the egg divides into two cells, four cells, etc. particular regional components come to lie in different daughter cells. These regional components could then initiate different patterns of DNA expression in each cell, leading to overt cell differentiation (Figure 1.3).

A variation of this theme is that regionalization of the egg is established at fertilization. On sperm entry, many eggs can be seen to regionalize: cytoplasmic

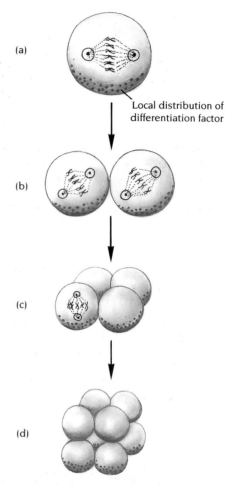

(a)

Local distribution of
differentiation factor

(b)

(c)

(d)

FIGURE 1.3 Cytoplasmic localization. Many eggs have localized patterns of contents before fertilization. (a) Diagrammatic view of an idealized egg, with darker pigmented material concentrated at the ventral aspect. (b) The first cleavage plane (shown from left to right on the page) divides the egg into two equivalent blastomeres, each containing pigment. (c) The second cleavage plane (perpendicular to the plane of the page) again gives four equivalent cells. (d) The third cleavage plane (up and down the page) gives eight blastomeres, four with pigment and four without. If the pigment then initiates the expression of particular genes, two outcomes will be followed by the cells. Although this is not thought to be a major factor in mammalian development, it cannot be ruled out.

components segregate from each other in a manner influenced by the point of sperm entry. Such components direct the development of the cells that come to include them subsequently (Figure 1.4)

Although such developmental strategies have been shown to be employed by many kinds of animal, they do not seem to play a major role in mammalian

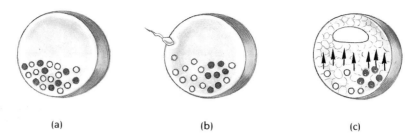

(a)   (b)   (c)

FIGURE 1.4   The point of sperm entry can also provide informational cues leading to differentiation. Here two substances, marked ○ and •, are evenly distributed in the ventral region of a diagrammatic amphibian egg (a). Sperm entry occurs near the equator of the egg (b), but otherwise is random. Once it has taken place (c), component • shifts its position to lie opposite the point of sperm entry. It is then enclosed in cells forming in this region, and can direct their further differentiation (see Box 2.1).

development. This is suggested by the featureless nature of mammalian eggs and may be deduced from the totipotency of early mammalian cells indicating that the early cells, at least, do not inherit different controlling factors from their progenitors. In some way, early mammalian cells can respond to changes in their cell–cell contacts by changing their behaviour. The advent of in vitro fertilization techniques for mammalian eggs has enabled early events to be studied directly. (See Special Topic 2, pp. 45–6.) It appears that the rules governing the development of all mammals are so similar that experimental animal systems can be used to explore the underlying mechanisms.

The influence of the cellular environment

After fertilization, the mammalian egg divides into two cells, then four, and so on, with the divisions quickly becoming asynchronous. A ball of apparently identical cells (known as a 'morula', from the Latin for mulberry) is formed (Figure 1.5). Next a cavity begins to form inside the ball, which is then known as the blastocyst (Figure 1.6). Now a critical event occurs: two different kinds of cells begin to be recognizable. The first overt differentiation event has occurred. These new cell kinds are the **trophectoderm**, which forms the outer layer, and the **inner cell mass**, clustered together inside the trophectoderm shell at one end of the cavity (Figure 1.7).

As indicated earlier, at the two-cell and four-cell stages all cells appear to be totipotent. It is possible that this totipotency extends a little further into development, but the later cells become very hard to examine because they decrease in size at each of the early divisions. This totipotency of the early cells actually plays a role in the normal development of some mammals: in the nine-banded

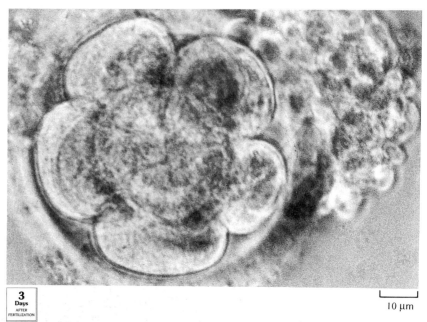

FIGURE 1.5 Human morula. (Photograph courtesy of Dr David Edgar, Ninewells Hospital, Dundee.)

armadillo, the initial embryo generally divides spontaneously to give rise to a litter of identical quadruplets. In humans, the totipotency of the early cells points to one of the ways in which twinning can occur (see Special Topic 3, pp. 62–8).

Another consequence of totipotency is that deficiencies can be regulated. If one cell is removed from the four-cell stage, the remaining three go on to form a

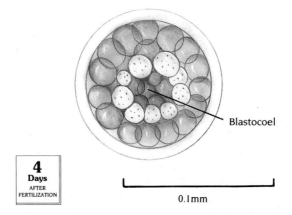

FIGURE 1.6 Early human blastocyst. A fluid-filled space (the blastocoel) begins to open up inside the ball of cells, not quite at the centre.

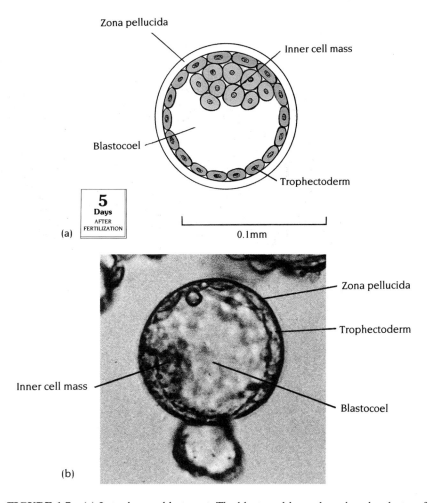

FIGURE 1.7 (a) Later human blastocyst. The blastocoel has enlarged, and a cluster of cells is found at one end of the internal cavity – the inner cell mass. The blastocoel is lined with the flattened cells of the trophectoderm. (b) Mouse embryo at equivalent stage to (a). (Photograph courtesy of Dr David Edgar, Ninewells Hospital, Dundee.)

normal embryo (see Special Topic 1, pp. 18–21). More surprising is the ability to regulate excesses. If two pre-embryos at the four-cell stage are pushed together, they will amalgamate to form a single double-sized pre-embryo. This in turn will form a double-sized blastocyst. If such a giant combination is placed in the uterus of a surrogate mother, it will give rise to an offspring that is normal in form and (fortunately for the mother) in size but which will be composed of two different kinds of cells mingled together in a **mosaic** manner and will have four different parents. An easy way to show this is to use mouse embryos from two strains with different coat colours. A patchwork mouse results, with regions of each coat

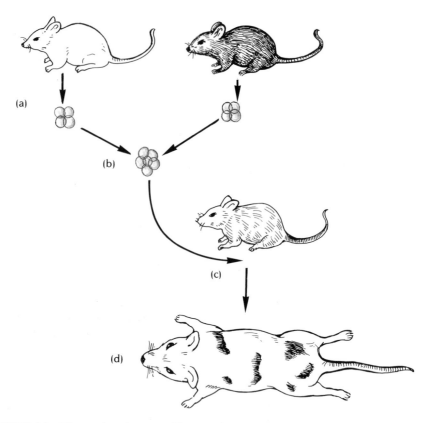

FIGURE 1.8   The patchwork mouse. If two early mouse morulae from mothers of different colour (a) are pushed together, they fuse to form an aggregate (b). This can then be placed in the uterus of a surrogate mother (c). In time she will give birth to a mouse normal in size and morphology, but visibly made from cells from each source (d) (see McLaren, 1976).

colour recognizably present in the skin (Figure 1.8). All the other organs in the body will be mosaic too, although this will not be visible to the naked eye. This process can occur spontaneously, though rarely, during human development. For example, two eggs may be fertilized and commence development; if by some accident they adhere, fusion may occur. The baby born following such a process is a mosaic. A number of cases of such mosiacs have been identified. They may face reproductive problems if their component conceptuses were not of the same sex.

This phenomenon of regulation of excess is the basis of a critical experiment that reveals how differentiation is controlled in the early mammalian embryo. Because the first differentiative decision on whether to form inner cell mass or trophectoderm is clearly not controlled by the DNA or by localized components in the egg, it was postulated that the choice was influenced by the relative position of cells within the morula. Perhaps 'internal' cells develop as inner cell mass, and 'external' cells become trophectoderm.

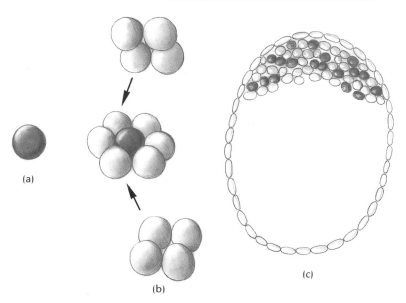

(a)

(b)

(c)

FIGURE 1.9 Influence of the cellular environment. A single marked eight-cell morula (a) is surrounded by otherwise identical unmarked morulae (b). The resulting giant morula will develop in culture into a giant blastula (c). The marked cells are largely confined to the inner cell mass.

This idea was tested in the following way. An eight-cell mouse embryo was labelled with a radioactive tracer, so that all the cells could be subsequently identified. (Labelled control embryos developed into normal blastocysts, with the normal proportions of trophectoderm to inner cell mass cells.) Each labelled embryo was then completely surrounded by normal unlabelled morulae at the same stage, so that it came to lie in the centre of a giant morula 15 times the normal size (Figure 1.9). This giant morula subsequently developed into a giant blastocyst with a trophectodermal shell and inner cell mass exactly as in a normal-sized embryo. When the labelled cells were identified, they were found to have contributed overwhelmingly to the inner cell mass. This demonstrates that the decision to become inner cell mass or trophectoderm is indeed controlled by the relative position of the cells. In fact, it seems that the key factor is the number of cell contacts each cell has: cells with many cell contacts become inner cell mass and cells with few become trophectoderm. An isolated single cell will recommence dividing until it reaches the appropriate number of contacts to re-enter the normal differentiative pattern, and hence develop into a normal embryo. The cellular environment is therefore revealed as the critical factor in determining the differentiative decisions of the cells. How the different environments interact with DNA to ensure that the particular patterns of gene expression appropriate to inner cell mass or trophectoderm are switched on remains unknown. (See also Box 1.2.)

This is not the only decision made in this way. As described in the next chapter, the inner cell mass will give rise to two further cell types – primitive ectoderm and primitive endoderm. Again, individual early inner cell mass cells can become either of these tissues, depending on where they are in the inner cell mass: those exposed to the blastocyst cavity become primitive endoderm and the others primitive ectoderm. The trophectoderm also has several options open to it: these are influenced by contact with the inner cell mass.

In these ways, a variety of different kinds of tissue can be generated by the influence of neighbouring cells.

Spatial arrangement of cells

The position of cells in the early embryo leads to their adoption of particular patterns of differentiation and gene expression, and this indicates an answer to the question of how cells first become different from each other. Once such differences have begun to be established, more complex interactions can arise. As part of the expression of their differentiated state, cells may begin to produce molecules capable of diffusing through the embryo. These diffusing substances may have a signalling function and may in turn effect more changes in cells belonging to other differentiation classes, even though they are some distance away. Such responses can be graded, so that the concentration of signal molecule determines the particular nature of the differentiative outcome. Complex patterns may develop as a result. As part of their differentiative state, some cells may become mobile, capable of ranging throughout the embryo until they come across other cells which inhibit their movement; mixed structures can arise in this way also. Through such processes, the level of complexity of the embryo gradually increases. At the same time, the options open to individual cells continually decrease as they make particular choices at each stage in development. Finally, most cells will reach a stable end state. As indicated earlier, only a few cell types retain a number of options: these remain relatively undifferentiated so that they can give rise to differentiated progeny on demand. This is usually because the fully differentiated progeny cannot themselves divide, and therefore cannot maintain their own numbers. Such **stem cell** populations are retained to replenish differentiated cells when they become depleted by accident or by normal wear and tear.

The concept of cell signalling leading to specific distributions of cells in space is explored in more detail in Chapter 5, where information on the underlying molecular mechanisms will also be discussed.

Box 1.2 Further consequences of cell interaction • 17

Box 1.2 Further consequences of cell interaction

The interactive abilities of early cells are extensive. If, for instance, an early mouse morula is pushed together with an early rat morula the two morulae fuse and, if the combination is placed in the uterus of a surrogate mother, a creature made of both rat and mouse cells will eventually be born. This is known as a 'chimaera', from the mythical animal of Greek legend, which was made from the parts of a number of other animals. It tends to resemble one or other of the donors, rather than being a mixture of both, but it is composed of a mosaic of cells from the different donors. This experiment indicates that early developmental signals operate across species boundaries: a similar result has also been obtained using sheep and goats as the chimaera sources.

An even more dramatic outcome is revealed by the use of teratocarcinoma cells. Teratocarcinomas are highly malignant tumour cells arising in the germ line (see Special Topic 10, pp. 384–5). An early mouse morula can be pushed together with a cluster of mouse teratocarcinoma cells and the aggregate placed in the uterus of a surrogate mother. The morula and cancer cells can be obtained from mice of different coat colours to aid identification. In time, a mouse will be born that is composed of both tumour and normal mouse cells: it is normal in morphology, though the coat colour patches reveal its hybrid nature (it therefore looks rather like the mouse in Figure 1.8). These cancer chimaeras are no more prone to develop cancer than normal laboratory mice: the cancer cells have been returned to normal behaviour by their exposure to early embryonic signals. The tumour-derived cells are present in all the organs of the body, including the gonads, where some germ cells are of tumour origin. This means that if the tumour-chimaera mouse is used for breeding, a proportion of its offspring will develop from tumour-derived gametes: these offspring will therefore have a tumour as one of their parents.

More practically, it has recently proved possible to develop culture regimes which prevent the cells of the early morula from differentiating. This relies on the presence of a protein factor known as differentiation inhibiting agent. In the presence of this agent, cells can be maintained in a totipotent condition for extended periods of time: when desired, they can be permitted to differentiate by removal of the agent and they will then give rise to normal embryos. In their non-differentiated condition they can be modified by, for example, insertion of particular genes into their genome. There is no reason to doubt that the same procedure could be carried out with human embryonic material, although ethical considerations apply to humans that do not apply to mice.

Special Topic 1 Diagnosis in the preimplantation embryo

The totipotency of the early blastomeres, as described earlier, has important medical implications for the detection of genetic abnormalities. These have arisen as a result of the development of in vitro fertilization, or IVF, techniques (see Special Topic 2, pp. 45–6). The pre-embryo can compensate completely for absent cells and this means that individual cells, or groups of cells, can be removed for testing. If these are found to be free of genetic abnormality the remaining cells can be placed in the mother's uterus to continue their development. This offers advantages over allowing a pregnancy to proceed in an at-risk mother up to the point where amniocentesis or chorionic villus sampling can be undertaken (see Special Topic 4, pp. 80–4), and the mother then being given the choice of an abortion if the fetus is found to be abnormal.

Cells for testing can be removed in a number of ways. At the early morula stage the zona pellucida can be wholly or partly removed and one or two cells detached from the others (Figure 1). These cells can then be examined for genetic defects. In practice, it might be more convenient to freeze the remaining two- or three-cell embryo and allow the sample to divide a number of times to increase the amount of material available. Another way of acquiring larger amounts of material would be to allow the embryo to develop inside its zona until it reaches the blastula stage. If a slit is now made in the zona some of the trophectoderm cells will bulge out, and these can be removed (Figure 2). As described in Chapter 3, these cells would have contributed to the extraembryonic membranes, rather than to the body of the embryo itself, and hence their removal should have no ill effects.

Cells removed in these ways may be assayed in a number of ways for genetic defects. The chromosomes could be examined directly for abnormalities of number (see Chapter 26) or the sex of the embryo could be determined from the chromosomes, which would be valuable in the case of sex-linked defects. At a greater level of sophistication,

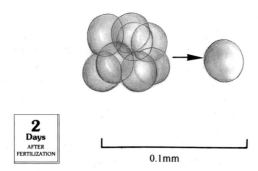

2
Days
AFTER
FERTILIZATION

0.1mm

FIGURE 1 Zona-free early human morula, from which one or two cells can be removed for examination.

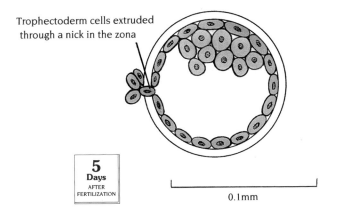

Trophectoderm cells extruded
through a nick in the zona

5
Days
AFTER
FERTILIZATION

0.1mm

FIGURE 2 Alternatively, a slit in the blastocyst could allow some trophectoderm cells to be obtained for sampling.

particular defects such as Duchenne muscular dystrophy and cystic fibrosis could be diagnosed, because the genes for these defects have been characterized. This fine level of analysis will be greatly aided by the use of the polymerase chain reaction (PCR), which can greatly amplify the number of copies of a particular gene. For this technique, a single cell may provide sufficient starting material.

(1) The DNA under examination (Figure 3(a)) is heated to separate the two helical strands into complementary single strands (Figure 3(b)).
(2) Two kinds of 'primer' – short oligonucleotides that bind specifically to particular regions of DNA – are added as the mixture cools (Figure 3(c)). One primer is designed to bind to the 'sense' strand and the other to the 'antisense' strand. These primers are selected so as to bind to regions near the desired genes.
(3) A DNA polymerase is next supplied, which begins to add nucleotides to the primers (Figure 3(d)). The primers are constructed in such a way that this occurs only in the direction of the desired gene. In this way two double-stranded copies of the desired gene are constructed (Figure 3(e)).

When sufficient time has elapsed for the polymerase to copy the gene steps 1–3 are repeated (Figure 3(f)), producing four copies of the gene for the next heating sequence, which then provides eight copies, and so on, in exponentially increasing amounts. In this way, one copy of a gene can be amplified to billions of copies in an afternoon: allowing the cell to divide in the conventional way would take more than a million years to give the same number of gene copies.

The PCR has already been used in practice (Handyside *et al.*, 1990). Many genetic conditions are X-linked, so males are at risk if the single X chromosome they inherit from their mother is affected. Handyside *et al.* carried out IVF with eggs from at-risk mothers, and removed cells from the pre-embryos at the six- to eight-cell stage. They then used PCR to amplify Y chromosome specific sequences (naturally, this could not occur if the donor pre-embryo was female). Because the female pre-embryos would be unaffected,

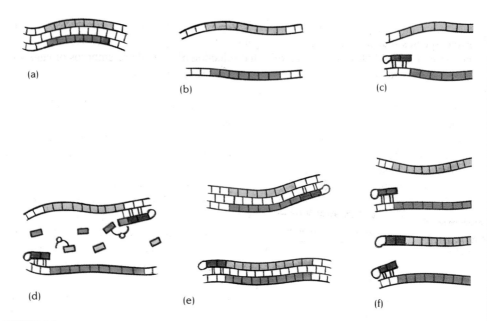

FIGURE 3 Polymerase chain reaction (see text for explanation).

only these were selected for reimplantation. Sex-selection to rule out a particular genetic defect has led to a successful pregnancy and birth.

In a similar way a particular gene – for a haemoglobin chain, for instance – could be amplified to reveal whether it was normal or abnormal, allowing implantation only of those pre-embryos which will not express the thalassaemias.

Undoubtedly, this selection of pre-embryos poses moral dilemmas. However, PCR has also been used to amplify a particular gene from the DNA in the first polar body present in the unfertilized egg (Chapter 2). The polar bodies of eggs taken from an at-risk mother who is heterozygous for a particular condition could be screened for the presence of the defective gene at this stage, before fertilization. If the copy in the polar body proved normal, the copy in the corresponding egg would be abnormal, and vice versa. In this way, only eggs that were normal would go forward for use in IVF.

An even less invasive technique is to analyse the biochemical status of the blastocyst by studying the proteins it secretes in culture, or the materials it takes up from the culture medium. However, this is likely to be limited in usefulness to only a few special circumstances, in which relevant genes are expressed very early in development, and where their abnormal function can be detected.

In time, preimplantation diagnostic techniques may reduce the frequency with which tragic diseases such as cystic fibrosis, Duchenne muscular dystrophy and the thalassaemias occur in the population.

It is even possible to foresee that defects will become routinely correctable at the level of the gene itself. Foreign DNA injected into a nucleus will incorporate into the host genome. Particular lengths of DNA can be targeted so as to insert into particular sites in the genome, so that in principle a missing or defective gene could be supplemented by insertion of a copy of the normal gene. The inserted DNA need not even be from the same species – it has been said that a gene from an orange could be inserted into the genome of a duck! However, it is likely that selection of normal pre-embryos or eggs will always be more economical than genetic engineering of this kind. And many promising science-fiction scenarios are rendered impossible by the multigenic nature of complex properties such as personality, intelligence, and even morphology. In addition, as described earlier in this chapter, there is a complex interaction between the genome and the environment in the expression of such properties, which makes them difficult to manipulate. Direct genetic engineering of the egg, as opposed to body cells, does not seem likely in the foreseeable future.

It is, however, possible to speculate that defects might be corrected by the use of 'chimaeras' created within a species (see Chapter 2). An abnormal pre-embryo, or even a fetus, might be rescued by addition of cells from a normal donor of the same stage and sex. Such a transplant before the time of onset of immunological function would subsequently be recognized as 'self' by the host. The resulting individual would be a mosaic of the two different donors, with the expression of the defect perhaps being alleviated by the non-defective cells.

However, IVF success rates are still comparatively low (see Special Topic 2, pp. 45–6), and this currently limits the usefulness of preimplantation diagnosis to only the most serious abnormalities, or to cases where the mother is already undergoing IVF treatment for other reasons.

Further reading

Barnett T., Pachl C., Gergen J.P. and Wensin, P.C. (1980). The isolation and characterisation of *Drosophila* yolk protein genes. *Cell*, **21**, 729–38

Braude P., Bolton V. and Moore S. (1988). Human gene expression first occurs between the four- and eight-cell stages of preimplantation development. *Nature*, **332**, 459–61

Gardner R.L. (1985). Manipulation of development. In *Reproduction in Mammals 2: Embryonic and Fetal Development* (Austin C.R. and Short R.V., eds.), pp. 159–80. Cambridge: Cambridge University Press

Gerhart J., Ubbels G., Black S. , Hara K. and Kirschner M. (1981). A re-investigation of the role of the grey crescent in axis formation in *Xenopus laevis*. *Nature*, **292**, 511–16

Gurdon J.B., Laskey R.A. and Reeves O.R. (1975). The developmental capacity of nuclei transplanted from keratinised skin cells of adult frogs. *J. Embryol. Exp. Morph.*, **34**, 93–112

Hillman N., Sherman M.I. and Graham C.F. (1972). The effect of spatial arrangement on cell determination during mouse development. *J. Embryol. Exp. Morph.*, **28**, 263–78

Hozumi N. and Tonegawa S. (1976). Evidence for somatic re-arrangement of immunoglobulin genes coding for variable and constant regions. *Proc. Natl Acad. Sci. USA*, **73**, 3628–32

Illmansee K. and Mahowald A. (1974). Transplantation of posterior plasm in *Drosophila*. Induction of germ cells at the anterior pole of the egg. *Proc. Natl Acad. Sci. USA*, **71**, 1016–20

Jeffrey W.R. (1985). Specification of cell fate by cytoplasmic determinants in ascidian embryos. *Cell*, **41**, 11–12

McLaren A. (1976). *Mammalian Chimaeras*. London: Cambridge University Press

Newport J. and Kirschener M. (1982). A major developmental transition in early *Xenopus* embryos. II. Control of the onset of transcription. *Cell*, **30**, 687–96

Uchida I.A., Freeman V.C. and Chen P. (1976). Detection and interpretation of two different cell lines in triploid abortions. *Clin. Genet.*, **28**, 489–94

Willadsen S.M. (1979). A method for culture of micromanipulated sheep embryos and its use to produce monozygotic twins. *Nature*, **277**, 298–300

Wolpert L. (1978). Pattern formation in biological development. *Sci. Am.*, **239**, 159–64

Wolpert L. (1991). *The Triumph of the Embryo*. Oxford: Oxford University Press

Box 1.1

Beisson J. and Sonneborn T.M. (1965). Cytoplasmic inheritance of the organisation of the cell cortex in *Paramecium aurelia*. *Proc. Natl Acad. Sci. USA*, **53**, 275–82

Brothers A.J. (1976). Stable nuclear activation dependent on a protein synthesized during development. *Nature*, **260**, 112–15

Hoffman M. (1991). Unraveling the genetics of Fragile X Syndrome. *Science*, **252**, 1070

Humphrey R.R. (1966). A recessive factor (o, for Ova Deficient) determining a complex of abnormalities in the Mexican Axolotl (*Amblystoma mexicanum*). *Devel. Biol.*, **13**, 57–76

Nelson E.M., Frankel J. and Jenkins L.M. (1989). Non-genic inheritance of cellular handedness. *Development*, **105**, 447–56

Oberle I., Rousseay F., Heitz D. *et al.* (1991). Instability of a 550-base pair DNA segment and abnormal methylation in Fragile X Syndrome. *Science*, **252**, 1097–102

Pruisner S.B. (1991). Molecular biology of prion diseases. *Science*, **252**, 1515–22

Box 1.2

Beddington R.S.P. and Robertson E.J. (1989). An assessment of the developmental potential of embryonic stem cells in the midgestation mouse embryo. *Development*, **105**, 733–7

Bradley A., Evans M., Kaufman M.H. and Robertson E. (1984). Formation of germ-line chimaeras from embryo-derived teratocarcinoma cell lines. *Nature*, **309**, 255–6

Gardner R.L. and Johnson M.H. (1973). Investigation of early mammalian development using interspecific chimaeras between rat and mouse. *Nature*, **246**, 86–9

Martin, G. (1981). Isolation of a pluripotent cell line from early mouse embryos cultured in medium conditioned by teratocarcinoma stem cells. *Proc. Natl Acad. Sci. USA*, **78**, 7634–8

Smith A.G., Heath J.K., Donaldson D.D. *et al.* (1988). Inhibition of pluripotential embryonic stem cell differentiation by purified polypeptides. *Nature*, **336**, 688–90

Stewart C.L. (1982). Formation of viable chimaeras by aggregation between teratocarcinomas and pre-implantation mouse embryos. *J. Embryol. Exp. Morph.*, **67**, 167–79

West J.D., Frels W.I., Papaioannou Karr J.P. and Chapman V.M. (1977). Development of interspecific hybrids of *Mus*. *J. Embryol. Exp. Morph.*, **41**, 233–43

Special Topic 1

Adinolfi M. and Polani P.E. (1989). Prenatal diagnosis of genetic disorders in pre-implantation embryos: invasive and non-invasive approaches. *Hum. Genet.*, **83**, 16–19

Handyside A.H., Kontogianni E.H., Hardy K. and Winston R.M.L. (1990). Pregnancies
from biopsied human preimplantation embryos sexed by Y-specific DNA amplification. *Nature*, **344**, 768–70

Monk M. (1990). Embryo research and genetic disease. *New Sci.*, **125**, 56–9

Monk M. and Holding C. (1990). Amplification of a β-haemoglobin sequence in individual human oocytes and polar bodies. *Lancet*, **335**, 985–8

Mullis K.B. (1990). The unusual origin of the Polymerase Chain Reaction. *Sci. Am.*, **260**,
36–43

2

The genesis of the individual: from fertilization to day 16

Human development is a repeating process from generation to generation and we could begin our account at any point. A convenient starting place is fertilization, when the sperm fuses with the egg. This process, occurring not in a moment but over a period of time, is taken by many to represent the beginning of 'life'. However, although this is an extremely important landmark event, both egg and sperm were alive before this time, and the term 'beginning of life' is thus used in a rather special sense. Another important candidate event for the beginning of being is the fusion of the pronuclei, when the genetic material of the individual that is to be born is assembled for the first time. Yet this does not necessarily correspond to the onset of individuality, because more than one individual may result from the zygote. Individuality is not irrevocably established until gastrulation, which offers another important stage in the development of being.

The onset of 'independent viability' is recognized in many societies as an important legal watershed in the acquisition of 'personality'. Birth itself, the end of infancy and the end of childhood are also steps in the progression towards full rights as an adult, and are given various forms of cultural and legal recognition within different societies. The technical advances described in the first four chapters of this book have moved such considerations from the realm of philosophy to that of urgent practical concern.

The mature oocyte (see Chapter 26) is shed into the peritoneal cavity. However, the upper end of the uterine tube is closely apposed to the ovary and its ciliated, finger-like projections help gather the oocyte into the ampulla of the tube.

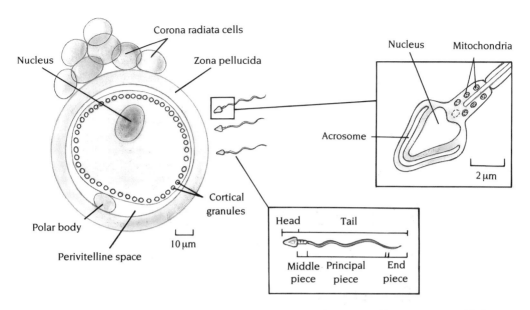

FIGURE 2.1 Diagram of human oocyte showing approaching sperm. Magnified sperm shown inset.

The oocyte is a large cell approximately 80 μm in diameter (see Figure 2.1). A layer of cortical granules lies in its cytoplasm beneath the oocyte membrane. The oocyte and the first polar body lie in the perivitelline space, inside the transparent, proteinaceous, acellular zona pellucida. Outside the zona a cloud of cells derived from the follicle walls adheres loosely to it. These are known as the corona radiata (see also cumulus oophorus cells, Chapter 26).

The spermatozoon is much smaller than the egg (Figure 2.1). The genetic material is contained in the posterior part of its head, while the anterior part contains the acrosome, an organelle containing digestive enzymes. The long tail provides motive force.

Fertilization

Fertilization usually takes place in the ampulla of the uterine tube (Figure 2.2). Sperm have a considerable distance to cover from their point of entry at the cervix and it is likely that only a few hundred of the many sperm (200–500 million on average, though this number can vary greatly) that begin the journey will even reach the ampulla. Newly ejaculated sperm cannot fertilize the egg: they first must undergo a process of maturation, known as **capacitation**. This occurs naturally in the uterus, and even in simple culture fluids: its nature is not completely

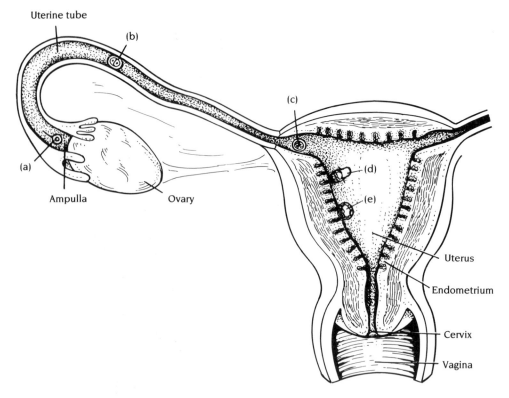

FIGURE 2.2 Ovary, uterine tube and uterus. (a) The ampulla of the uterine tube, where fertilization of the oocyte occurs. (b) First cleavage of the egg, approximately 24–36 hours after fertilization. (c) The morula, 3–4 days after fertilization. (d) The blastocyst 'hatching' from the zona pellucida, approximately 5 days after fertilization. (e) Implantation of the blastocyst into the uterine wall, 6 days after fertilization.

clear but may involve removal of proteins from the head of the sperm to reveal specific binding molecules underneath and an increase in swimming activity.

Mammalian sperm, unlike those of many animals, do not 'home in' on the egg but rely on chance encounters. When a sperm does meet an egg it passes through the corona cells, which seem to pose no real barrier, and adheres to the zona. The zona is composed – certainly in mice, and probably in humans – of three glycoprotein types. One of these, ZP3, functions as a specific receptor for complementary molecules on the head of the sperm, which explains why fertilization of one species by another is unlikely.

Once binding has occurred the acrosome membrane begins to fuse with the outer sperm membrane and the digestive enzymes thus released start to break down the zona. The binding receptor, ZP3, is responsible for initiating this process. Several sperm may bind to one egg and engage in a race to digest their way through the zona, a process that may take 15–20 minutes in humans (Figure

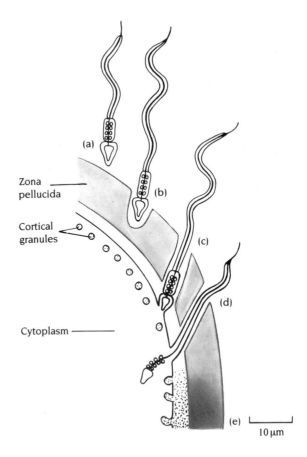

FIGURE 2.3 (a) Sperm approach the zona pellucida and bind specifically to it. (b) The acrosome enzymes enables the sperm to digest its way through the zona in a 'race' to fertilize the egg. (c) The head of the sperm fuses with the oocyte cell membrane. (d) The sperm nucleus and components of the motile apparatus make their way into the cytoplasm. (e) When the sperm binds to the oocyte membrane the cortical granules fuse with the oocyte membrane and release their contents into the perivitelline space. The zona responds by becoming incapable of binding sperm.

2.3). Once a sperm reaches the perivitelline space it may swim briefly in it before binding to the oocyte membrane, not by its tip, but by the remaining region of acrosome around the middle of the head. It is then engulfed by the oocyte.

In many invertebrates binding of the sperm to the egg is followed within seconds by a membrane depolarization, which prevents **polyspermy** (more than one sperm fertilizing the egg). This 'fast' block to polyspermy lasts about a minute. During this time, the cortical granules begin to fuse with the egg membrane and release their contents into the perivitelline space, where they alter the zona pellucida so that no more sperm can penetrate it – the 'slow' block to polyspermy. It is not yet clear if the 'fast' blocking step occurs in mammals but the slow block certainly does. The cortical granules release an unknown material that alters ZP3 in the zona so that it is no longer able to bind sperm heads.

Fusion also permits the oocyte to complete its second meiotic division (see Chapter 26), and the second polar body is expelled into the perivitelline space.

The maternal and paternal DNA each contribute to the formation of a pronucleus: the two pronuclei then fuse to form a single nucleus (see Figure 1.1). In humans this process may take as long as 11 or 12 hours.

Fusion of the pronuclei marks the conclusion of the process of fertilization and the definitive formation of the zygote. It is more difficult, however, to define unequivocally when fertilization began: it could be taken as the moment when the sperm approaches the egg, when it binds to the zona, or when it binds to the oocyte membrane. Diagnostic criteria for fertilization are generally taken to be the presence of two or more polar bodies in the perivitelline space, the presence of two pronuclei in the cytoplasm of the egg *and* the presence of sperm flagellar material in the egg cytoplasm.

Formation of the morula and blastocyst

The fertilized egg – the **zygote** – first divides 24–36 hours after fertilization (Figure 2.4). As no net growth has taken place, the resulting daughter cells or **blastomeres** are half the size of the zygote and as successive divisions continue

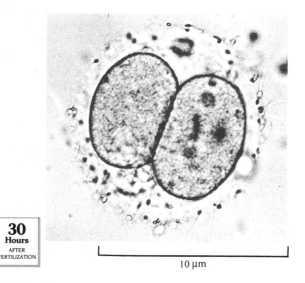

30 Hours AFTER FERTILIZATION

10 μm

FIGURE 2.4   Two-cell human pre-embryo. (Photograph courtesy of Dr David Edgar, Ninewells Hospital, Dundee.)

Zona pellucida —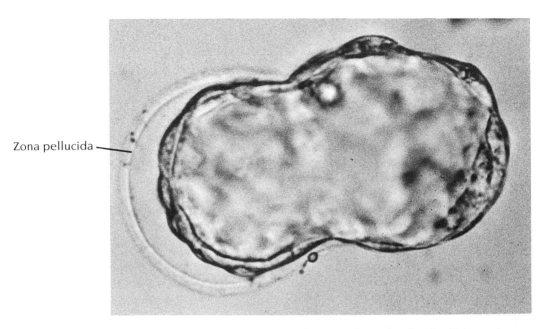

FIGURE 2.5 Human blastocyst 'hatching' from the zona pellucida. (Photograph courtesy of Dr David Edgar, Ninewells Hospital, Dundee.)

they become smaller and smaller. Eventually, 3–4 days after fertilization, they form a cluster of cells (the morula) (see Figure 1.5). The morula is still enclosed inside the zona at this stage. It has by now made its way down the uterine tube almost to the uterus, aided by the movement of cilia in the wall of the uterine tube and by peristalsis of the tube itself (Figure 2.2).

Approximately 4 days after fertilization, when about 32 cells are present, a space begins to form inside the morula. This space lies off-centre in the morula and is created by the cells moving apart and pumping fluid into the forming cavity. The cavity is known as the **blastocoel** (see Figure 1.7(b)), and this stage of development is known as the **blastocyst**.

As the blastocyst forms it begins to emerge from the zona pellucida (Figure 2.5), and enlarges. It is likely that its cells are taking up uterine fluid at this stage. However, the most important event as blastocyst formation proceeds is the appearance of two recognizably different cell types (see Figure 1.7(b)): an outer shell of **trophectoderm** cells and an eccentrically placed internal cluster of cells known as the **inner cell mass** (the mechanism underlying these events is discussed in Chapter 1). The trophectoderm cells will contribute only to the extraembryonic membranes: the inner cell mass will contribute both to the extraembryonic membranes and to the body of the embryo itself (Figure 2.6).

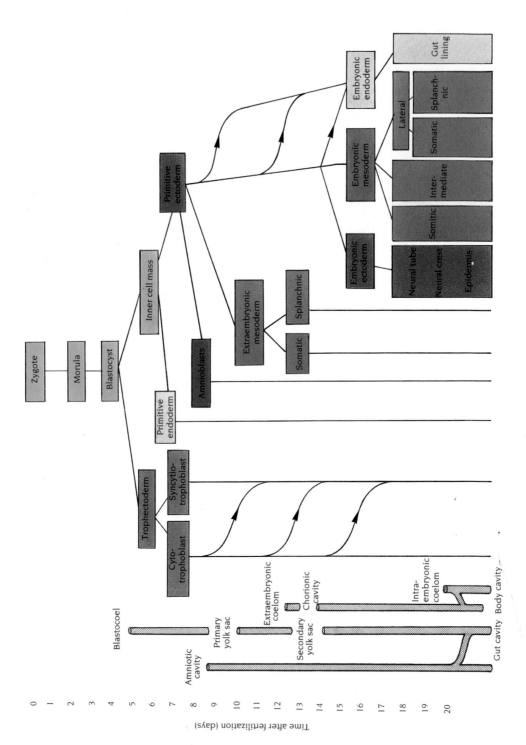

FIGURE 2.6 Tissue and cavity lineages in the early stages of human development (see text for details).

Implantation

Human embryos at implantation are difficult to identify in the uterus and there are still uncertainties as to exactly what is taking place. The account given below is based on morphological studies of human and animal embryos, and on experimental studies, mostly in the mouse.

Around 6 days, after the blastocyst has emerged from the zona, it begins to adhere to the uterine wall (Figure 2.7). Exactly how this occurs is not clear. The inner cell mass is generally found near the attachment site, which might be a consequence of either active migration round the inside of the blastocyst or because the trophoblast cells are induced by the underlying inner cell mass cells to begin differentiation in a way appropriate to promoting adhesion. However, the inner cell mass certainly plays a role in the next differentiative event in which some of the trophoblast cells begin to form a **syncytium**. The nuclei of the syncytium share a common cytoplasm, possibly because repeated nuclear division occurs without corresponding cell division.

The syncytial tissue is known as **syncytiotrophoblast** and the corresponding non-syncytial trophectoderm cells are known as **cytotrophoblast**. Close to the

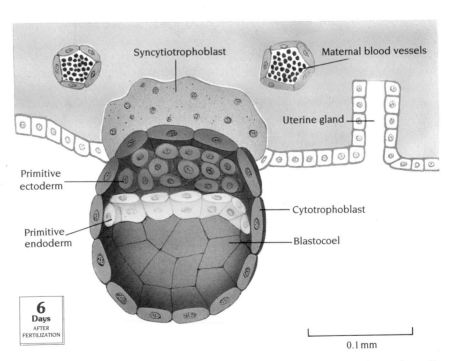

FIGURE 2.7 At about 6 days after fertilization the blastula adheres to the uterine wall. The trophectoderm layer has given rise to cytotrophoblast and syncytiotrophoblast. The syncytiotrophoblast cells then begin to invade the uterine endometrium. The inner cell mass has produced primitive ectoderm and endoderm.

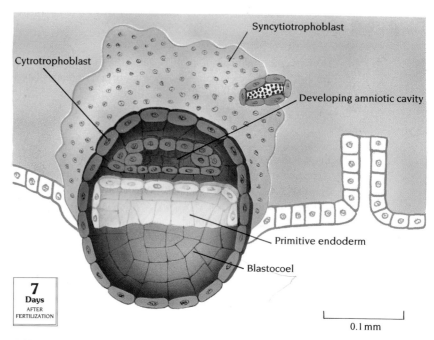

FIGURE 2.8 At about 7 days after fertilization the amniotic cavity begins to form.

inner cell mass the cytotrophoblast cells seem to become capable of giving off syncytiotrophoblast and acting as a stem cell population, but further from the inner cell mass the trophoblast cells remain as cytotrophoblast. This can be demonstrated in mice by placing an extra inner cell mass at the opposite end of the blastocyst cavity: the overlying trophoblast cells respond by producing syncytial cells.

Syncytiotrophoblast cells appear to be highly invasive and begin to 'eat' their way into the uterine wall. The blastocyst is now no longer dependent on its stored supplies of yolk: it receives nourishment from the maternal tissue and begins to grow rapidly. Eventually the blastocyst will sink completely into the uterine wall.

At the same time, the inner cell mass cells are also undergoing differentiation (Figure 2.7). Those cells exposed to the blastocyst cavity flatten to form a single layer: which is referred to as **primitive endoderm** (or **hypoblast**). The remaining inner cell mass cells are known as **primitive ectoderm** (or **epiblast**). It seems likely that hypoblast formation is induced by exposure to the blastocyst cavity.

Approximately 7 days after fertilization, the amniotic cavity appears (Figure 2.8). Exactly how this forms in humans is not known, but it probably arises from a cavity in the epiblast layer, in much the same way as the blastocyst cavity develops. The **amnioblasts** that line the amniotic cavity are therefore epiblastic in origin.

Meanwhile, the hypoblast cells migrate round the inside of the blastocoel cavity (Figure 2.9): and by about 9 days come to line it completely. These cells form the **extraembryonic endoderm**. A thin basement membrane lies between these cells and the cytotrophoblast. During this process some of the gaps created

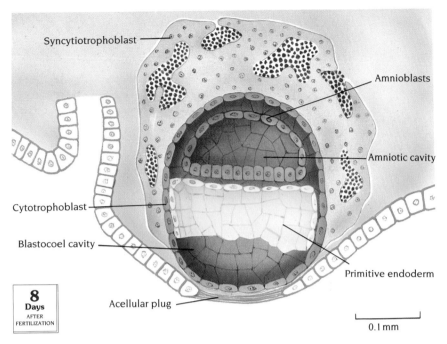

Syncytiotrophoblast

Amnioblasts

Amniotic cavity

Cytotrophoblast

Blastocoel cavity

Primitive endoderm

8
Days
AFTER
FERTILIZATION

Acellular plug

0.1 mm

FIGURE 2.9   At about 8 days after fertilization the conceptus has almost sunk into the uterine wall. The amniotic cavity is well formed. The primitive endoderm continues to migrate round the inside of the blastocoel. The syncytiotrophoblast has engulfed uterine blood vessels. A plug of acellular material closes off the opening to the uterine cavity.

in the hypoblast may be filled by cells from the epiblast. The disc of tissue that lies between the amniotic cavity and the blastocoel can be described as the **embryonic disc**. From this disc the embryo itself will develop.

Once the extraembryonic endoderm has completely lined the blastocoel, the endoderm cells expand and become reticulated, enclosing extensive fluid-filled spaces, largely occluding the original blastocoel cavity. The cavity remaining underneath the embryonic disc is now known as the **primary yolk sac** (Figure 2.10).

Appearance of the main body axis and mesoderm

The embryonic disc presents no obvious sign of orientation in the first days of its existence, but perhaps the most important single event in the whole developmental process is about to take place: the development of the main body axis. This will establish where the head and tail will lie, and because the dorsoventral axis

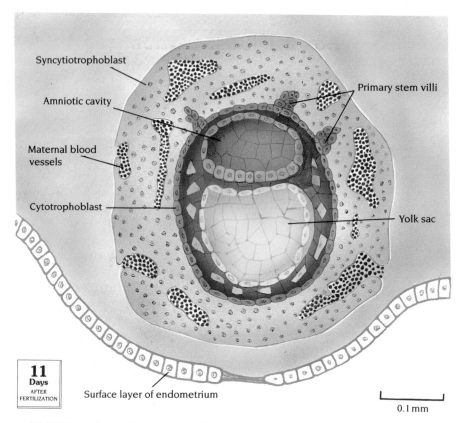

FIGURE 2.10 At about 11 days after fertilization the primary yolk sac detaches from the surrounding cytotrophoblast. Loose cells, perhaps endodermal in origin, are scattered round the yolk sac. An acellular basement membrane may also form here. Villi of cytotrophoblast cells begin to extend into the syncytiotrophoblast.

is defined by the relative positions of epiblast and hypoblast it also establishes left and right. The mechanisms underlying this event in humans have not been fully elucidated but a good understanding has been achieved of amphibian axis formation and, given the universality of developmental mechanisms, it is likely that a similar mechanism determines the axis in humans (see Box 2.1). Only the appearance of the axis can be described at present.

Approximately 13–14 days after fertilization, at the caudal end of the embryo, the first sign of the **primitive streak** appears in the epiblast (Figure 2.11), initially as a thickening at the margin of the epiblast which then extends towards the centre of the disc. A midline groove (known as the **primitive groove**) develops in the streak as seen from the amniotic cavity. At the cranial end of the groove a distinct **primitive node** or pit also forms.

At the primitive groove the process of **gastrulation** is taking place (see Box 2.1), in which cells from the epiblast migrate into the groove then detach

Box 2.1 Gastrulation • 35

Box 2.1 Gastrulation

The embryonic disc is radially symmetrical until gastrulation begins, then one definitive axis normally develops. This axis could form in any orientation on the disc: certainly, in experimental studies, it can be induced to appear in a variety of positions. Axis formation may even begin in two different places simultaneously, which may result in identical twins sharing one amniotic cavity (see Special Topic 3, pp. 62–8): however, there is also a possibility that the embryonic axes will approach each other or cross at some point (Figure 1), perhaps resulting in conjoined twins. A spectrum of such twinning is observed, from minor joining of the superficial layers (whereby twins are separable by surgery) to the sharing of major organs (which makes separation impossible).

Associated intimately with the process of axis formation is the formation of the embryonic mesoderm. Primitive ectoderm cells begin to move towards the primitive streak (Figure 2) and at the primitive groove they detach ventrally from the epiblast and move into the space between the epiblast and hypoblast. The cells travel laterally under the epiblast, forming the intermediate layer known as the embryonic mesoderm.

The primitive pit or node represents an area of cranial and lateral movement of the mesoderm cells. The node originates at the most cranial

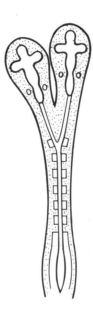

FIGURE 1 Bifurcated embryonic axis seen during the development of the chick (from specimen in author's collection).

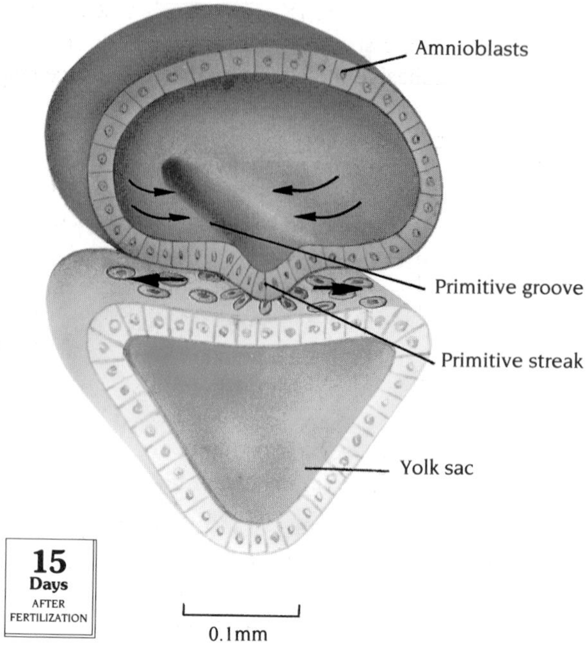

FIGURE 2   Mesoderm formation at the primitive streak during gastrulation.

end of the primitive streak but gradually shifts its relative position caudally down the body axis.

Mechanisms of gastrulation

There are two aspects to gastrulation: what happens, and what makes it
happen. The favoured embryos for investigation of gastrulation are those
of birds and amphibians. Mammalian embryos are much less well studied,
and at first appear very different from birds and amphibians because of the
very small amounts of yolk present in their eggs. However, the great unification of developmental biology that has occurred in the last 10 years
seems to justify the prediction that the information gained from birds and
frogs will be applicable to mammals, particularly at the molecular level.

Main cellular events

A number of cell behaviours are involved in gastrulation.

(1)   Cells move towards the primitive streak as a continuous sheet rather
       than as individuals. This movement may be driven by cell division
       in the epiblast and by conversion of the epiblast from a structure
       several cells thick to a single layer.

Box 2.1 Gastrulation • **37**

(2)   Passage through the primitive streak is associated with changes in cell shape and adhesiveness, modulated by the cytoskeleton and by adhesive molecules on the cell surface respectively.

(3)   Subsequent spreading out of the mesoderm cells is under the influence of a network of extracellular fibrils secreted by the epiblast cells.

These can be carried out by isolated fragments of tissue: in other words the behaviours are part of the intrinsic repertoire of the cells at that stage in their differentiation, and they merely need to be organized to carry them out in the correct spatial orientation. An understanding of the mechanism behind this 'organization' has long been ardently pursued by developmental biologists: answers are slowly being found, at least to the problem of the induction of mesoderm differentiation.

Mechanisms behind events

The amphibian egg before fertilization has a recognizable distribution of components from dorsal to ventral (compare with Figure 1.3) and fertilization occurs near the equator of the egg. On fertilization, cytoplasmic rearrangements occur, which result in the appearance of the 'grey crescent': a distinct region lying rather more towards the vegetal pole than the animal, and opposite the point of sperm entry. As cleavage proceeds and the embryo converts itself into a ball of cells, the grey crescent area proves to be the region at which gastrulation will begin.

It has long been known that the dorsal and ventral cells of the blastula need to interact to form mesoderm. If separated they form ectoderm and endoderm respectively, but mesoderm can be generated at the interface only when they are combined. The molecular mechanism behind this is becoming clear. The scheme described below is based on a number of research approaches and, although it is preliminary in nature, provides an explanation in principle of all the key features of gastrulation and axis formation. Future research may result in this model being modified in detail, rather than being completely rejected.

An essential key step was the discovery of classes of molecule that possess mesodermal-inducing properties. When presumptive ectodermal cells are exposed to these factors in culture, they convert into mesoderm cells. The particular type of mesoderm formed depends on the concentration and precise nature of the inducing factors. Three such families of factors have been identified:

- molecules of the transforming growth factor beta (TGF-β) family, which includes activins A and B, and bone morphogenetic protein 4;
- molecules related to the fibroblast growth factors (FGFs) (which will reappear as angiogenic factors);
- members of the Wnt family.

Identifying which of these are active in the egg is not easy: it is necessary to establish that the candidate molecule is present in the correct

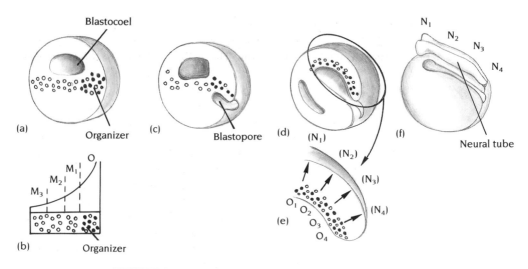

FIGURE 3 Gastrulation in the amphibian *Xenopus laevis* (compare with Figure 1.4). Molecules of the TGF-β family are shown as •, and those of the FGF family as ○. After fertilization, differential localization of molecules of the TGF-β family occurs in a specialized region close to where the 'grey crescent' will form. (a) This special region, known as the organizer (b), is believed to signal to the remaining mesoderm, creating a gradient which the mesodermal cells interpret by differentiating into different kinds of mesoderm (labelled M_1, M_2, M_3). (c) Invagination begins at the grey crescent region. Surface cells begin to pass to the inside via the blastopore. (d,e) As they pass through the organizer region in sequence, they acquire positional values (labelled O_1 to O_4). These values then influence the overlying ectoderm, conveying positional values labelled as N_1–N_4. (f) Positional values N_1–N_4 are interpreted by the cells as the craniocaudal differentiation states of the neural tube.

amounts at the right time and place, and as yet no unequivocal candidate has emerged. This is perhaps because complex interactions between the molecules are involved. However, a speculative explanation is as follows.

Maternal mRNAs for the TGF-β family and protein and mRNAs for the FGF family are believed to be present in the unfertilized amphibian egg. The TGF-β-like mRNA precursors are known to be concentrated in the ventral region of the egg. Fertilization activates microtubules and other cytoskeletal elements to transport various factors (perhaps mRNA precursors, or perhaps activators of mRNA transcription) throughout the cytoplasm and as a result differential activity of TGF-β-like molecules is believed to commence opposite the point of sperm entry, in the grey crescent region (Figure 3). Cleavage proceeds and the egg gradually forms a ball of small cells (the morula), which goes on to develop an internal cavity (the blastula). At some point before gastrulation the TGF-β-like and FGF-like molecules become active and induce mesoderm formation in the

Box 2.1 Gastrulation • 39

overlying cells. Both types of molecule can perform this role in culture but the TGF-β-like molecules in the grey crescent seem to induce formation of a particular kind of mesoderm. The cells overlying the grey crescent become 'organizer' cells, capable of signalling to the other cells of the mesoderm (Figure 3(b)). The strength of this signal is highest near the organizing region and falls off across the embryo. The undifferentiated mesoderm responds by producing different types of mesoderm, in accordance with the level of signal to which it is exposed. In this way a variety of mesodermal cell types are induced. Gastrulation is induced at the grey crescent region where the level of signal is at its strongest.

During gastrulation in amphibians cells flow from the outside to the inside of the organism via an opening known as the blastopore (Figure 3(c)) causing the 'organizer' tissue to be distributed underneath the surface ectoderm (Figure 3(d)). The overlying ectoderm is in turn induced to form particular regions of the brain and neural tube, generating the craniocaudal pattern of the central nervous system (Figure 3(e)).

In this way, a simple regional difference induced by fertilization initiates a cascade of events determining the morphology of the whole organism.

Mesoderm-inducing factors have been shown to activate particular classes of genes containing a sequence known as the **homoeobox**. This is of great importance to our understanding of pattern formation, and is dealt with in Special Topic 6 (pp. 174–7). In addition, retinoic acid, an agent with morphogenetic action in a number of developing organ systems, appears to influence the expression of neural tube regional specificity, and activates homoeobox-containing genes. This will be discussed fully in Chapter 18.

and drop off to lie between the epiblast and hypoblast. These cells give rise to a new tissue: the **embryonic mesoderm**. As it forms, the primitive ectoderm or epiblast is more conveniently described as **embryonic ectoderm**. Similarly, the primitive endoderm or hypoblast contributes to the **embryonic endoderm**, although this is also thought to derive, at least in part, by invagination from the embryonic ectoderm at the primitive groove. These are the three definitive **germ layers**: each will give rise to a characteristic set of tissues in the embryo and fetus.

Extraembryonic mesoderm and the chorionic cavity

Some mesodermal cells begin to appear close to the embryonic disc just before the primitive streak is evident and spread out along the inside of the cytotrophoblast lining cells to form **extraembryonic mesoderm**, named to reflect its position. However, it is likely that the extraembryonic mesoderm arises in the

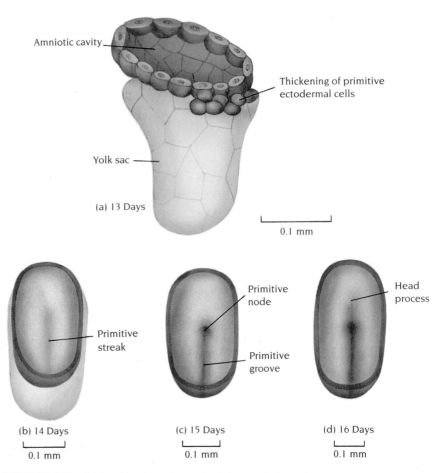

FIGURE 2.11 (a) In this view, the roof of the amniotic cavity has been removed. A thickening begins to form in the primitive ectoderm. The surrounding cytotrophoblast, and the mesoderm when it forms, are not shown: see Figure 2.12 for the arrangement of these structures. (b) Looking down into the amniotic cavity, the primitive streak can be seen forming in the primitive ectoderm. (c) The primitive groove forms in the midline of the streak. The node can be seen at the cranial end of the groove. (d) The head process forms, underlying the ectoderm and extending towards what will be the cranial end of the embryo (compare with Figure 2.13).

same general manner as the definitive embryonic mesoderm and it makes sense to believe that it forms in the region where the primitive streak will first appear. While it is forming, the primary yolk sac collapses, producing the **secondary yolk sac** and **extraembryonic coelom** (Figure 2.12). There is a high probability that vesicles of yolk sac and strands of extraembryonic endoderm tissue will be left behind in the space thus formed. As the extraembryonic mesoderm creeps round the cytotrophoblast cells to line the space formed by the collapse of the

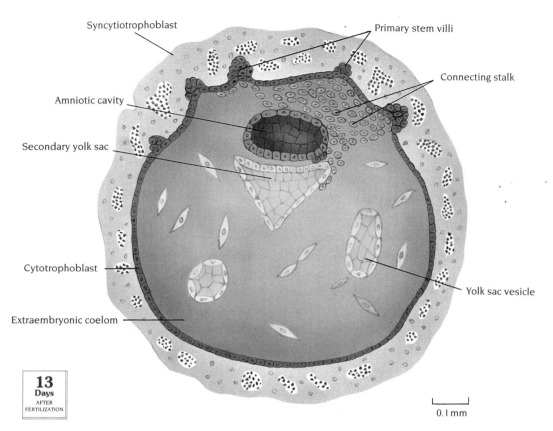

Syncytiotrophoblast

Primary stem villi

Connecting stalk

Amniotic cavity

Secondary yolk sac

Cytotrophoblast

Yolk sac vesicle

Extraembryonic coelom

13 Days AFTER FERTILIZATION

0.1 mm

FIGURE 2.12 At about day 13 after fertilization, cells begin to appear in the extra-embryonic space at the presumptive tail end of the amniotic vesicle. These are probably extraembryonic mesoderm cells derived from the primitive ectoderm and they will form a 'connecting stalk' to the cytotrophoblast, around which they will migrate. The extra-embryonic space has expanded considerably from that shown in Figure 2.10, while the yolk sac may also have contracted. This new space is initially known as the extraembryonic coelom.

primary yolk sac, so it completes a tissue structure in three layers: extraembry-onic mesoderm, cytotrophoblast and syncytiotrophoblast. This structure is known as the **chorion**, and the cavity it surrounds as the **chorionic cavity**. Eventually the extraembryonic mesoderm will not only cover the secondary yolk sac and amnion completely but it will also form a **connecting stalk**, which joins the caudal end of the embryo to the wall of the chorionic cavity (Figure 2.13).

Chorionic villi

Meanwhile, the syncytiotrophoblast has continued to invade unevenly into the maternal uterine tissue in the form of small processes known as **chorionic villi**

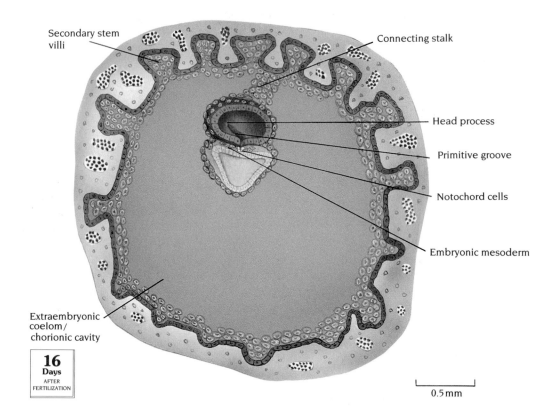

FIGURE 2.13 Mesoderm has migrated all the way round the extraembryonic coelom, which can now be known as the chorionic cavity. Note the change in scale.

(Figure 2.10). Small maternal blood vessels may be engulfed by the syncytiotrophoblast cells, forming blood-filled spaces within the syncytiotrophoblast. At roughly 9 days, cytotrophoblast villi also begin to push into the syncytial layer. At first these are composed of cytotrophoblast cells only but, subsequently, extraembryonic mesoderm cells will come to lie at their core (Figure 2.13). Finally, they will become highly branched and ramified, with blood vessels in the central mesoderm. These three stages are described as representing primary, secondary and tertiary stem villi respectively. Their purpose is to increase the surface area available for interchange with the maternal tissue. They will continue to ramify and come to interconnect during the embryonic stage.

During this time, the whole conceptus (that is, everything produced by fertilization) continues to sink into the uterine wall. It will eventually disappear beneath the surface and the syncytiotrophoblast will grow around it. A plug of cellular and acellular material remains at the surface to mark the site of implantation (Figure 2.10).

The conceptus can now grow rapidly as it receives nutrients by diffusion from the maternal blood vessels, which have been engulfed by syncytiotrophoblast cells.

Maternal immune suppression

The conceptus is genetically unique foreign tissue: why then is it not rejected by the mother in the same way that a tissue graft from the child would be rejected after birth? A variety of answers have been proposed to this riddle, but the answer appears to lie in the mode of expression of antigens of the major histocompatibility complex (MHC) by syncytio- and cytotrophoblast cells. These are cell-surface molecules that are recognized by T cells in immune reactions, and are responsible for the rejection of grafts between individuals. In trophoblast-derived tissues the expression of MHC antigens seems to be suppressed or confined to non-immunogenic categories by control mechanisms operating at the level of protein transcription. Further understanding of this mechanism could have important implications for suppression of immunity in organ transplantation.

Defects of conception

Hydatidiform mole This is an invasive mass of cytotrophoblast and syncytiotrophoblast cells, which might be part of the normal placenta or might replace the conceptus completely (**partial** and **complete** hydatidiform mole respectively). The appearance is often described as reminiscent of a bunch of grapes (Figure 2.14). The mole may fill the uterine cavity, growing faster than a normal conceptus, and is likely to dislodge spontaneously during the pregnancy. These abnormalities are believed to originate very early in development, immediately after partial and complete hydatidiform fertilization. Both types of mole are associated with an abnormal complement of DNA, which can arise either from the penetration of two sperms into the egg or from the abnormal duplication of the paternal genetic material immediately after fertilization. In the complete form the maternal chromosomes are absent and only paternal chromosomes are present; in the partial form the maternal chromosomes remain in the cell, so the resulting individual is triploid.

In complete hydatidiform mole, no fetal material develops and there is a high probability – perhaps as much as one in 12 – that the mole will give rise to a choriocarcinoma (see below). Partial hydatidiform mole may be present in association with fetal material in a variety of forms. It is even possible for a triploid individual to be born alive, though none has survived longer than a few

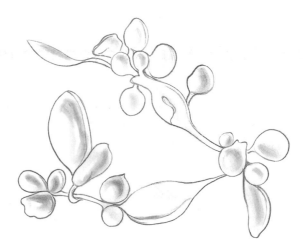

FIGURE 2.14 Hydatidiform mole.

months. A partial hydatidiform mole may also give rise to a choriocarcinoma, although this is less likely than with the complete form. The incidence of condition varies with social and genetic factors. It can be as high as one in 80 pregnancies in very deprived areas such as the Philippines, compared with one in 2500 in North America.

Choriocarcinoma This is a highly invasive tumour of the uterine wall, associated with hydatidiform mole. The tumour invades the underlying uterine muscle. Its presence can be recognized by the persistently high levels of human chorionic gonadotrophin in the maternal blood. This type of tumour was once almost invariably lethal but it can now be treated by chemotherapy.

Ectopic pregnancy When the egg is fertilized, it lies in the ampulla of the uterus. The zygote, dividing as it goes, is moved towards the uterus. Implantation cannot occur until the trophoblast has developed, so normally it cannot implant before reaching the uterus. However, if the passage of the blastula is delayed it may implant in the uterine tube. Alternatively, fertilization may have occurred in the abdominal cavity or the fertilized egg may have fallen into the cavity, and implantation has been known to take place in the mesodermal cavity lining – an **ectopic** pregnancy. It is very rare for the embryo to survive, because the implantation site is not a proper endometrium. However, the erosive capabilities of trophoblast cells may expose and damage blood vessels, causing persistent, and sometimes fatal, bleeding. A tubal pregnancy (an ectopic pregnancy in the uterine tube) is likely to cause the tube to rupture during the second month of pregnancy. Warning signs of an ectopic pregnancy include vaginal bleeding and abdominal pain.

Special Topic 2 In vitro fertilization

In vitro fertilization (IVF) and embryo transfer of human eggs was unknown before 1978: by 1989, it had been responsible for the birth of perhaps 12 000 children world-wide and had become an everyday term. IVF has revolutionized the outlook for infertile couples, who represent perhaps one in ten of all couples. The technique is most appropriate for those women whose oviducts cannot transmit eggs from the ovary to the uterus, due to scar damage caused by pelvic infection or ectopic pregnancies, or for women who have had an ovary removed for cancer-related conditions. However, a number of other conditions, including low functional sperm counts, can also be alleviated by its use.

As women usually produce only one egg per cycle, which is insufficient to offer a reasonable chance of conception by IVF, the first step is to increase the number of eggs released. This can be done using the oestrogen agonist clomiphene or gonadotrophins. Follicle development can be followed by ultrasound visualization techniques and, when the woman is approaching ovulation, the eggs can be removed by aspiration with a fine needle inserted through the abdominal wall, aided by fibre-optic viewing devices.

The eggs removed in this way are surrounded by cumulus cells (which would normally become the corona radiata – see Chapter 26). These may be removed by gentle agitation or by mild chemical treatments, although fertilization is not hindered if a few cumulus cells remain: indeed, the cumulus cells may have a role in nutrition of the egg, and their presence may be an advantage.

A sperm sample is obtained from the man, and the sperm are capacitated (as discussed earlier in this chapter) by maintaining them for a short time in culture medium containing one of a number of non-specific agents. Sperm may be concentrated and resuspended in smaller volumes of medium, which can improve the fertilization rate for men with low sperm counts or high numbers of abnormal sperm.

The oocytes and sperm are combined for 4–24 hours, often in a small drop of culture medium under a layer of paraffin oil, which inhibits the loss of gases from the culture medium. After fertilization, the zygotes are maintained in a culture tube and their progress through the early stages monitored.

Pre-embryos past the four-cell stage are placed in the uterus or uterine tube via the vagina and cervix, using a narrow catheter. A substantial number of pre-embryos fail to implant, although this may reflect the natural situation (where many, perhaps most, fertilizations fail to lead to pregnancy), rather than being a deleterious effect of in vitro fertilization itself. Therefore it is customary to return more than one fertilized egg to the uterus. This in turn means that the overall number of multiple pregnancies is high. A reasonable compromise between the risk of having no resulting pregnancy and that of having a multiple pregnancy is to place three pre-embryos in the uterus.

Although success rates vary from clinic to clinic, approximately 25–30% of all women entering an IVF programme have a successful pregnancy. Negative outcomes such as stillbirth or abnormality are increased in IVF pregnancies, although this seems to be a consequence of the increased number of multiple pregnancies rather than the procedure itself.

An alternative to IVF and embryo transfer is gamete intrafallopian transfer (GIFT), in which sperm and eggs are placed together in the uterine tubes of the intended mother. This is technically rather simpler than achieving fertilization in vitro.

Sperm or fertilized eggs may be deep frozen for later use. During freezing it is essential to avoid the formation of ice crystals in the cells. This can be done by adding a cryoprotectant such as dimethylsulphoxide or glycerol and gently lowering the temperature to a point at which the specimen can be immersed safely in liquid nitrogen. Freezing lowers the chances of subsequent development by about half but any non-implanted embryos can be stored for later use if the first attempt at fertilization is unsuccessful. In addition, a fertilized pre-embryo can be frozen while a few of its cells are being tested for genetic defects (see Special Topic 1, pp. 18–21).

Freezing embryos can pose a variety of unusual ethical and legal problems: for example when the 'parents' of a frozen embryo were killed in a plane crash, an extensive legal argument ensued over the rights of the frozen embryo, as opposed to living next of kin, to inherit its parents' property.

Further reading

Bagshawe K.D., Lawler S.D., Paradinas F.J., Dent J., Brown P. and Boxer G.M. (1990). Gestational trophoblastic tumours following initial diagnosis of partial hydatidiform mole. *Lancet*, **335**, 1074–6.

Bellairs R. (1986). The primitive streak. *Anat. Embryol.*, **174**, 1–14

Brackett B.G., Seitz H.M., Rocha G. and Mastroianni L. (1972). The mammalian fertilisation process.In *Biology of Mammalian Fertilization and Implantation* (Moghissi, K.S. and Hafez, E.S.E., eds), pp.165–84.Springfield Il: Thomas

Copp A.J. (1978). Interaction between inner cell mass cells and trophectoderm of the mouse blastocyst. 1. A study of cellular proliferation. *J. Embryol. Exp. Morph.*, **48**, 109–25

Edwards R.G. (1972). Fertilization and cleavage in vitro of human ova. In *Biology of Mammalian Fertilization and Implantation* (Moghissi, K.S. and Hafez, E.S.E., eds), pp. 263–78. Springfield Il: Thomas

Edwards R.G. (1980). *Conception in the Human Female*. London: Academic Press

Edwards R., Crow J., Dale S., Macnamee M., Hartshorne G. and Brinsden P. (1990). Preimplantation diagnosis and recurrent hydatidiform mole. *Lancet*, **335**, 1030–1

Gardner R.L. (1985). Manipulation of development. In *Reproduction in Mammals* Vol. 4. (Austin C.R. and Short R.V., eds), pp. 159–80. Cambridge: Cambridge University Press

Hertig A.T. (1968). *Human Trophoblast*. Springfield Il: Thomas

Kawata M., Parnes J.R. and Herzenberg L.A. (1984). Transcriptional control of HLA A B, C antigens in human placental cytotrophoblasts isolated using trophoblast and HLA specific monoclonal antibodies and the fluorescence activated cell sorter. *J. Exp. Med.*, **160**, 633–51

Kovats S., Elliot K.M., Librach C., Stubbleline M., Fisher S.J. and DeMars R. (1990). A class I antigen, HLA-G, expressed in human trophoblasts. *Science*, **248**, 220–3

Luckett W.P. (1975). The development of primordial and definitive amniotic cavities in early rhesus monkey and human embryos. *Am. J. Anat.*, **144**, 149–68

Luckett W.P. (1978). Origin and differentiation of the yolk sac and extra-embryonic mesoderm in pre-somite human and rhesus monkey embryos. *Am. J. Anat.*, **152**, 59–97

Novak E.R. and Woodruff J.D. (1974). *Novak's Gynecologic and Obstetric Pathology*. Philadelphia: W.B. Saunders

O'Rahilly R. and Muller M. (1987). *Developmental stages in human embryos*. Carnegie Institute of Washington Publication 637

Sathananthan A.H., Trounson A.O. and Wood C. (1986). *Atlas of Fine Structure of Human Sperm Penetration, Eggs, and Embryos Cultured in vitro*. New York: Praeger

Soupart P. and Strong P.A. (1974). Ultrastructural observations on human oocytes fertilised in vitro. *Fertil. Steril.*, **24**, 462–78

Tesarik J. (1986). From the cellular to the molecular dimension: the actual challenge for human fertilisation research. *Gamete Res.*, **13**, 47–89

Tesarik J., Kopecny V., Plachot M., Mandelbaum J., DaLage C. and Flechon J.-E. (1986). Nucleologenesis in the human embryo developing in vitro: ultrastructural and autoradiographic analysis. *Dev. Biol.*, **115**, 193–203

Wassarman P.M. (1987). The biology and chemistry of fertilisation. *Science*, **235**, 553–60

Wassarman P.M. (1988). Fertilisation in mammals. *Sci. Am.*, **279**, 52–8

Box 2.1

Boucaut J.-C., D'Arribere T., Li S.D., Boulekbache H., Yamada K.M. and Thierry J.P. (1985). Evidence for the role of fibronectin in amphibian gastrulation. *J. Embryol. Exp. Morph.*, **89** (suppl.), 211–27

Keller R.E. (1980). The cellular basis of amphibian gastrulation. In *Developmental Biology: a Comprehensive Synthesis*. Vol. 2. (Browder, L., ed.), pp. 241–327. New York: Plenum Press

Slack J.M.W. (1983). *From Egg to Embryo. Determinative Events in Early Development*. Cambridge: Cambridge University Press

Slack J.M.W., Isaacs H.V. and Darlington B.G. (1988). Inductive effects of fibroblast growth factor and lithium ion on *Xenopus* blastula ectoderm. *Development*, **103**, 581–90

Smith J.C. (1989). Mesoderm induction and mesoderm inducing factors in early amphibian development. *Development*, **105**, 665–77

Smith J.C. and Howard J.E. (1992). Mesoderm-inducing factors and the control of gastrulation. In *Gastrulation. Development Supplement* (Stern C.D. and Ingham P., eds), pp. 127–36. Cambridge: The Company of Biologists Ltd.

Smith J.C., Yaqoob M. and Symes K. (1988). Purification, partial characterisation and biological effects of the XTC mesoderm-inducing factor. *Development*, **103**, 591–600

Special Topic 2

Asch R.H., Balmaceda J.P., Ellsworth L.R. and Wong P.C. (1985). Gamete intrafallopian transfer (GIFT). A new treatment for infertility. *Int. J. Fertil.*, **40**, 41–5

Cohen J., Fehilly C. and Edwards R. (1986). Alleviating human infertility. In

Reproduction in Mammals 5: Manipulating Reproduction (Austin, C.R. and Short, R.V., eds), pp. 148–75. Cambridge: Cambridge University Press

Edwards R.G. (1981). Test-tube babies, 1981. *Nature*, **293**, 253–6

Edwards R.G. and Purdy J.M., eds (1982). *Human Conception in vitro*. London: Academic Press

Leese H. (1988). *Human Reproduction and in vitro Fertilisation*. London: Macmillan

Singer P., Kuhse H., Buckle S., Dawson K. and Kasimba P. (1990). *Embryo Experimentation*. Cambridge: Cambridge University Press

Steptoe P.C. and Edwards R.G. (1978). Birth after the implantation of a human embryo. *Lancet*, **ii**, 366

Trounson A. and Mohr L. (1983). Human pregnancy following cryopreservation, thawing and transfer of an eight-cell embryo. *Nature*, **305**, 707–9

3

From the gastrula to the early embryo

Gastrulation is perhaps the most important single event in animal development: the orientation of the body is laid down and the progenitor tissues for much of the body are established. The events immediately following the onset of gastrulation continue these themes of establishment of the main body axis and origination of major tissue types. However, the increasing complexity of the tissue arrangements makes it difficult to describe these stages in strict chronological sequence, and it is less confusing to follow the development of individual tissues.

The notochord

While the primitive streak indicates the main line of the body axis it does not contribute to any of the axial structures and eventually it will degenerate and disappear. From the primitive node at its cranial end, however, a structure will be laid down in a cranial direction. This is the notochord, at first composed of mesodermal-like cells arranged in the form of a rod (Figure 3.1). The notochord forms a tube and fuses with the underlying endoderm. Finally, a rod-like structure is re-formed, lying underneath the neural tube (see below). The exact cellular origin of the notochord remains obscure (Figure 3.2).

The notochord extends cranially to the region where the mouth will appear. Here, the advancing mesoderm cells do not invade between the ectoderm and

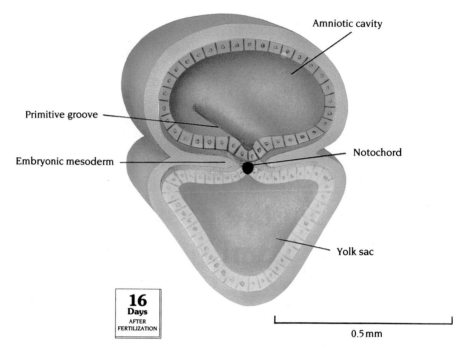

FIGURE 3.1   Notochord cells underlie the primitive groove (see Figure 2.13).

endoderm, which therefore remain closely apposed to each other (Figure 3.2). A similar situation applies in the region in which the anus will develop.

The notochord cells produce extracellular matrix molecules such as collagen, so the notochord becomes cartilaginous in nature. It underlies the developing neural tube, which it may help to induce in the ectoderm. In humans, the notochord will eventually degenerate, contributing only to the nuclei pulposi of the intervertebral discs.

EVOLUTION OF THE NOTOCHORD

The notochord is a very primitive vertebrate feature: it is one of the defining features of the class Chordata, which includes all the vertebrates. Originally it served to stiffen the body during swimming movements – a function carried out in modern vertebrates by the spine. Its continued presence in the embryos of higher vertebrates may hint at a role during development: it is believed to act as an inducer of the neural plate, and may convey the information that helps to regionalize the neural tube as it develops. It may also assist in the physical extension of the neural region as it forms.

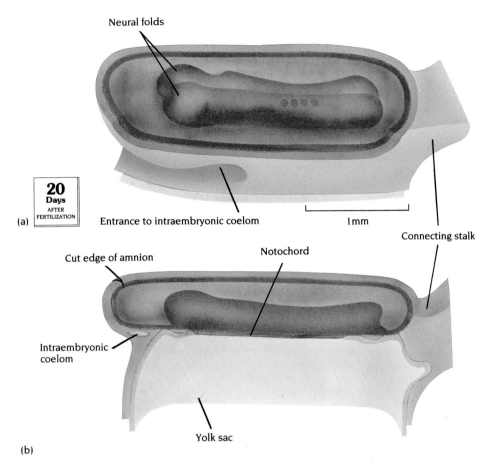

Neural folds

20
Days
AFTER
FERTILIZATION

(a)

Entrance to intraembryonic coelom

1mm

Connecting stalk

Cut edge of amnion

Notochord

Intraembryonic coelom

Yolk sac

(b)

FIGURE 3.2 (a) View of 20-day embryo, with the amniotic cavity and yolk sac cut away. (b) Diagrammatic midline sagittal section through the figure shown in (a). The notochord underlies the neural axis, and its cells are continuous with the endoderm. Mesoderm has separated the ectoderm and endoderm except in the regions where the mouth and anus will form.

The intraembryonic coelom

Spaces or openings begin to appear in the intraembryonic mesoderm, in a manner reminiscent of the formation of the blastocoel and the amniotic cavity (Figure 3.3(a)). These spaces coalesce to form the **intraembryonic coelom** (Figure 3.3(b)), which runs forwards (in the form of tunnels in the mesoderm) on either side of the main body axis and crosses in front of the developing forebrain (see Figure 3.2), to give a horseshoe shape. At the base of the legs of the horseshoe the intraembryonic coelom opens out into the chorionic cavity.

The intraembryonic mesoderm lateral to the main body axis is separated by the intraembryonic coelom into two leaflets (Figure 3.3(b)). The more dorsal of

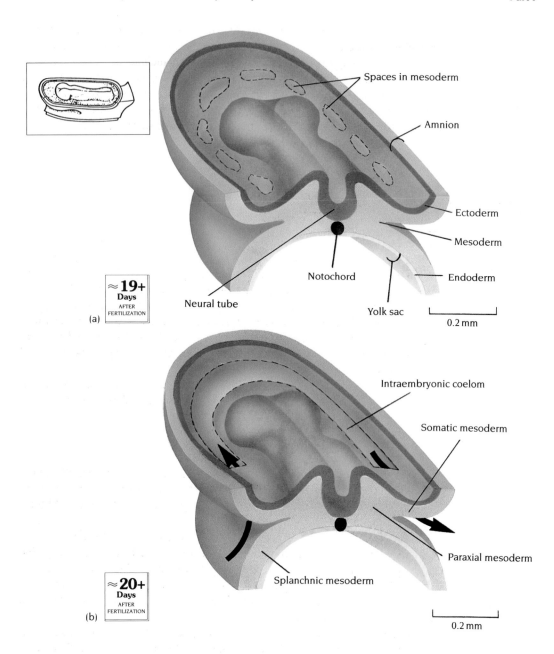

FIGURE 3.3 (a) Transverse section through an embryo slightly younger than that in Figure 3.2(a), looking forward towards the cranial end. Spaces begin to appear in the mesoderm and gradually coalesce to form a horseshoe shaped cavity opening out to the chorionic cavity. This later arrangement is shown in Figure 3.2(b), with the roof of the intraembryonic coelom removed. The fully formed intraembryonic coelom separates the mesoderm into two leaflets described as somatic and splanchnic mesoderm.

these is known as the somatic (body) mesoderm; the more ventral as the splanchnic (visceral) mesoderm. Somatic mesoderm is associated with ectoderm, and together are called the **somatopleure**; splanchnic mesoderm is associated with endoderm, and these two together are correspondingly named the **splanchnopleure**. The somatic and splanchnic mesoderms are initially similar in appearance and potential but will give rise to different structures because they are exposed to different influences from various neighbouring tissues.

Germ layer derivatives

The three layers of tissue thus formed – ectoderm, mesoderm and endoderm – can be followed throughout development. In general terms, the ectoderm will give rise to the surface layer of the skin and neural tissue. The endoderm will give rise to the lining of the gut and will contribute to many of the organs derived from the gut. The mesoderm, intermediate between these layers, will lead to the development of muscle, bone, connective tissue and blood, amongst others. However, these divisions are far from inviolable. The germ layers are conceptually useful as an organizing idea, rather than as a rigid description of tissue lineages.

In the following sections, the axial derivatives of the germ layers (the neural tube, the somites and the intermediate mesoderm) will be considered

Neurulation

In human embryos neurulation begins at about 17 or 18 days after fertilization. Influenced by the underlying tissues, the ectoderm along the axis starts to thicken to form the **neural plate**. Almost any region of the ectoderm could form the neural plate: it is intrinsic to all ectodermal cells at this time. The neural plate elongates in the craniocaudal axis, narrowing laterally. Cell division, cell rearrangement and changes in cell shape all play a role in this reshaping. The neural plate then begins to fold, with ridges arising on either side of the axis (Figure 3.4). This folding appears to be related to the formation of hinge points (one medially and one on each side (Figure 3.5)), which are associated with local changes in cell shape.

Changes in cell shape may be caused by local action of the cytoskeleton within each cell. Cells of the developing neural tube often have rings of microfilament at their apex, and these may be capable of contracting (Figure 3.6). As a cell may be considered to be of constant volume in the short term, this inevitably causes the cell to become wedge-shaped, which in turn influences the shape of the sheet of cells in which it lies.

Eventually the folds on either side of the neural plate come into contact with each other and fuse (Figure 3.7). This fusion does not take place simultane-

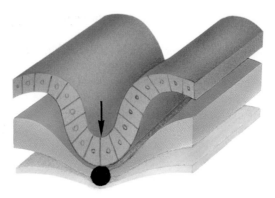

FIGURE 3.4 The ectoderm begins to roll up parallel to the primitive streak to form neural ridges.

ously along the whole length of the forming tube: it begins in the region between the developing hindbrain and upper neck, at about 22 days after fertilization. (regionalization of the brain is evident almost from the earliest appearance of the neural tube), and extends out towards the head and tail (Figure 3.8). The tube closes completely at the cranial end 3 or 4 days later, with the tail end closing several days subsequently. Failure of fusion leads to a variety of defects (see Chapter 6).

Along the dorsal edges of the fusing neural tube another category of differ-entiated cell begins to appear; the **neural crest** cells (Figure 3.7), which will

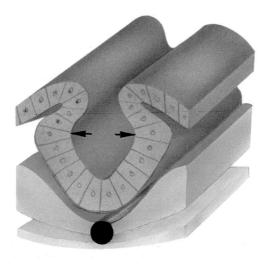

FIGURE 3.5 Neural hinge points.

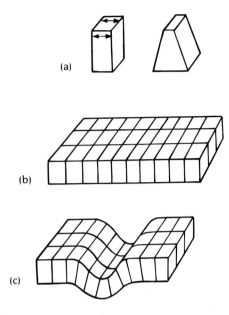

FIGURE 3.6 (a) Contraction of microfilaments at the apex of a single neural plate cell of constant volume can lead to cell shape changes. A sheet of such cells (b) showing shape changes of this kind will undergo deformation (c).

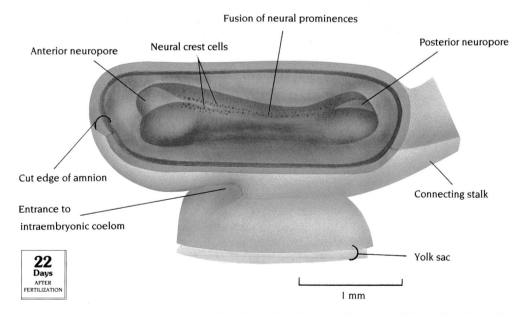

FIGURE 3.7 Diagram of 22-day embryo in the amniotic cavity. Neural ridge fusion first occurs in the presumptive hindbrain/cervical region. Note the considerable growth the caudal part of the neural tube will therefore have to undergo to reach adult proportions.

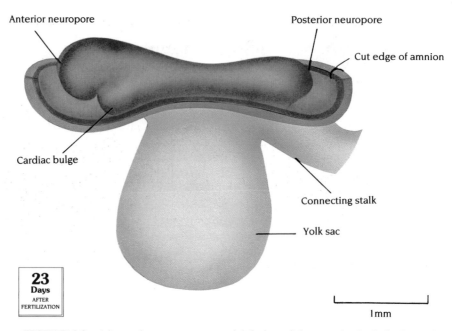

FIGURE 3.8 After a day or two, sequential fusion of the neural tube in both cranial and caudal directions has occurred.

give rise to an extraordinary variety of cell types (see Chapter 11), although in this chapter we are concerned only with their contribution to the nervous system. The neural crest cells detach from the neural folds and migrate into the meso-derm. At first they form a continuous sheet: later, they form clusters which fore-shadow the appearance of particular neural ganglia (see Chapter 11). Cells are also contributed to some of these ganglia from ectodermal thickenings or pla-codes that form in the side of the head (see Chapter 11).

Somitogenesis

The mesoderm near the neural tube is not divided into somatic and splanchnic parts because the intraembryonic coelom does not penetrate to the midline (Figure 3.3(b)). This **paraxial mesoderm** forms the **segmental plate** and the **intermediate mesoderm**. From the segmental plate **somites** will form (Figure 3.9), which are paired aggregations of mesoderm cells in the form of rounded cuboids, separated from each other by clefts. They form in craniocaudal sequence, beginning at 18–19 days after fertilization in humans. Before becoming fully recognizable, somites can be detected by cellular swirls or condensations visible under the stereoscopic scanning electron microscope. These precursors to the fully formed somites are called **somitomeres**. The most

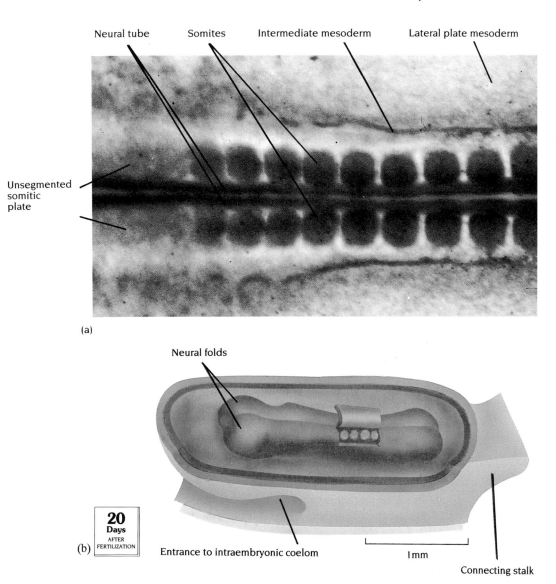

Neural tube   Somites   Intermediate mesoderm   Lateral plate mesoderm

Unsegmented somitic plate

(a)

Neural folds

20 Days AFTER FERTILIZATION

(b)   Entrance to intraembryonic coelom   1mm

Connecting stalk

FIGURE 3.9 (a) Somites from a chick embryo. (b) The same embryo as Figure 3.2 (a) with the ectoderm peeled back over the forming somites.

cranial somitomeres do not develop as far as the somite stage, but do play a highly significant role in head development (see Special Topic 6, pp. 174–7).

The sequential emergence of the paired somitomeres and somites from the unsegmented segmental plate is one of the most dramatic events in vertebrate development. It has inspired active theorizing and experimentation, but a definitive explanation remains elusive. At the cellular level somitogenesis involves

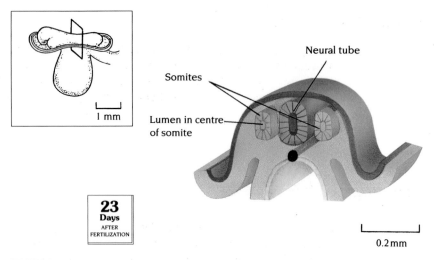

FIGURE 3.10   Section through 23-day embryo, showing somites developing a central lumen.

changes in cellular adhesive properties and in the secretion of extracellular matrix components such as fibronectin and glycosaminoglycans. As the somite condenses the cells become epithelial in appearance, surrounding a lumen (Figure 3.10). The ventral part of each somite will lose this epithelial organization to become a loose association once again: this is known as the **sclerotome**, and gives rise to the vertebrae (see Chapter 9). The remaining dorsolateral region of the somite is known as the **dermomyotome**. The most dorsal part of the dermomyotome will contribute to the dermis (Chapter 10, p. 133) and the remainder to striated skeletal muscle cells that migrate throughout the body (Chapter 8). The somites are therefore important not only as structures in themselves but also as the source of a variety of other cells.

A subtle distinction, probably caused by different cell-surface molecules, exists between the cranial and caudal parts of the somites. Cells from cranial regions do not mix with cells from caudal regions: however, they do mix readily with cells from the cranial region of another somite.

The arrangement of the somites may impose a segmental pattern on other body tissues. Segmental nerve outgrowth from the spinal cord (Chapter 6) and segmental blood vessel outgrowth from the aorta are both related to the initial segmental pattern of the somites.

In the human, somitogenesis proceeds until there are 42–44 pairs of somites. The most caudal 5–7 somites disappear and those cranial to this fuse to form the coccyx, except in very rare individuals when a tail-like structure exists at birth.

Intermediate mesoderm

A strip of unsegmented mesoderm, the **intermediate mesoderm**, lies lateral to the somites on each side between the somites and the extraembryonic coelom in the intermediate mesoderm. A primitive excretion system will form which in time will initiate the development of the kidney (see Chapter 24).

Folding of the embryo

As these events proceed a major shift in the relative position of the body tissues becomes evident. Until now, development of the body axis has occurred largely in the flat plane of the embryonic disc that forms the floor of the amniotic cavity: now what is recognizable for the first time as the body of the embryo begins to rise up from this plane and project into the amniotic cavity (Figure 3.11) as a result of the appearance of folds lateral to the body axis. At the same time, the formation of head and tail folds causes the head and tail to project forward over the embryonic disc as the flanks become evident (Figure 3.12). This combination of events could be viewed as a folding of the tissues around the embryo body axis, but equally could be regarded as the amniotic cavity sweeping round the embryo axis. Surprisingly little is known about the mechanics of this important event.

The embryo remains attached in the ventral region (Figure 3.12(c)); the attachment gradually narrows relative to the length of the body until a 'stalk' of tissue covered with amniotic ectoderm is formed containing the connecting stalk and the remnant of the yolk sac, which has been shrinking in relative size. The whole structure represents the beginning of the **umbilical cord** (Figure 3.13).

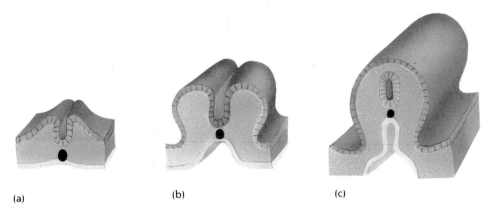

(a) (b) (c)

FIGURE 3.11 Diagrammatic view of how the body of the embryo rises to project into the amniotic cavity during folding.

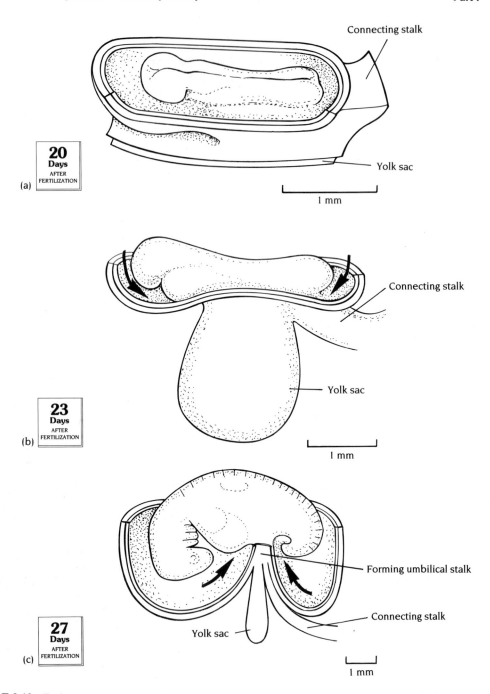

Connecting stalk

20 Days AFTER FERTILIZATION

(a)

Yolk sac

1 mm

Connecting stalk

23 Days AFTER FERTILIZATION

(b)

Yolk sac

1 mm

Forming umbilical stalk

Connecting stalk

27 Days AFTER FERTILIZATION

(c)

Yolk sac

1 mm

FIGURE 3.12   Embryos at 20, 23 and 27 days, showing the effect of folding on the head and tail regions of the embryo.

FIGURE 3.13 (*opposite*)   Folding can also be seen as the amniotic cavity sweeping round the embryo. (a) A section through a 23-day embryo, at a level corresponding to Figure 3.10. (b) and (c) Sections through a 27-day embryo, at the positions marked b and c respectively in the inset. The ventral attachment of the embryo, covered in ectoderm, represents the early stages of umbilical cord formation.

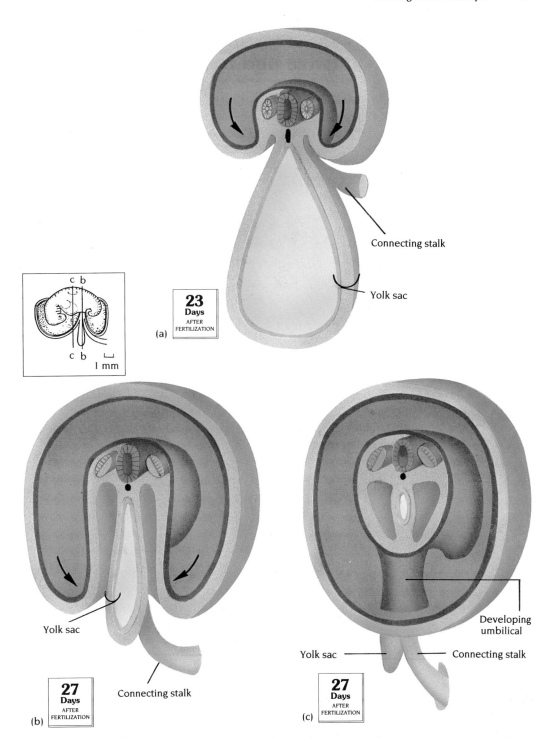

(a) **23** Days AFTER FERTILIZATION

Connecting stalk

Yolk sac

c b

c b
⌞___⌟
1 mm

(b) **27** Days AFTER FERTILIZATION

Yolk sac

Connecting stalk

(c) **27** Days AFTER FERTILIZATION

Yolk sac

Developing umbilical

Connecting stalk

Special Topic 3 Twins and multiple births

Twinning is relatively common in humans, although its incidence varies markedly between groups with different genetic and environmental backgrounds. Frequencies ranging from 60 per 10 000 to 330 per 10 000 pregnancies have been reported (note that this is not per live birth!). However, the figure for England and Wales in 1960 (before the introduction of superovulation and in vitro fertilization) of 115 per 10 000 pregnancies is probably a more typical indication of natural frequency (Bulmer, 1970). These figures are used as a baseline for the frequencies given below, but must not be thought of as exact.

There are two main types of twinning. Twins may result from fertilization of two oocytes at about the same time. These are known as **dizygotic twins** (because two zygotes are formed), and the twins will be no more alike than other siblings. Alternatively twins can result from one zygote. These are **monozygotic twins**: they have the same genotype and are described as 'identical' twins, although there may be differences between them due to their slightly different maternal environments and to chance events during development.

Dizygotic twins

Dizygotic twins are more common than monozygotic twins by just over two to one. This means they occurred overall in 80 or so pregnancies per 10 000 in the study cited above. The marked variability in overall twinning frequencies is almost entirely due to variation in dizygotic twinning: frequency is influenced both by environmental factors and by the genotype of the mother (but not, apparently, of the father).

Because dizygotic twins develop separately they have separate amniotic and chorionic cavities; they also begin with separate placentae, but in just under half of all cases of dizygotic twinning these subsequently fuse (Figure 1).

Variations

A variety of curious forms of dizygosity occur very infrequently. For example, the two zygotes may be fertilized by different males, if both inseminate the female within a short space of time. Two ova may be fertilized at consecutive menstrual cycles, so that the twins are one month apart in their developmental age (superfetation). It is also possible for a polar body to be fertilized and begin further development.

Monozygotic twins

Monozygotic twins show much less variability in occurrence, occurring in 30–40 pregnancies per 10 000. Three different kinds are observed, depending on exactly when division of the zygote occurred (Table 1).

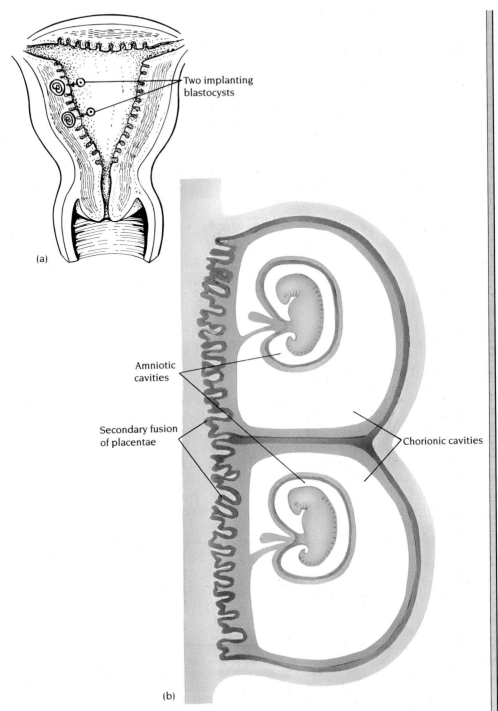

(a)

Two implanting blastocysts

Amniotic cavities

Secondary fusion of placentae

Chorionic cavities

(b)

FIGURE 1 Dizygotic twins implant separately (a) and develop separate amniotic and chorionic cavities (embryos not to scale). However, there is a good chance that their placentae will fuse (b).

Division at morula stage

At the morula stage, separation of blastomeres will result in identical twins with separate amniotic and chorionic cavities (hence described as diamniotic, dichorial). Two separate placentae are also formed, but these may fuse secondarily with approximately the same frequency as in dizygotic twins (see Figure 1). Dichorial, diamniotic splitting accounts for about 30% of monozygotic twins (approximately 10–12 per 10 000 pregnancies).

Division of inner cell mass

The most frequent time for division of the zygote occurs at the inner cell mass stage. This will produce twins sharing a placenta and chorionic cavity but with separate amniotic cavities because the amniotic cavity had not formed at the time of splitting (Figure 2). This monochorial, diamniotic condition represents about two-thirds of all monozygotic twins (about 20–25 per 10 000 pregnancies overall).

Division after amniotic cavity formation

Twins may originate after amniotic cavity formation, and therefore share amniotic and chorionic cavities (being in consequence monochorial, monoamniotic) (Figure 3); they also share a placenta. This is believed to occur in only about 4% of monozygotic twins, representing 1–2 occurrences in 10 000 pregnancies. Presumably, gastrulation begins at two separate sites on the embryonic disc (see Chapter 2).

Variations

Just as with dizygotic twins there are a number of unusual variations of monozygotic twinning. Perhaps the most dramatic of these is conjoined (or Siamese) twins, which develop inside one amniotic cavity. Although it is often suggested that conjoined twins result from incomplete division of the inner cell mass, it seems just as likely, on the basis of information gained from animal studies, that they arise when gastrulation begins at two places simultaneously, as in monochorial, monamniotic twins, but that the two axes cross each other or approach each other very closely and then fuse. This fusion can occur in a variety of ways. In some cases it is possible to separate conjoined twins after birth. Such twins pose intriguing problems concerning the identity of the individual.

Another unusual phenomenon is that of the 'included fetus' or 'fetus-in-fetu'. In this condition, further fetus-like structures develop within the body of the main fetus. However, it is not clear if this arises from an abnormality of monozygotic twinning or from the occurrence of a teratoma (see Box 1.2, p. 17 and Special Topic 10, pp. 384–5).

TABLE 1 Incidence of different types of twinning.

Type	Incidence (percentage of pregnancies)	Amniotic cavities	Chorionic cavities	Placentae
Dizygotic	0.8	Two	Two	Two (may then fuse)
Monozygotic	0.3–0.4			
diamniotic, dichorial	0.1	Two	Two	Two (may then fuse)
diamniotic, monochorial	0.2–0.25	Two	One	One
monoamniotic, monochorial	0.04	One	One	One

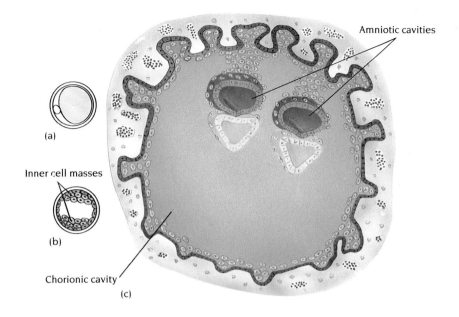

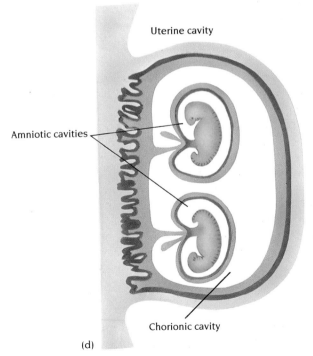

FIGURE 2 The fertilized egg (a) may produce a blastula with two inner cell masses (b). These develop in a combined chorionic cavity, but have separate amniotic cavities (c). Such monochorial, diamniotic twins share a placenta (d).

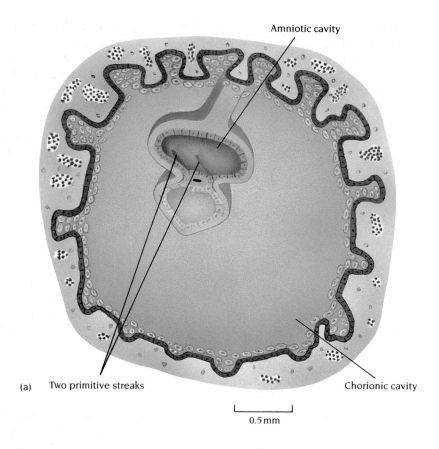

Amniotic cavity

(a)   Two primitive streaks

Chorionic cavity

0.5 mm

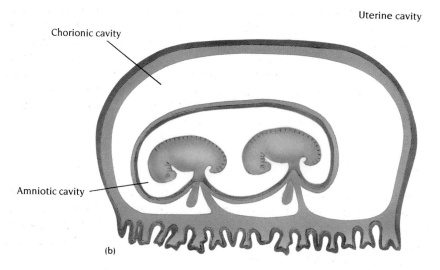

Uterine cavity

Chorionic cavity

Amniotic cavity

(b)

FIGURE 3 If two primitive streaks develop in the blastodisc (a), two embryos will develop inside a shared amniotic cavity (b).

Monozygotic twins inherit identical genetic information and grow in almost identical environments, and so are generally very similar, but they need not be identical. For instance, abnormalities may affect one twin but not the other. This may reflect slight differences in their environment or it may be due to chance. On occasion monozygotic twins possess different genetic information, for example, after the splitting of the zygote one twin may suffer from non-disjunction of chromosomes. These individuals usually die but, as we have seen, trisomy 21 and most sex chromosome trisomies are non-lethal, so an affected twin *may* survive. In the case of Turner's syndrome, in which one sex chromosome is inactivated (see Chapter 26), this may mean that of two 'identical' twins one is male and one female.

Such an event could explain at least some 'vanishing twin' episodes, in which one of the twins dies before birth. In one extensive American study, one of the twins died in 5% of multiple gestations. This does not seem to affect the survivor very greatly, although the implications are not entirely clear.

Monozygotic, monochorionic twins often share a blood system. This may lead to 'twin transfusion syndrome', which usually arises when an artery of one fetus supplies a placental cotyledon drained by the vein of the other fetus. Blood is shunted from one to the other, often to the detriment of both as one twin becomes severely anaemic and undernourished while the other may develop an enlarged heart and liver and polyhydramnios. Marked differences in birth weight may be observed. This syndrome may occur in 15–30% of monochorial twins, but is rare in dichorial twins.

Importance of classification

Classification of whether a pregnancy is monozygotic or dizygotic is of some importance, because monozygotic twins make excellent mutual transplant donors. This is because they do not recognize each other's body tissue as foreign. Generally, the fetal membranes provide sufficient information to determine the twin type: genetic fingerprinting will also determine their relationship. It *is* possible for dizygotic twins to acquire mutual transplant tolerance during development, for example if a connection develops between the vascular systems of dizygotic twins via a fused placenta. This leads to an interchange of blood, which causes the immune system to come to recognize the twin tissue as 'self'. It is interesting to speculate on the medical and ethical implications that would arise if it were possible to routinely transfuse fetuses in utero with blood from their siblings, so that they might be able to act as organ donors if necessary in later life.

Higher-order births

Higher-order multiple births are proportionately less likely to occur than twins. Triplets occur naturally with a frequency of about 1.2–1.4 per 10 000 pregnancies, while quadruplets occur with a frequency of about 0.017 per 10 000 (1.7 per 1 000 000). Monozygotic triplets and quadruplets, and every possible combination down to trizygotic triplets and tetrazygotic quadruplets, have been known.

Induced higher-order births now occur frequently with the use of superovulation and in vitro fertilization.

More problems arise during the development of twins than with the equivalent number of singleton fetuses, possibly because of lack of space and the division of nutrients between the fetuses. There is thus a higher incidence of abnormalities in twins than in singletons. The return of multiple pre-embryos to the uterus following in vitro fertilization results in a higher than normal incidence of multiple pregnancies, and abnormality rates following IVF are correspondingly increased. This difference vanishes when abnormality rates are corrected for the incidence of twins.

Further reading

Bard J.L. (1990). *Morphogenesis*. Cambridge: Cambridge University Press

Bellairs R., Ede D.A. and Lash J.W., eds (1986). *Somites in Developing Embryos*. New York: Plenum Press

Bleischmidt E. (1961). *Stages of human development before birth*. Philadelphia: W.B. Saunders

Keynes R.J. and Stern C.D. (1991). Mechanisms of vertebrate segmentation. *Development*, **103**, 413–29

Meier S. (1979). Development of the chick embryo mesoblast. Formation of the embryonic axis and establishment of the metameric pattern. *Dev. Biol.*, **73**, 25-45

Muller F. and O'Rahilly F. (1986). The development of the human brain and the closure of the rostral neuropore at stage 11. *Anat. Embryol.*, **175**, 205–22

Schoenwolf G.C. and Smith J.L. (1990). Mechanisms of neurulation: traditional viewpoint and recent advances. *Development*, **109**, 243–70

Tuckett F. and Morriss-Kay G.M. (1985). The kinetic behaviour of the cranial neural epithelium during neurulation in the rat. *J. Embryol. Exp. Morph.*, **85**, 111–19

Wilson D.B. and Finta L.A. (1980). Fine structure of the lumbrosacral neural folds in the mouse embryo. *J. Embryol. Exp. Morph.*, **55**, 279–90

Special Topic 3

Allen M.S and Turner U.G. (1971). Twin births – identical or fraternal twins? *Obstet. Gynecol.*, **37**, 538–42

Benirschke K. and Kim C.K. (1973). Multiple pregnancy. *N. Engl. J. Med.*, **288**, 1276–84, 1329–36

Bieber F.R., Morton C.C., Nance W.E. *et al.* (1981). Genetic studies of an acardiac monster: evidence of polar body twinning in man. *Science*, **213**, 775–7

Bulmer M.G. (1970). *The Biology of Twinning in Man*. Oxford: Clarendon Press

Corner G.W. (1955). The observed embryology of human single ovum twins and other multiple births. *Am. J. Obstet. Gynecol.*, **70**, 933–51

Edwards R.G., Mettler L. and Walters D.E. (1986). Identical twins and in vitro fertilisation. *J. in Vitro Fertiliz. Emb. Transfer*, **3**, 114–7

Filler R.M. (1986). Conjoined twins and their separation. *Semin. Perinatol.*, **10**, 82–91

Gedda L. (1961). *Twins in History and Science*. Springfield IL: Thomas

Groseld J.L., Stepita D.S., Nance W.E. *et al.* (1974). Fetus in fetu. *Ann. Surg.*, **180**, 80–4

Hill A.V. and Jeffreys A.J. (1985). Use of minisatellite DNA probes for determination of monozygosity at birth. *Lancet*, **ii**, 8467–70

Johnson S.F. and Driscoll S.G. (1986). Twin placentation and its complications. *Semin. Perinatol.*, **10**, 9–13

Johnson S.F., Barss V. and Driscoll S.G. (1986). Incidence and impact of single intrauterine death in multiple gestation. *Lab. Invest.*, **54**, 29A

Jones K.L. and Benirschke K. (1983). The developmental pathogenesis of structural defects: the contribution of monozygotic twins. *Semin. Perinatol.*, **7**, 239–43

Little J. and Bryan E. (1986). Congenital anomalies in twins. *Semin. Perinatol.*, **10**, 50–64

MacGillivray I. (1986). Epidemiology of twin pregnancy. *Semin. Perinatol.*, **10**, 4–8

Page E.W., Villee C.A. and Villee D.B. (1981). *Human Reproduction: Essentials of Reproductive and Perinatal Medicine.* Philadelphia: W.B. Saunders

Robertson E.G. and Neer K.J. (1983). Placental injection studies in twin gestation. *Am. J. Obstet. Gynecol.*, **147**, 170–4

Wenk R.E., Brooks M. and Houtz T. (1986). Heteropaternal dizygotic twinning: evidence of superfecundation. *Lab. Med.*, **17**, 526–8

Wittman B.K., Baldwin V.J. and Nichol B. (1981). Antenatal diagnosis of twin transfusion syndrome by ultrasound. *Obstet. Gynecol.*, **58**, 123–7

4

Extraembryonic structures

The mammalian embryo develops in an intimate relationship with its mother, necessitating the development of specialized tissues to mediate this interaction. These are derived partly from the mother and partly from the conceptus. Because these tissues derived from the conceptus do not contribute to the embryo proper, they are described as 'extraembryonic'. A variety of other extraembryonic tissues play various roles during development, which can only be properly understood in the context of the evolutionary history of the vertebrates. In accordance with the adaptive nature of evolution, tissues have been continually modified as old purposes became redundant and new needs arose.

EVOLUTION

To promote the use of large amounts of stored yolk products in the egg, our fish-like ancestors evolved the **yolk sac**, *a tissue that surrounds the yolk, and actively absorbs nutrients from it. As a result it is highly vascularized.*

When the vertebrates colonized the land, they evolved a tough shell surrounding their eggs to provide mechanical support and inhibit water loss, enabling eggs to survive out of water. The fluid environment of the sea was recreated by a liquid-filled sac, the **amnion**, *in which the developing embryo floated. However, the shell also prevented the loss of poisonous waste products by diffusion. This problem was solved by the evolution of an impermeable out-*

*pouching from the hindgut – the **allantois**. Wastes could be safely sequestered in this during development and left behind at hatching.*

*Oxygen and carbon dioxide exchange was also inhibited by the shell, so a highly vascularized membrane was developed by the fusion of the allantois to the surrounding **chorionic mesoderm**. This **chorioallantoic membrane** functioned as a kind of external lung pressed against the interior of the shell until hatching.*

*The evolution of true mammals is associated with retention of the developing embryo inside the mother's uterus. The shell becomes unnecessary, as does the yolk, because the embryo obtains nutrients from the uterine wall. In advanced mammals, this interchange of nutrients is obtained via the **placenta**, which is formed by fusion of a modified chorioallantoic membrane with the uterine wall.*

Although their original functions are now redundant, the yolk sac and the allantois still develop in human embryos in much the same way as in our ancestors, before being adapted to new uses.

The amnion

As indicated in Chapter 2, the amniotic cavity first appears in humans at about 7 days after fertilization. Specimens of this age are difficult to obtain, and the dynamic processes involved in forming all the extraembryonic membranes in humans are not fully documented. However, the development of other mammals offers valuable clues to human development.

The available evidence suggests that the amnion appears by the expansion of a space in the epiblast or primitive ectoderm. Initially, the cavity is surrounded by primitive ectoderm cells (see Figure 2.11), although it may open briefly to communicate with the cytotrophoblast. Soon the primitive ectoderm cells become flattened and extend all the way around the cavity (Figure 4.1); at this stage, and thereafter, they are known as **amnioblasts**. The amnioblast layer is continuous with the primitive ectoderm, and with the definitive ectoderm when this forms at gastrulation.

The cells of the primitive ectoderm secrete fluid from their amniotic cavity surfaces. This **amniotic fluid** is essentially a saline solution, but contains proteins and other components that may provide important clues to the condition of the embryo (see Special Topic 4, pp. 80–4). When the neural tube forms, the lining ectoderm will also secrete a fluid. Once the neural tube closes this may be described as **cerebrospinal fluid**, but at first it is similar to early amniotic fluid.

As the extraembryonic coelom forms (see Figures 2.12 and 2.13), the outside of the amnion becomes covered with mesoderm, giving it an inner ectodermal layer and an outer mesodermal layer. The amniotic cavity continues to expand, and in time sweeps round the forming body of the embryo (see Figures 3.12 and 3.13). As the amniotic cavity expands the volume of amniotic fluid also

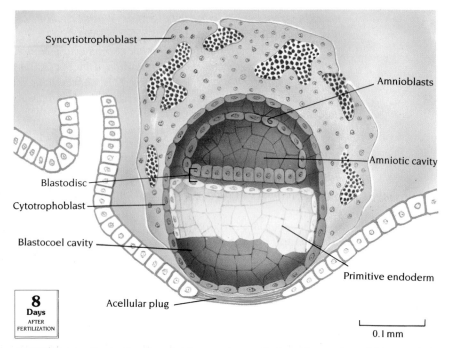

Syncytiotrophoblast

Amnioblasts

Amniotic cavity

Blastodisc

Cytotrophoblast

Blastocoel cavity

Primitive endoderm

8
Days
AFTER
FERTILIZATION

Acellular plug

0.1 mm

FIGURE 4.1   Gradually, the primitive ectoderm cells form flattened amnioblasts, which roof over the amniotic cavity. The primitive ectoderm in contact with the primitive endoderm contributes to a roughly circular, two-layered blastodisc.

increases, and this may drive the expansion. At about 10 weeks the volume has become 30 ml; by 20 weeks 350 ml; by 37 weeks 1000 ml. There is subsequently a slight decrease up to the time of birth. The embryo begins to swallow amniotic fluid in the early fetal period, and in consequence also begins to excrete fluid via the urogenital system. An equilibrium between swallowing and excretion is usually established. Inability to swallow amniotic fluid (due perhaps to a blockage in the foregut – see Chapter 23) will lead to an excess of amniotic fluid (polyhydramnios); conversely, kidney defects (see Chapter 24) may lead to a reduced fluid volume (oligohydramnios). These conditions are not only warning signs of defects (see Chapters 23–25), but may also cause problems in their own right: polyhydramnios may induce premature labour, while oligohydramnios may compress the embryo inside the amniotic sac, causing abnormalities of limb position and development and possibly also palatal abnormalities.

The continuing expansion of the amnion inside the chorionic cavity will eventually bring it into contact with the walls of the cavity (Figure 4.2). These walls are lined with mesoderm on their *inner* surface and this fuses with the outer mesoderm of the amnion. Continuing fetal growth and expansion of the chorioamnion eventually lead to the almost complete obliteration of the uterine

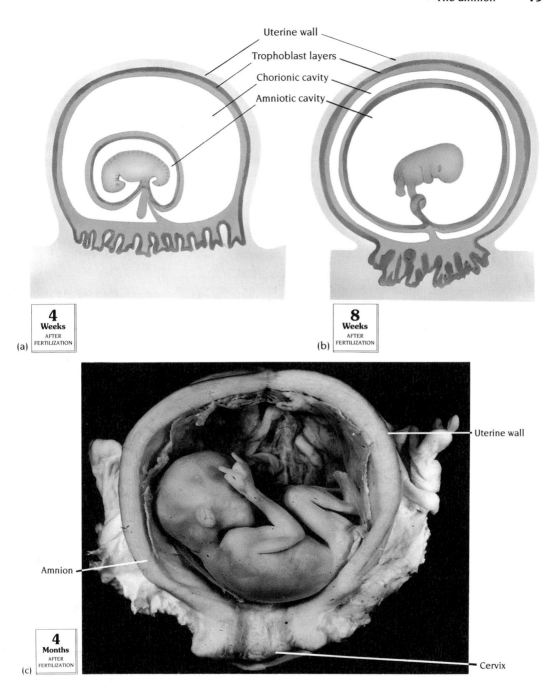

FIGURE 4.2 (a) At first the amniotic sac occupies a small proportion of the chorionic cavity. (b) As the amnion expands it will occlude the chorionic cavity. The amnion has mesoderm on its external aspect, while the chorionic cavity has mesoderm on its inner aspect. When these meet they will fuse. (In both these figures, cyto- and syncytiotrophoblast are shown as a single layer.) (c) Human fetus in utero at about 4 months after fertilization. (From the Anatomy Museum, University of St Andrews, by permission.)

cavity. The combined chorioamniotic membrane ruptures shortly before birth, releasing the amniotic fluid (the 'breaking of the waters').

The amniotic fluid serves as a buffer to protect the embryo or fetus from shock and may regulate temperature changes. In addition, because the developing child is floating freely in the amniotic fluid it is not exposed to powerful compressive forces that could distort its form and perhaps bring about adhesions of one body part to another. However, being immersed in amniotic fluid during the relatively long human gestation period poses problems of its own, because tissue continually soaked in fluid tends to macerate. The solution to this problem is discussed in Chapter 10.

The yolk sac

The origin of the yolk sac in human embryos is a matter of some dispute: although of considerable scientific interest, the details may seem of little clinical relevance. Surprisingly often, however, important biological discoveries prove later to have unguessed clinical applications. The account given below follows the studies of Luckett (1978) and of lineage studies in other mammalian embryos.

As described in Chapter 2, the primary yolk sac is formed when primitive endoderm cells migrate round the inside of the blastocoel cavity. It is likely that the primitive ectoderm is able to continue to generate primitive endoderm cells for some time, to replace migrating cells. Subsequently (13 or 14 days after fertilization), the primary yolk sac contracts to form the secondary yolk sac, leaving a space filled with extracellular material and endodermal cells (Figure 2.12). Vesicles of yolk sac may also be formed during this process. This space will form the chorionic cavity.

The extraembryonic mesoderm (Chapter 2) migrates round the inside of the chorionic cavity and, also, comes to cover the secondary yolk sac (Figure 2.13). By day 16 after fertilization, 'blood islands' begin to form in this yolk sac mesoderm (see Chapter 7). Generation of blood cells is thought to be one of the major functions of the yolk sac, and this may account for its persistence so long after its original function in evolutionary terms has disappeared.

Another very unexpected derivative of yolk sac mesoderm cells is the primordial germ cell line, which will give rise to the next generation (Chapter 26).

With the folding of the embryo the definitive gut begins to form at the cranial and caudal ends (Figure 4.3(a)). The gut is lined with endodermal cells, derived in part from the endoderm of the yolk sac but also originating from the primitive streak during gastrulation. At first, the yolk sac represents a substantial proportion of the gut length but later, as the embryo grows, the yolk sac decreases in relative importance (Figure 4.3(b)) until it is attached to the gut only by a narrow stalk (Figure 4.3(c)). It will eventually be incorporated into the umbilical cord (see Chapter 23).

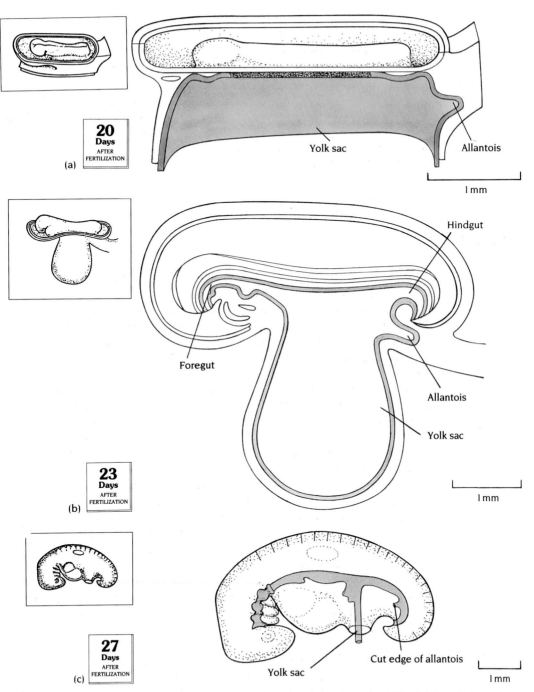

FIGURE 4.3 Endoderm derivatives are shown in yellow. The folding of the embryo alters the initial arrangement of the yolk sac (a) by first defining foregut and hindgut (b), and then establishing midgut as the relative size of the yolk sac decreases (c).

The allantois

The allantois develops as an outgrowth from the hindgut during the third week after fertilization and projects into the mesoderm of the connecting stalk (Figure 4.3). It never functions as a waste store in human embryos. Eventually it will contribute to the bladder (see Chapter 24). The blood vessels running to the allantois, one on each side, will become the umbilical arteries when the connecting stalk becomes enfolded in the umbilical cord.

The umbilical cord

As the embryo folds the connecting stalk and yolk sac become engulfed by amniotic ectoderm (see Chapter 2). The outer aspects of the connecting stalk and yolk sac are covered with mesoderm, as is the outer aspect of the amnion. Mesodermal layers in contact with each other tend to fuse (see Chapter 19) so gradually the contents of the umbilical cord inside its ectodermal covering fuse together. The mesoderm will in time alter its nature to form a mucus-like connective tissue known as Wharton's jelly, in which the blood vessels run.

Of the two original umbilical arteries the right one will disappear during the early months of pregnancy. The umbilical cord lengthens markedly but variably during pregnancy, averaging 50 cm, but ranging between 20 and 120 cm in length.

The placenta

At 16 days after fertilization a view from inside the chorionic cavity would show the amnion and the yolk sac both covered by mesoderm and jointly connected to the mesoderm lining the chorionic cavity by the connecting stalk (Figure 4.4).

The wall of the chorionic cavity (from its inner surface outwards) is composed of:

- extraembryonic somatopleural mesoderm – the chorionic plate;
- cytotrophoblast;
- syncytiotrophoblast, through which maternal blood is flowing;
- maternal tissue. This is part of the uterine wall.

As development proceeds the chorionic villi begin to form (Chapter 2) and blood vessels form in the extraembryonic mesoderm of the chorionic plate. These run back to the embryo via the connecting stalk (which lies in the developing umbilical cord) where they will connect with the heart. When the heart begins to beat at about the fourth week after fertilization, embryonic blood can be pumped round the circuit.

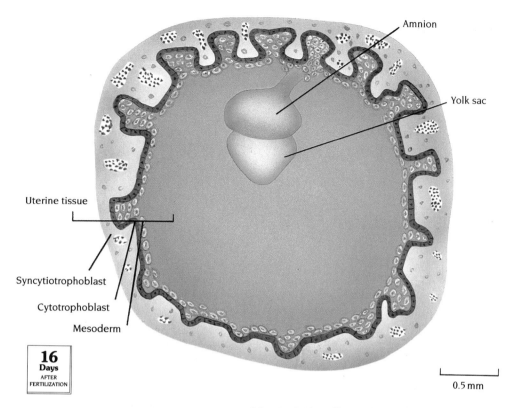

Amnion

Yolk sac

Uterine tissue

Syncytiotrophoblast

Cytotrophoblast

Mesoderm

16
Days
AFTER
FERTILIZATION

0.5 mm

FIGURE 4.4   The components of the chorionic wall.

The cytotrophoblast component of the villi is dominant, and makes its way through the syncytiotrophoblast. The villi sprout protrusions or **villus trees** that project into the maternal blood-filled spaces or **blood lakes**. The blood of the embryo never mixes with that of the mother.

The embryonic pole always undergoes these processes more markedly than the non-embryonic pole, and is therefore described as the **bushy chorion** or **chorion frondosum** (Figure 4.5). The opposite pole is the **smooth chorion** or **chorion laeve**.

As the conceptus embedded in the uterine wall expands, the uterine space is occluded. The uterine wall over the conceptus will eventually fuse with the opposite wall. Meanwhile, the placenta generally becomes confined to one site but this is by no means inevitable: many mammals have multiple placentae and perhaps in consequence the human placenta is sometimes divided into several parts. Eventually it will normally be about 20cm in diameter, and about 7cm deep. It is subdivided into smaller units, known as **cotyledons** (Figure 4.6).

Functions

The most important functions of the placenta are exchange of vital gases and supply of nutrients to the embryo, and removal of waste products. In addition,

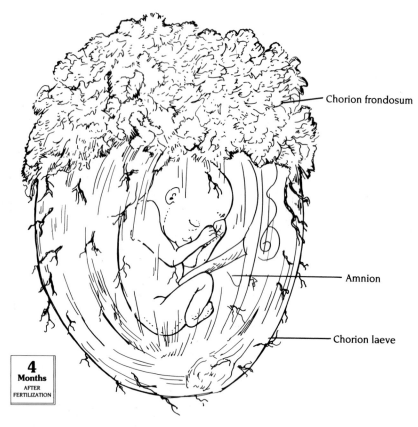

Chorion frondosum

Amnion

Chorion laeve

4 Months AFTER FERTILIZATION

FIGURE 4.5 View of the chorion frondosum and chorion laeve in the fetus (see Figure 4.2 for an earlier view).

maternal antibodies are taken up by pinocytosis to confer a degree of passive immunity on the fetus. The placenta produces hormones such as progesterone, oestrogen and human chorionic gonadotrophin, which mediate pregnancy (see Chapter 27), and human placental lactogen, which gives the fetus priority over the mother for blood glucose.

Defects of the placenta

The placenta occurs in a variety of sizes and forms, but it is unclear whether this causes or reflects abnormalities of the fetus. A serious problem arises if the blastocyst implants near the cervical exit of the uterus (Figure 4.7) because the placenta may cover the opening of the cervix. This is known as placenta praevia, and creates the risk of severe bleeding during birth. Placenta praevia occurs in approximately 50 pregnancies per 10 000 (0.5%).

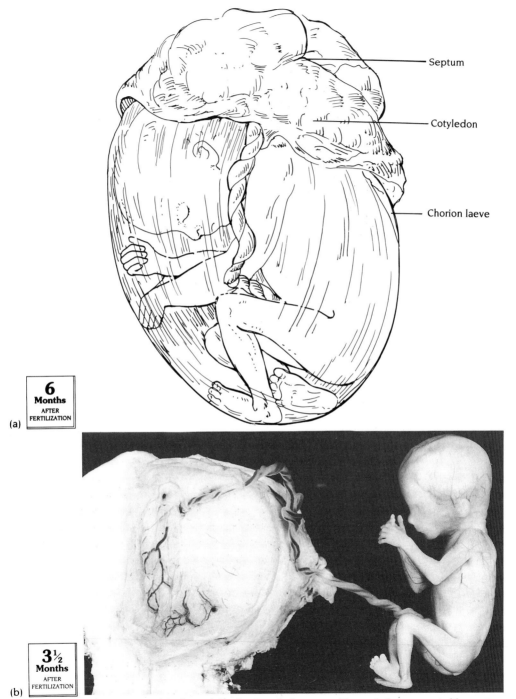

FIGURE 4.6 (a) View of the developed placenta, with cotyledons separated by septae; (b) human 3½-month fetus, showing placenta. (From the Anatomy Museum, University of St Andrews by permission.)

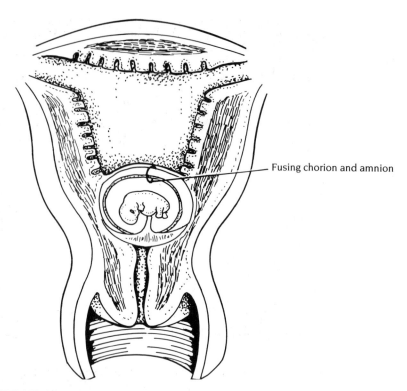

Fusing chorion and amnion

FIGURE 4.7 Implantation in the lower part of the uterus may lead to the placenta covering all or part of the cervical canal. This condition is known as placenta praevia.

Special Topic 4 Diagnosis in the postimplantation embryo

During the last 10 years methods for monitoring the process of development after implantation, and of detecting abnormalities, have radically improved so that clinical decisions can be more confidently made. Such decisions may include termination of pregnancy, early induction of birth or administration of particular treatments to the mother, fetus or both.

Ultrasonography

By far the most widely used and successful diagnostic technique during pregnancy is visualization using ultrasonography (Figure 1).

Gross abnormalities that can readily be detected by ultrasonography include neural tube defects, hydrocephaly, microcephaly, anencephaly, heart defects, limb defects, kidney anomalies and gastrointestinal anomalies.

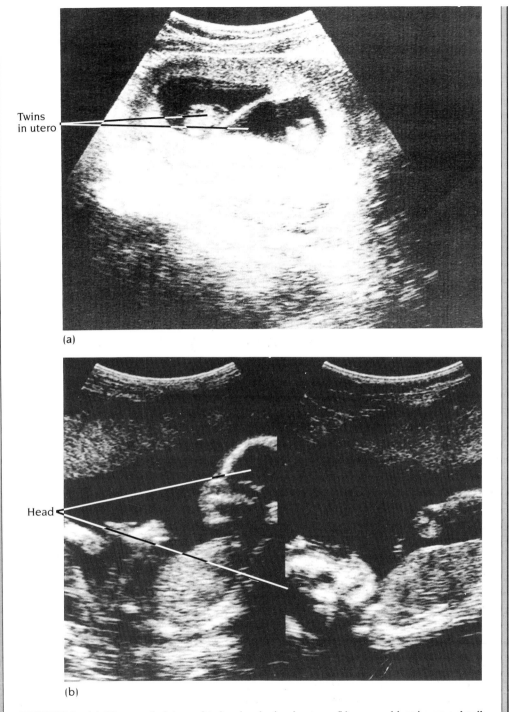

(a)

(b)

FIGURE 1 (a) Ultrasound picture of twins developing in utero; (b) same subject in more detail. (Photographs courtesy of Dr Martin Milner and Ninewells Hospital, Dundee.)

Ultrasonography is also useful for estimating fetal age and growth because it allows direct measurement of crown–rump length, foot size, head diameter, long bone length and many other parameters. Not only may age after fertilization be estimated quite accurately by these means, but also repeat measurements give evidence of growth rate, which may be affected in certain conditions.

Another use of ultrasonography is in analysis of Doppler effects. The Doppler effect is familiar as the change in note of the sound from an object such as a train as it approaches and passes; in the same way, a beam of ultrasound directed at a fetal blood vessel reflects a signal that varies according to the velocity of flow in that vessel. This technique can be used to give information on hypoxia in the fetus.

Amniocentesis

In amniocentesis, a needle is introduced into the amniotic sac via the lower abdomen, with the aid of real-time ultrasonography (Figure 2), and a sample of amniotic fluid is withdrawn. This sample may be analysed directly for the presence of biochemical components associated with particular kinds of defects (for instance, levels of α-fetoprotein are markedly raised in cases of open neural tube defects). The amniotic fluid also contains cells shed by the developing fetus and the amniotic lining. It is possible to culture such cells until they are sufficiently numerous for chromosomal and metabolic analysis. Unfortunately, about one million cells are required, and this may take several weeks to achieve. If the chromosomes are then found to be abnormal, as in trisomy 21 (Down's syndrome), the decision of whether to terminate the pregnancy needs to be made. However, the later in pregnancy a termination is carried out the more dangerous and traumatic it tends to be. Amniocentesis itself carries a risk of inducing spontaneous abortion: the rate of this is variable but may represent an additional procedure-related loss rate of 0.5%.

Amniocentesis can be performed under local anaesthesia with only slight discomfort to the mother from 16 weeks of gestation (14 weeks after fertilization) onwards: before this time the small amount of amniotic fluid present makes the procedure difficult.

Chorionic villus sampling

This can be carried out before 12 weeks of pregnancy, earlier than amniocentesis is generally considered practicable. A needle is inserted via the cervix or, less commonly, through the abdominal wall into the chosen placental site, guided by ultrasonographic visualization (Figure 2). A tissue sample containing fetal villus tissue is collected. Sufficient numbers of dividing fetal cells are obtained to conduct chromosome analysis for defects immediately, so not only can this procedure be carried out earlier than amniocentesis, but it also gives results within a few hours. Unfortunately, it appears to be associated with increased rates of miscarriage, and possibly with increased incidence of fetal abnormalities.

Coelocentesis

It is also possible to withdraw fluid from the extraembryonic coelom, and this has been done in a clinical setting. The fluid from this cavity is quite different in composition and

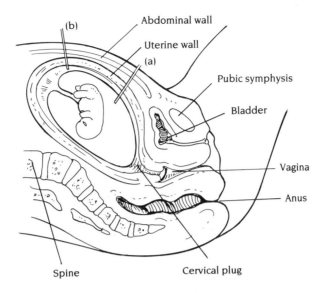

FIGURE 2 The uterus in pregnancy lies close to the abdominal wall, so amniocentesis (a) and chorionic villus sampling (b) can be carried out by this route; alternatively, a transcervical approach can be made.

colour from amniotic fluid. Fetal sexing was successfully carried out from the samples.

No information is yet available on the risk associated with this procedure. However, it can be performed early in development (between 6 and 10 weeks), and may well prove as valuable as amniocentesis and chorionic villus sampling, if it can be carried out safely.

Fetoscopy and cordocentesis

In addition to, or instead of, introducing a needle into the amniotic fluid during amniocentesis, a fibre-optic fetoscope may be introduced, allowing the fetus to be examined directly. However, after 20 weeks' gestation, the amniotic fluid becomes so turbid with fetal cells that it is difficult to see the fetus. Tissue samples may be taken directly from the fetus or the umbilical cord by this means. Once again, however, these procedures are associated with significant rates of miscarriage.

Maternal blood sampling

Certain kinds of fetal abnormality are associated with detectable changes in the maternal blood. For example, levels of α-fetoprotein in the maternal serum are raised above normal values for that gestational age in cases where the fetus has an open neural tube defect. Once the age of the child has been checked by ultrasonography mothers with high levels of α-fetoprotein may be recommended for amniocentesis. The optimum time for these tests seems to be 16–18 weeks into the pregnancy.

Future prospects

Magnetic resonance imaging (MRI)

Nuclear magnetic resonance (NMR) is a phenomenon employing the absorption of electromagnetic radiation in the form of a magnetic field by certain energy transitions inside
molecules. It can be used to build up an image in a similar way to the use of X-rays in
computed tomography (CT). Unlike CT scans, however, the radiation to which the fetus
is exposed seems to be harmless. Not only can this give a valuable direct picture of the
fetus, but MRI can also be used to give information on physiological processes in the
fetus by using marker molecules that change their NMR absorptive properties while
undergoing particular chemical reactions.

Fetal cell sampling from maternal blood

Fetal cells detach from the chorionic villi and circulate in the maternal blood. If these
cells could be isolated by, for example, the use of a fluorescent antibody that identified
fetal cells, followed by fluorescence-activated cell sorting, then the fetal cells could be
studied directly for abnormalities, particularly in association with the PCR (see Special
Topic 1, pp. 18–21).

Surgical intervention

The early detection of defects raises the hope that they could be treated rather than that a
termination of pregnancy will result. This is made the more feasible by the nature of fetal
tissue, which heals better, and scars less, than postnatal tissue but there are a number of
difficulties in such procedures, including the tendency of the uterus to begin premature
contractions if it is wounded. However, successful attempts have been made to treat
hydrocephaly and urinary obstructions by the insertion of shunts to relieve fluid pressure
on the brain and bladder respectively, and to operate on heart abnormalities.

Further reading

Boyd J.D. and Hamilton W.J. (1970). *The Human Placenta*. Cambridge: Heffer

Boyd P.A. (1987). The placenta. In *Fetal and Perinatal Pathology* (Keeling, J.W., ed.),
pp. 45–76. Berlin: Springer-Verlag

Enders A.C., Schlafke S. and Hendrickx A.G. (1983). Differentiation of the embryonic
disc, amnion, and yolk sac in the rhesus monkey. *Am. J. Anat.*, **177**, 161–85

Gardner R.L. (1985). Manipulation of development. In *Reproduction in Mammals* Vol. 5.
(Austin C.R. and Short R.V., eds), pp. 159–80. Cambridge: Cambridge University
Press

Gasser R.F. (1982). *Atlas of Human Embryos*. Hagerstown, Maryland: Harper & Row

Hamilton W.J., Boyd J.D. and Mossman H.W. (1962). *Human Embryology* 3rd edn.
Cambridge: Heffer

Hildebrand M. (1982). *Analysis of Vertebrate Structure* 2nd edn. New York: John Wiley & Sons

Luckett W.P. (1975). The development of primordial and definitive amniotic cavities in early rhesus monkeys and human embryos. *Am. J. Anat.*, **144**, 149–68

Luckett W.P. (1978). Origin and differentiation of the yolk sac and extraembryonic mesoderm in presomite human and rhesus monkey embryos. *Am. J. Anat.*, **152**, 59–98

Novak E.R. and Woodruff J.D. (1974). *Novak's Gynecologic and Obstetric Pathology*. Philadelphia: W.B. Saunders

O'Rahilly R. and Muller F. (1987). *Developmental Stages in Human Embryos*. Carnegie Institution of Washington Publication 637

Sandler M. (ed.) (1981). *The Amniotic Fluid and its Clinical Significance*. New York: Marcel Dekker

Winter R.M., Knowles S.A.S., Bieber F.R. and Baraitser M. (1988). *The Malformed Fetus and Still Birth*. New York: John Wiley & Sons

Special Topic 4

Ager R.P. and Oliver R.W.A. (1986). *The Risks of Midtrimester Amniocentesis*. Bramhall: Harboro Publications

Archer L.N.J. *et al.* (1988). Cerebral artery Doppler ultrasonography for prediction of outcome after perinatal asphyxia. *Lancet*, **i**, 1116–18

Ferguson-Smith M.A. (ed.) (1983). Early prenatal diagnosis. *Br. Med. Bull.*, **39**, 301–408

Hansen J.T. and Sladek J.R. Jr. (1989). Fetal research. *Science*, **246**, 775–9

Jurkovic D., Jauniaux E., Campbell S., Pandya P., Cardy D.L. and Nicolaides K.H. (1983). Coelocentesis: a new technique for early prenatal diagnosis. *Lancet*, **341**, 1623–4

Liu D.T.Y., Jeavons B., Preson C. and Person D. (1987). A retrospective study of spontaneous miscarriage in ultrasonically abnormal pregnancy and relevance to chorionic villus sampling. *Prenat. Diagn.*, **7**, 223–7

Ward R.H., Modell B., Petrou M., Karagoxlu M. and Douratsos L. (1983). A method of chorionic villus sampling in the first trimester of pregnancy on the real time ultrasound guidance. *BMJ*, **286**, 1542–44

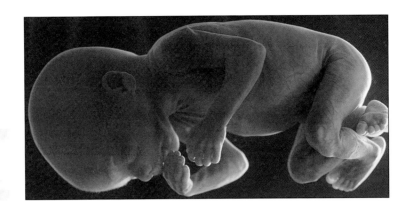

PART II

Systematic embryology

5

Positional information: establishing position in the embryo

In Part I, the events from fertilization to the appearance of the early embryo were considered. An answer was suggested for part of the central enigma of how complexity arises from apparent simplicity: cells differentiate from each other on the basis of their relative position. During the embryonic period, however, the complexity of tissue organization increases very dramatically and this simple answer is insufficient. In particular, we must address the problem of how differentiated cells become arranged in patterns in space.

A valuable concept in considering this mystery is that of positional information, as formulated by Lewis Wolpert, but before explaining the concept it is necessary to describe some of the experimental evidence on which it is based.

Balancers and suckers in amphibians

The first set of experiments concerns amphibian development, and in particular grafts between early embryos of particular species of frog and newt. As adults these species can be distinguished by two dramatic morphological features of the ectoderm in the head region (Figure 5.1). The newts possess a balancer – an elongated structure protruding from each side of the head. Frogs do not possess balancers but do, however, possess suckers – modified regions of epithelium in

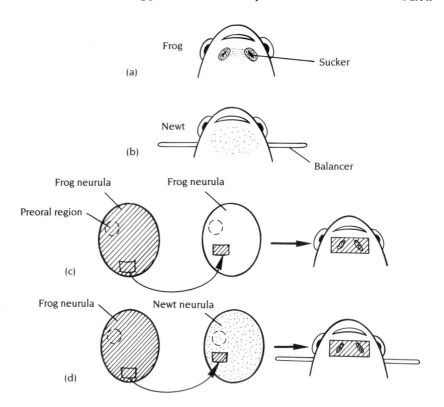

FIGURE 5.1 The sucker apparatus of the frog (a) and the balancer apparatus of the newt (b) provide conveniently recognizable examples of regionalization in the amphibian embryo. Belly ectoderm from the early frog neurula grafted to the mouth region responds by differentiating in a way appropriate to its new position by forming suckers (c). However, the same ectoderm grafted to the mouth region of a newt also differentiates as suckers (d), showing that it is not responding to a specific 'sucker induction' signal but rather to a signal giving its position in the body.

the area of the mouth, which secrete mucus. During development, at the amphibian equivalent of the neurula stage, no trace of these structures can be seen in either species.

During experiments aimed at exploring the differentiative capacity of embryonic tissues, ectoderm from the prospective belly region of a neurula-stage frog was grafted to the oral region of another frog neurula. This grafted belly ectoderm contributed to the formation of a normal sucker. In a corresponding experiment newt neurula belly ectoderm grafted to the lateral head region of a host newt neurula gave rise to a balancer. These experiments indicate that the ectoderm was not irreversibly determined to differentiate as belly at the time of the graft: it could respond to a shift in position by differentiating in a manner appropriate to its new position. It might have been suspected that something in the area of the frog mouth (the mesoderm, for instance) had induced the frog belly ectoderm to turn into a sucker. Equally, something in the lateral head region of the newt could have induced the newt belly ectoderm to turn into a balancer. However, a second series of experiments showed that this was not the case.

Belly ectoderm pieces from frog neurulae were grafted to the side of the head *and* to the oral region of newt neurulae. Frog ectoderm grafted to the mouth region of the newt developed into a structure like a sucker but that grafted to the side of the newt's head did *not* form a balancer.

The reciprocal grafts, of newt neurula belly ectoderm to frog lateral head and mouth, were also carried out. The newt ectoderm showed reciprocal behaviour: in the lateral frog head region it formed balancers, even though this region of the frog normally shows no such structures, while in the region of the mouth it behaved like newt mouth ectoderm.

These results are profoundly revealing. They show that frog ectoderm placed in the mouth region of a newt differentiates *as if it were in the mouth region of a frog*. There can be no specific 'sucker-inducing' signal coming from the newt, because it does not possess a sucker: the frog ectodermal graft has somehow detected that it has been moved to 'mouth region' (albeit that of a newt), and has differentiated accordingly. In other words, there is some whole-body reference system in the newt that the frog ectoderm can interpret, and that is therefore common to them both. Once the frog ectoderm has detected its position it differentiates accordingly. The same argument applies to the transplanted newt ectoderm.

Frogs and newts are both amphibians, and it is interesting, but not astonishing, that they share some positional reference system. However, other experiments extend the common positional reference system across very different animal groups.

Ectoderm differentiation in birds and mice

As we will see in Chapter 17 the ectoderm in the eye region differentiates into the cornea, which is unusual in being transparent. This provides a convenient, and distinctive, marker for its differentiation state. In birds, the flank ectoderm differentiates into feathers, and the leg ectoderm differentiates into scales. These three structures are readily distinguished.

Head ectoderm from a chick embryo was combined (1) with chick optic cup (which normally underlies it: see Chapter 17); (2) with mesoderm from the flank of a chick embryo; and (3) with chick leg mesoderm. In experiment (1) the head ectoderm became cornea-like, in (2) it contributed to feather germs and in (3) it contributed to scales: in other words it formed the structures associated with each kind of mesoderm. However, a further experiment revealed that this was not due to a specific 'inductive' influence of the underlying mesoderm.

Chick embryo head ectoderm was combined with mouse embryo flank mesoderm (mice, of course, are furred in this region, rather than feathered!) and the chick head ectoderm attempted to form feathers in this graft combination rather than fur or any other chick ectoderm derivative. Once again the chick embryo ectoderm had responded to the position from which the mesoderm had been taken and had differentiated accordingly. But this information on position was obtained from a mouse embryo, which suggests that the mouse positional signalling system, whatever it might be, is functionally identical to that in the chick.

Lewis Wolpert formulated the concept of **positional information** to explain the phenomena in these experiments. This suggests that there are universal coordinate systems in vertebrate embryos that tissues, or rather the cells that compose the tissues, detect in order to establish where their position lies within the embryo. Once a group of cells has established their position, they differentiate appropriately. Of course, the 'appropriate' differentiation depends upon their evolutionary history: chick cells respond to the information that they are in 'flank' position by forming feathers, not fur as a mouse might do, or scales as a fish might do.

Early in development, such differentiation decisions are reversible and a piece of tissue moved from one location to another can respond by differentiating according to its new position. This flexibility is gradually lost and eventually cells and tissues become committed to forming one type of tissue – say an arm or a leg. Within the arm or leg they may still be able to respond to signals that influence which part of the limb they form, but they can no longer change the limb to which they belong. Their developmental, as well as their evolutionary, history has reduced their options. The concept of 'positional information' could therefore be summarized as: 'Cells determine their differentiation on the basis of their position and history', although this bald statement appears to understate its profundity.

One consequence of this concept is that cells of the same differentiation class may have different 'positional values'. For example, the cartilage cells that form the precursor of the femur are very similar to those that form the precursor of the big toe, yet they lie in different positions. Positional differences may be interpreted in terms of patterns of cell behaviour, such as the likelihood of dividing, lifespan, amount of material secreted, and so on, to give rise to the different morphologies of these elements.

The nature of the coordinate system

If there is a coordinate system throughout the embryo, what form does it take? One possibility is that it is established in terms of gradients. If particular regions differentiate to form 'sources' of diffusible substances early in development, gradients of these substances could be established across the embryo. Cells could then detect the local level of the diffusible substance and use this as a clue to exactly where they lie, particularly if several gradients are operating simultaneously. Results of investigative studies of the development of limbs are consistent with the idea that such gradients exist and a candidate molecule for the diffusible substance itself has been suggested (see Chapter 18). In the last 10 years, positional information has changed from a brilliant intellectual concept to a practical guide to the mechanisms of development.

Further reading

Coulombre J.L. and Coulombre A.J. (1971). Metaplastic induction of scales and feathers in the corneal anterior epithelium of the chick. *Dev. Biol.*, **25**, 464–78

Crick F. (1970). Diffusion in embryogenesis. *Nature*, **225**, 420–2

Lewis J.H., Slack J.M.W. and Wolpert L. (1977). Thresholds in development. *J. Theoret. Biol.*, **65**, 579–90

Spemann H. and Schotte O. (1932). Uber xenoplastische transplantation als mittel zur analyse der embryonalen induction. *Naturwissenschaften*, **20**, 463–7

Wolpert L. (1969). Positional information and the spatial pattern of cellular determination. *J. Theoret. Biol.*, **25**, 1–47

Wolpert L. (1978). Pattern formation in biological development. *Sci. Am.*, **239**, 159–64

Wolpert L. (1981). Positional information and pattern formation. *Philos. Trans. R. Soc. Lond. (Biol.)*, **295**, 441–50

Wolpert L. (1991). *The Triumph of the Embryo*. Oxford: Oxford University Press

6

The nervous system

Three sources contribute to the tissues of the nervous system:

- neural tube
- neural crest, and
- a series of localized thickenings (or placodes) in the ectoderm.

The neural tube gives rise to the brain and spinal cord. These represent the **central nervous system** (CNS). In addition, axons grow out from the neural tube to innervate muscles throughout the body. These form the motor component of the **peripheral nervous system**. The neural crest cells produce the sensory component of the peripheral nervous system. Epithelial placodes (Figure 6.1) lying lateral to the main body axis will develop into the sensory cells of the ear and nose and into sensory neurons.

Neural tube

Even before the neural tube begins to fuse (see Chapter 3) it is divided into different regions down its length (Figure 6.2). Fore-, mid- and hind-regions are evident in the developing brain (see Chapter 12), and caudal to this lies the spinal cord. It can be concluded from animal studies that the information for this cran-

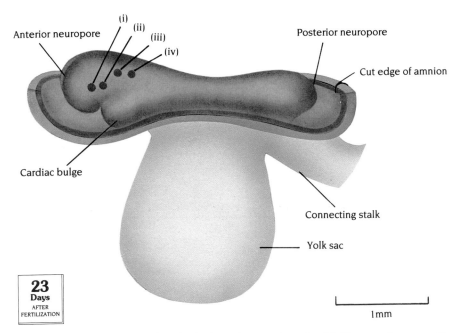

Anterior neuropore
(i)
(ii)
(iii)
(iv)
Posterior neuropore
Cut edge of amnion
Cardiac bulge
Connecting stalk
Yolk sac

23
Days
AFTER
FERTILIZATION

1mm

FIGURE 6.1 Epithelial placodes in the embryo at about day 23. These are known as (i) placode V, (ii) placode VII, (iii) placode VIII (the otic placode), and (iv) placode IX–X.

iocaudal regionalization is derived from the underlying mesoderm, which in turn acquires craniocaudal regional values at gastrulation (see Box 2.1, p. 35). Once induced, the differentiation state of the regions of the brain is comparatively stable: if a transverse slice of brain is removed and dissociated to single cells, and these cells are recombined in culture, they will spontaneously reform the same region of brain.

The spinal cord will develop a highly segmental appearance. This segmentation corresponds to the basic segmentation of the body evident in the formation of the somites.

At first the neural tube is a simple single-layered structure and all the cells are capable of dividing. Gradually it will become more complex, and cells will lose their ability to divide as they differentiate into neurons. In time all the neural cells of the CNS will lose this ability, and the only way their numbers will change is by cell death.

At division the cells move to the inner aspect of the neural tube (Figure 6.3(a,b)). This may happen several times, but eventually a terminal division takes place and the resulting daughter cells take on the characteristic appearance of the non-dividing neurons. This happens on one particular day for any neuron and is spoken of as its 'birthday'. 'Birthdays' do not fall randomly throughout the early developmental period: they occur in waves that pass down the axis in a craniocaudal direction.

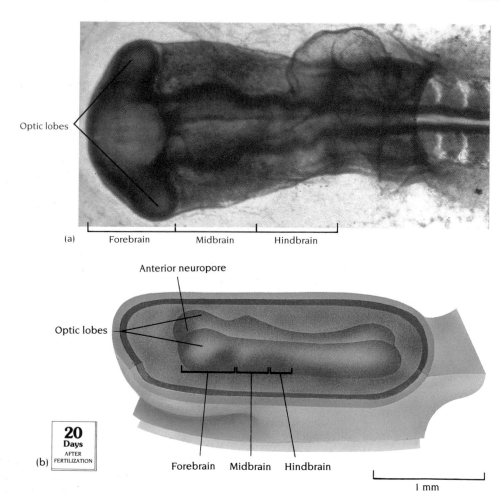

FIGURE 6.2   (a) Brain of 2-day chick embryo (approximately equivalent to human 23-day embryo) showing regionalization; (b) human embryo before neural fold fusion, showing regionalization.

After their 'birthday', the differentiating neurons begin to migrate to partic-ular parts of the neural tube and to take on particular functions. The migration occurs along long thin **glial cells** that stretch from side to side of the neural tube (Figure 6.3(b,c)). These are the columnar cells, which originally formed the epithelium of the neural tube. Neurons use these cells to haul themselves along through the surrounding layers.

Where the neurons go and what they turn into is related to their 'birthday'. In the cerebral cortex of the brain, for instance, cells at one level born on a par-ticular day migrate out to form a layer of large pyramidal cells and there is then a pause until the next wave of mitosis arrives: cells born on this 'birthday' push out past the large pyramidal layer to form a small pyramidal layer, and so on,

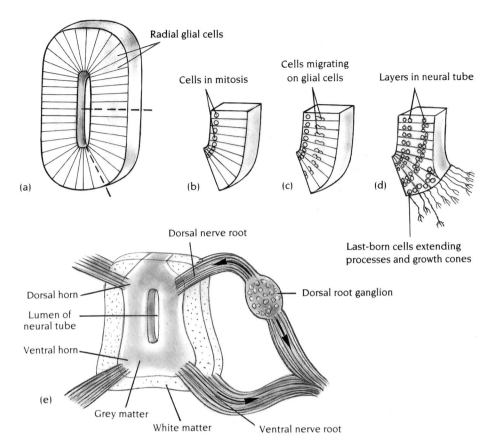

FIGURE 6.3 (a) Generalized view of a slice through the neural tube. The elongated radial glia cells can be seen stretching from the lumen to the outside wall. (b) Part of the ventral neural tube as marked in (a). Cells entering cell division round up and move to the lumenal wall of the neural tube. (c) After their 'birthday' cells migrate along the radial glial cells to the position appropriate to their type. The next wave of dividing cells is shown at the lumenal surface. These will migrate past the first wave. (d) The last wave of cells form the ventral horns. They then extend long processes which will carry the motor nerve impulses. (e) The neural crest-derived cells of the spinal ganglia grow towards the dorsal horns and join with the motor nerves. Axons running along the craniocaudal axis form the 'white matter'.

until all the layers of the cortex are formed. In this way, the single-layered neural tube gradually converts itself into the multilayered central nervous system (Figure 6.3(d)).

The origin of the motor nerves can be understood most clearly in the spinal cord rather than in the more complex brain. Late waves of 'birthdays' produce the motor neurons, which migrate to the outside of the spinal cord, not concentrically, but instead forming outpushings called 'horns' (Figure 6.3(d,e)). The aggregating nerve cell bodies in the sensory dorsal horn and the motor ventral horn are known as the **alar plate** and **basal plate** respectively. The neurons put out 'roots' – dendritic connections to neighbouring cells – and in the ventral horn put forth a single 'shoot' – an axon that grows out to provide motor innervation to a muscle somewhere in the body (Figure 6.3(d)). This axon possesses a growth cone at its tip.

A key question is: how do the nerve axons find the right muscles? The origin of muscles is discussed in Chapter 8, and the formation of neuromuscular connections in Special Topic 5 (pp. 153–7). Areas where the cell bodies lie appear grey in histological section, hence they are known as the **grey matter**. Outside the grey matter, myelinated axons establishing connections up and down the neural tube appear white, and are known as the **white matter**.

A number of biochemical defects affect cell migration; for instance, the function of the molecules mediating cell adhesion may be inhibited, which results in abnormal migration of the cells in the CNS. The mechanism of cell migration depends on a large number of components, and defects of this kind can occur in many ways. Epilepsy may result from such abnormalities.

Neural crest

Neural crest cells develop into many types of cell, and are therefore given a chapter of their own (Chapter 11). Here we will refer only to their role in the sensory nervous system.

The neural crest originates from the dorsal cells of the neural tube, from which it must detach. In the region of the brain it forms four major aggregations on each side, which move down to contribute to major ganglia (Figure 6.4(a)). The mechanisms underlying this event are dealt with in Special Topic 6 (pp. 174–7). Over the remainder of the neural tube the crest develops a 'scalloped' appearance, each outpushing of which corresponds to a somite (Figure 6.4(b)). The individual outpushings will develop as segmental ganglia. From each of these, processes will grow towards the spinal cord in one direction, entering via the dorsal horn (Figure 6.3(e)) and in the other direction processes grow out which meet and follow the motor neurons (see Special Topic 5, pp. 153–7). Sensory inputs are thus transmitted via the spinal ganglia to the dorsal horn of the spinal cord.

Neural crest cells also migrate to form the autonomic ganglia, which control the peristaltic actions of the gut.

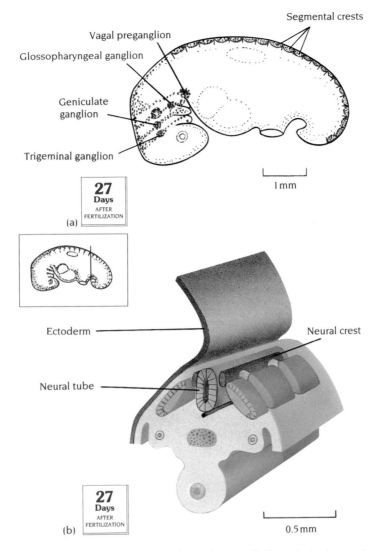

FIGURE 6.4 (a) Distinct streams of neural crest cells from the brain contribute to ganglia, among other structures; (b) neural crest cells along the neural tube show a scalloped appearance corresponding to the body segmentation.

Placodes

Closely associated with the neural crest ganglia in the region of the head are substantial ectodermal placodes, also four on each side, which also contribute to the parts of the sensory ganglia discussed above. The separate origin of these cells means that they respond to nerve growth factors in a different way from those cells deriving from neural crest, and this may have important therapeutic implications. The progress of neurodegenerative conditions such as Alzheimer's and Parkinson's diseases is slowed by the factors that contribute to the growth and maintenance of neurons in the embryo. The differential sensitivity of placode-derived and neural crest-derived neurons to such factors may be of importance in tailoring the combination of drugs to use.

The origin of the sensory apparatus mediating hearing and balance is discussed in Chapter 17.

Meninges

The brain and spinal cord are initially surrounded by loose mesoderm, which begins to condense around the central nervous system and eventually forms three distinct layers: the **pia mater** next to the brain and spinal cord, the **arachnoid mater** and the outer **dura mater** (Figure 6.5). There may be a contribution from the neural crest to the pia and arachnoid maters but these meningeal layers are shown as mesodermal in the diagrams. The pia mater is the vascular layer and is separated from the arachnoid mater by the **subarachnoid space**. The arachnoid mater is separated from the dura mater by the **subdural space**. The outer aspect of the dura mater gives rise to connective tissue and cartilage. Finally, another space can be found between the dura and the surrounding bone: this is the **epidural space**. As nerves leave the neighbourhood of the spinal cord the three meningeal layers approach each other more and more closely until the dura, the arachnoid and the pia become the epineurium, perinerium and endoneurium respectively.

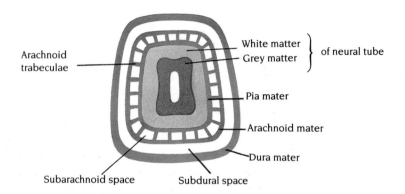

FIGURE 6.5 The meningeal layers.

Relationship with the spine

As described in Chapter 9, the vertebrae develop from the sclerotomal parts of the somites which originally lie on either side of the spinal cord. Sclerotomal projections from each segment develop on either side of the neural tube and eventually meet over the dorsal surface to enclose the spinal cord.

At first, the spinal cord occupies the entire vertebral canal but after the third month of development the vertebral column grows faster than the cord so there is a relative shift in the position of the cord. As a result of this the cord does not reach to the end of the column: at birth its end is at the level of the third lumbar vertebra. The spinal nerves must therefore run obliquely down to their original foramina, forming a structure known as the **cauda equina**.

Abnormalities of spinal cord morphology are often paralleled by abnormalities of the vertebrae, as discussed below.

The general result of the formation of the vertebrae is that the spinal cord comes to be clad in a flexible bony sheath. The brain's bony covering is discussed in Chapter 13.

Nerve regeneration

If it were possible to identify the factors controlling innervation in the embryo it might prove possible to re-evoke it in the adult and accentuate the healing of nerve damage. In spinal cord injuries – over 10 000 of which are recorded each year in the USA alone, mostly in young people – it might prove possible to alleviate or even cure the paralysis that often ensues.

Various 'growth factors' are believed to accelerate nerve sprouting and to influence the movement of nerve axons (see Special Topic 5, pp. 153–7). The clinical use of such growth factors has already been attempted, and has been reported to have therapeutic value even in severe spinal cord damage.

Defects in neurulation

The neural tube may fail to close completely, or may reopen secondarily after closing, giving rise to a family of conditions described as 'dysraphic' abnormalities ('raphe' is derived from the Greek word for a seam). In Europe generally, the baseline incidence of these defects is about 20 per 10 000 pregnancies, although something like one-quarter of affected fetuses die spontaneously during development. In regions where good prenatal diagnostic techniques are available, and where therapeutic abortion is permitted, a further 50% of affected fetuses are legally terminated.

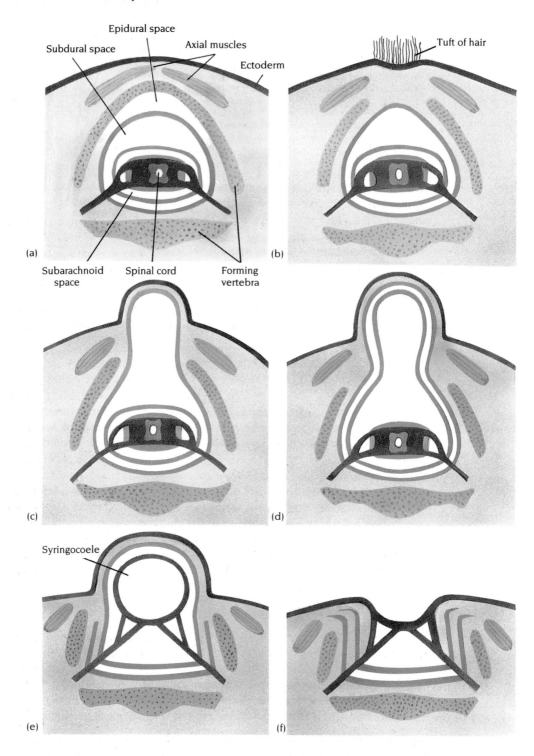

Within these overall figures are marked regional variations. In Europe, Wales, the west of Scotland and Ireland are particularly severely affected: for 1980–86, the rates per 10 000 pregnancies for Glasgow, Dublin and Paris were 37.3, 35.4 and 10.7 respectively. In Glasgow and Paris therapeutic termination of pregnancy is allowed and, after subtracting fetal deaths at all centres, the incidence per 10 000 live births was 10.6 in Glasgow, 24.6 in Dublin and 2.8 in Paris.

The observed baseline variations may be due to a combination of environmental and genetic factors. Use of vitamin supplementation in women intending to become pregnant seems to exert a beneficial effect (see Special Topic 9, pp. 369–74).

Spina bifida The most common dysraphic condition is spina bifida ('divided spine'). This may occur at any level of the neural tube, although it is most common caudally. The degree of severity also varies (see Figure 6.6). In the most severe cases, the spinal cord is exposed and abnormal, leading to neural dysfunction below the level of the lesion. The mortality rate is high in such children. Spina bifida detected at birth consistently represents just over 50% of dysraphic anomalies.

Spina bifida occulta Very minor forms of spina bifida such as spina bifida occulta, in which the vertebrae fail to fuse completely over the spinal cord, may be symptomless and may remain undetected in as many as 15% of the population.

Anencephaly This is slightly less common than spina bifida, but together the two conditions make up the bulk of the dysraphic abnormalities. In general, anencephaly occurs in about 10 per 10 000 pregnancies and in one region (South Wales) it has been as common as 100 per 10 000 pregnancies. In this condition the neural tube has failed to close in the region of the forebrain, although the subsequent lesion may extend all the way down the spine. The cerebral hemispheres (see Chapter 12) fail to form and the cerebral tissue degenerates, although the brain stem may be present. The neurocranium (see Chapter 13), whose development is strongly influenced by the brain, fails to form altogether. Anencephaly is incompatible with survival after birth. It can be detected prenatally by ultrasonography, and usually such a pregnancy is terminated but in at least one case the mother has carried the child to term so that its organs could be used for transplantation.

Severe dysraphic conditions are associated with increased levels of α-fetoprotein in the amniotic fluid and in the maternal blood: this can be used as a sign for further investigation.

FIGURE 6.6 (*opposite*)   (a) Normal arrangement of tissues around the spinal cord; (b) spina bifida occulta. The bony tissues have not fused over the spinal cord; (c) where the meninges alone protrude through the opening in the vertebral column the condition is described as a meningocoele. Here the dura is involved; (d) meningocoele in which arachnoid and dural layers of the meninges project through the vertebral opening; (e) where the neural tissue is included in the projecting mass, this is described as meningomyelocoele. Here the central cavity of the spinal cord is greatly enlarged, forming a syringocoele; (f) complete exposure of the interior of the spinal cord is known as rachischisis. The spinal cord will deteriorate as a result of its exposure on the surface.

Further reading

Adler R. (1973). Cell interactions and histogenesis in embryonic neural aggregates. *Dev. Biol.*, **21**, 403–23

Anon (1991). Epilepsy and disorders of neuronal migration. *Lancet*, **336**, 1035

Bergsma D. (1979). *Birth Defects Compendium* 2nd edn. London: Macmillan

Campbell I.R., Dayton D.H. and Nance W.E. (1986). Neural tube defects: a review of human and animal studies on the etiology of neural tube defects. *Teratology*, **34**, 171–87

Cowan C.M. (1979). The development of the brain. *Sci. Am.*, **242**, 106–17

D'Amico-Martel A. and Noden D.M. (1983). Contributions of placodal and neural crest cells to avian cranial peripheral ganglia. *Am. J. Anat.*, **166**, 445–68

Edelman G.M. (1984). Cell adhesion molecules: a molecular basis for animal form. *Sci. Am.*, **250**, 80–91

Garber B.B., Huttenlocher P.R. and Larramendi L.H.M. (1980). Self-assembly of cortical plate cells in vitro within embryonal mouse cerebral aggregates: Golgi and electron microscopic analysis. *Brain Res.*, **201**, 255–78

Geisler F.H., Dorsey F.C. and Coleman W.P. (1991). Recovery of motor function after spinal cord injury – a randomised placebo controlled trial with GM-1 ganglioside. *N. Engl. J. Med.*, **324**, 1829–38

Hyman C., Hofer M., Bard Y.-A. *et al.* (1991). BDNF is a neurotrophic factor for dopaminegic receptors of the substantia nigra. *Nature*, **350**, 230–2

Lechat M.F. (1989). *Eurocat Report 3. Surveillance of congenital anomalies. Years 1980-86*

Lindsay R.M., Thoenen H. and Barde Y.-A. (1985). Placode and neural crest-derived sensory neurones are responsive at early developmental stages to Brain-Derived Neurotrophic Factor. *Dev. Biol.*, **112**, 319–28

Marx J. (1990). NGF and Alzheimer's: Hopes and Fears. *Science*, **247**, 408–10

Purves D. and Lichtman J.W. (1985). *Principles of Neural Development.* Sunderland MA: Sinauer

Rakic P. (1972). Mode of cell migration to the superficial layers of the fetal monkey neocortex. *J. Comp. Neurol.*, **145**, 61–84

Saluja P. (1988). The incidence of spina bifida occulta in a historic and a modern London population. *J. Anat.*, **158**, 91–3

Winter R.M., Knowles S.A.S., Bieber F.R. and Baraitser M. (1988). *The Malformed Fetus and Still Birth*. New York: John Wiley & Sons

7

The vascular system

The vascular system comprises the heart, the blood and lymphatic vessels, the blood and the lymph (the heart is discussed in Chapter 21). It is perhaps the first organ system to become functional in the body because it is needed to pump blood through the embryonic and extraembryonic circulations to provide nutrients for rapid growth and to remove the resulting waste products. As a consequence, blood vessels in the early embryo and fetus are very much larger relative to body size than they are in the adult.

Development of the vascular system begins in the mesoderm of the yolk sac adjacent to the endoderm, at about 17 days after fertilization. Curiously, a common feature of blood formation in early development is that it occurs in mesoderm close to endoderm. It may well be that some endodermally produced factor induces the mesoderm to differentiate in this way. The vascular system is first evident in the form of **blood islands**, aggregations of cells of which the central cells will differentiate into red blood cells and the outer cells will form a flattened endothelial layer. These blood islands are visible as red spots in the mesoderm of the yolk sac wall (Figure 7.1).

Gradually, the blood islands of the yolk sac mesoderm fuse, until a loose branching network is formed. A rather similar sequence of events in the mesoderm of the floor of the intraembryonic coelom leads to the formation of the heart precursors (see Chapter 21) and the major paired blood vessels. Endothelial cells arise from the mesoderm, and form vesicles that gradually join up to form tubes which may not initially contain blood cells. Vessels formed in this way include the dorsal aortae, the cardinal veins and the major umbilical

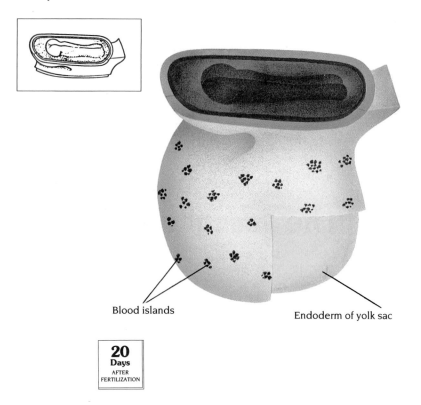

Blood islands

Endoderm of yolk sac

20 Days AFTER FERTILIZATION

FIGURE 7.1 Blood islands developing in yolk sac mesoderm. These will coalesce to form a net of arteries and veins running over the yolk sac.

arteries and veins. A network of blood vessel precursors also forms in the chorionic mesoderm.

Over the following week, more and more epithelial cavities form in the embryonic and extraembryonic mesoderm: again, these do not necessarily contain blood cells. Together the cavities form a loose connecting network of chambers and vessels in the mesoderm. The heart begins to beat at about 21 days after fertilization. At first blood washes back and forth in the loose connecting net of blood vessel tubules, but slowly takes on a patterned flow. It is likely that the flow of blood through any particular path in the network will lead to its further differentiation as a blood vessel, so that the blood vessel pattern takes on its definitive form partly as a result of fluid dynamic effects. Vertebrate embryos will survive briefly in the absence of a heart, but without blood flow the network of epithelial vessels remains undifferentiated. Blood vessel pattern is highly variable at early stages in vertebrates and there is a considerable degree of flexibility in the system. If one blood vessel is blocked, flow passes through the surrounding net of small vessels and in time one of these reforms as the major vessel (Figure 7.2). This ability survives in the adult and leads to anastomoses forming round obstructions.

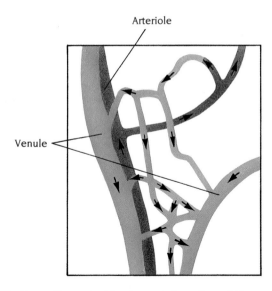

Arteriole

Venule

FIGURE 7.2 Even after major blood vessels have formed fine capillaries link the vessels. The network connecting two small veins and an artery are shown. Flow directions are marked with arrows. Obstruction of any of the small vessels cause the flow through the others to increase and they will begin to differentiate further.

Development of the blood vessel pattern

As the heart begins to beat (Figure 7.3), blood is pumped dorsally through blood vessels that form in the developing **branchial arches** (Chapter 14). It enters the **dorsal aortae** (paired at this stage), from which the precursors of the **internal carotid artery** run forwards to supply the head, but the main direction of blood flow in the aortae is towards the tail. **Intersegmental arteries** begin to develop as sprigs running between the developing somites. At the level of the gut an arterial complex branches off to connect with the site of blood formation in the yolk sac network: in time this complex will form the **vitelline arteries**. Towards the tail, the aortae form a plexus from which the single **umbilical artery** emerges to run in the connecting stalk to the chorionic wall, where the placenta is developing. Blood returns from the placenta via paired **umbilical veins**, which also pick up blood from the yolk sac, through what will become the **vitelline veins**. Blood then enters the **sinus venosi** before reaching the heart, to be pumped around the body once more. Blood from the head region runs through the **head veins**, which lie just lateral to the neural tube. Together these form a functional, though rudimentary, embryonic circulation connecting with the extraembryonic vessels in the chorionic mesoderm.

Within a few days (Figure 7.4) the **superior cardinal veins**, which drain the cranial portion of the body, have developed. Similarly, the **inferior cardinal**

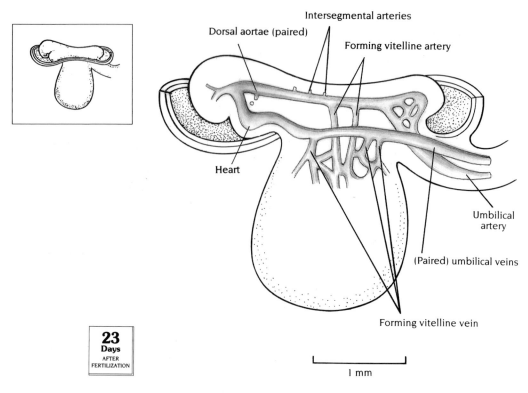

FIGURE 7.3 Embryonic circulation at 23 days.

veins drain the caudal embryo. The vitelline arteries and veins are now also distinct. The paired dorsal aortae have fused from the mid-cervical region caudally, becoming the definitive **dorsal aorta**. In the sacral region this gives rise to the **common iliac arteries**, which continue as the umbilical arteries to join the original umbilical artery in the connecting stalk. The common iliac arteries are derived from arteries supplying the allantois.

Changes to the umbilical and vitelline veins

Subsequent changes in the drainage of blood back to the heart are complex: indeed, they may seem sufficiently complicated to make them incomprehensible. However, certain general rules may help make these events clearer.

- The veins are part of a network, so anastomoses between left and right are frequent and can be readily exploited.
- The route to the heart involving the least work is the one that will be favoured in terms of blood flow, and vessels will differentiate accordingly.
- The embryo becomes increasingly asymmetric about the axis during the embryonic period (see Special Topic 8, pp. 295–6). As we will see, the branchial arch arteries, the heart, and the gut become different on each side of

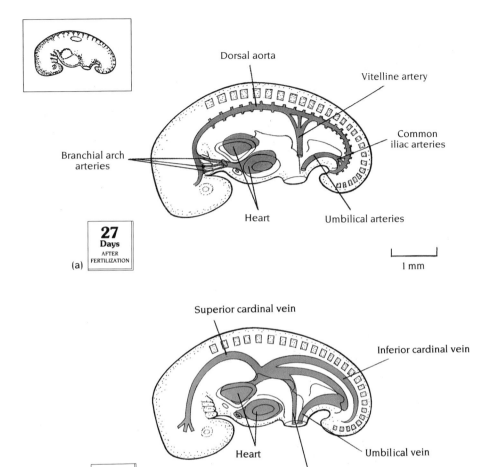

FIGURE 7.4   Embryonic circulation at 27 days.

the body. This affects the blood vessels, and often the shortest route to the heart.

Initially the vitelline veins and umbilical veins run on either side of the gut (Figure 7.5(a)). As the liver bud expands (see Chapter 23) it engulfs the vitelline veins (Figure 7.5(b)) and then the umbilical veins (Figure 7.5(c)). These form a common plexus of sinusoid vessels running through the liver. At the same time, the gut is becoming displaced to the right (see Chapter 23) and anastomoses between the vitelline veins become of importance, particularly those shown in Figure 7.5(b). As the gut continues to twist, the original right and left vitelline veins form an acute angle to the the blood flow, the main stream of which now loops round the gut via the original anastomoses (Figure 7.5(c)). This new route represents the formation of the hepatic portal vein.

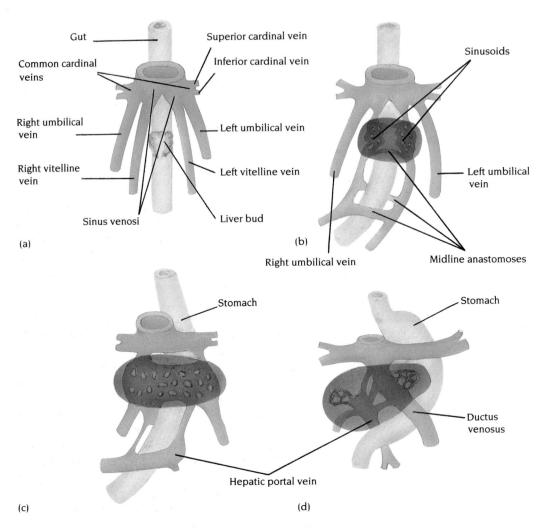

FIGURE 7.5 View of the inflow vessels into the heart, as seen in ventral view weeks 4–8 after fertilization. (a) Initially the liver lies between the vitelline veins. (b) As it enlarges it comes to incorporate the vitelline veins which form a plexus of blood vessels. Anastomoses across the midline become important. (c) The liver also encompasses the umbilical veins, and the vitelline veins are converted into the hepatic portal artery. (d) The right umbilical vein decreases in size, and the newly formed ductus venosus carries the blood to the right side of the heart.

These events may also be affected by progressive diminution of the left umbilical and vitelline veins where they enter the left sinus venosus (Figure 7.5(c)). Entry to the heart eventually shifts to the right and the blood from the caudal part of the left umbilical vein finds a new route to the heart through the plexus (Figure 7.5(d)).

Changes to the cardinal veins

The changes to the cardinal veins are even more complex than those to the umbilical and vitelline veins. It suffices here to say that blood from the left side is diverted via anastamoses to the right and that the right posterior cardinal vein, in association with other vessels, forms the inferior vena cava while the right anterior cardinal vein also undergoes many changes before contributing to the superior vena cava.

Interactive vascular development

As the body form begins to emerge so the blood vessel pattern begins to alter accordingly. As new organs are formed, sprig-like outgrowths from existing blood vessel walls begin to push out towards them to provide their blood supply. Possible mechanisms for inducing this are discussed in Special Topic 5 (pp. 153–7). For the moment we can note that when the most caudal branchial arch arteries form they will send out sprigs towards the developing lungs (see Chapters 14 and 20). Similarly, the segmental nature of the somite row (which has such a marked effect on the nervous system: see Chapter 6) continues to result in the development of intersegmental arteries from the dorsal aorta (30–40 small branches on each side of the embryo). Branching also occurs to supply the structures that develop from and in association with the gut (Chapter 23). When the hind limbs form, a branch artery will develop from each umbilical artery to provide its blood supply.

Conversely, the blood supply will diminish to structures that decrease in size. As already mentioned, the vitelline arteries are at first substantial (indicating the evolutionary importance of the yolk sac) but as the yolk sac reduces in relative size the vitelline arteries also diminish in importance, and will eventually disappear. A fused remnant, however, takes on the task of supplying the midgut and will become the **superior mesenteric artery**.

The circulatory system is also capable of shutting off major blood vessels over a very short timespan, as seen in the dramatic changes in the circulation at birth.

The lymphatic system

The lymphatic system returns fluid from the tissues to the veins and develops in the fifth week, after the first appearance of the major veins. Its exact mode of origin remains unclear, but it may arise as sacs from vein endothelial cells. The first pair of these are apparent near the junction of the anterior and posterior cardinal veins. Thereafter, further paired and midline sacs develop and interconnect in a rather variable manner. Lymph nodes develop from sacs following mesodermal invagination.

Blood-forming organs

The earliest site of blood formation is the yolk sac but as this diminishes in size this role is gradually adopted by the liver (Chapter 23). It is possible that blood-forming stem cells migrate to the liver from the yolk sac. The liver commences blood formation at about 6 weeks after fertilization.

During the later embryonic period the spleen also becomes a site of blood cell production (this forms during weeks 4–5 in the dorsal mesentery of the gut (see Chapter 23), dorsal to the greater curvature of stomach when it lies in the midline). Although the spleen is entirely mesodermal in origin it lies close to the endoderm of the gut and forms initially as thickenings in the mesoderm suspending the gut, which then coalesce to form a discrete structure. The spleen gives rise to lymphocytes and red blood cells, commencing later than the liver but persisting into the fetus and after birth.

In the fetal period the bone marrow begins to contribute to blood formation and, later still, peripheral lymphoid tissues (including the thymus) become sites of haematopoietic differentiation. In the adult the bone marrow, the spleen, the thymus and the lymph nodes are the main sites of haematopoiesis.

Blood cell differentiation

All blood cells are believed to derive from a single kind of progenitor stem cell. This can renew its own population numbers, but also gives rise to the progenitors of differentiated cells, which can be classed as **lymphoid** or **myeloid** cells. The former give rise to T and B lymphocytes, the latter to further stem cells, which will variously produce red blood cells, platelets (formed by the fragmentation of larger 'megakaryocytes'), monocytes, macrophages and granulocytes. Once a daughter cell has entered into one of these differentiation pathways it is apparently committed to it. As it embarks on the sequential programme of differentiation, a cell multiplies very rapidly to boost its numbers: it seems likely that all the blood cells in circulation at any one time are descendants of only a few stem cells.

The mechanisms that switch cells from being stem cells to becoming differentiated and lead to them making particular kinds of differentiation decisions are of major importance; when they go wrong they can give rise to a number of serious disorders including leukaemias. A variety of growth factors are known to be involved, often showing complex mutual interactions. Inhibitors help to keep production in equilibrium; the physical microenvironment of cells also plays a role. Signals from further down the differentiative chain influence the stem cells, so that excesses or deficiencies of particular kinds of cells can be adjusted and changing physiological circumstances accommodated.

Circulation changes at birth

In the adult blood leaves the left ventricle of the heart for the systemic circulation via the aorta (Figure 7.6(a)). Branches leave to supply the head and upper limbs and the blood from these regions returns to the heart via the superior vena cava. Further down, the dorsal aorta branches supply the liver and the gut and further down still branches supply the lower limbs. The blood returning from the legs enters the inferior vena cava, where it is joined by blood from the midgut arriving via the hepatic portal vein, and by blood via the veins from the liver. The inferior vena cava and superior vena cava enter the right atrium. Blood from here passes to the right ventricle, is pumped through the pulmonary circulation and finally returns to the left atrium.

This is rather different from the situation in the fetus (Figure 7.6(b)). The umbilical arteries carry blood from the level of the lower limbs to the placenta. The oxygenated blood returns via the left umbilical vein and the ductus venosus to the developing inferior vena cava, and enters the right atrium. Here, however, a considerable proportion crosses to the *left* atrium via the patent foramen ovale (see Chapter 21) and enters the left ventricle for recirculation through the aorta, where it is joined by much of the blood from the right ventricle via the ductus

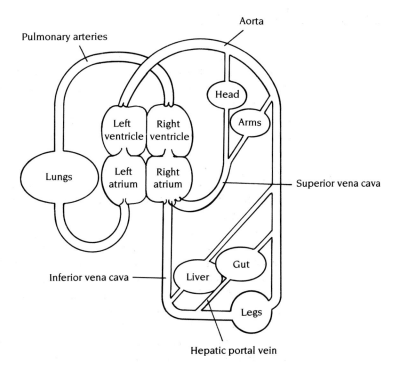

FIGURE 7.6 (a) Blood circulation in the adult.

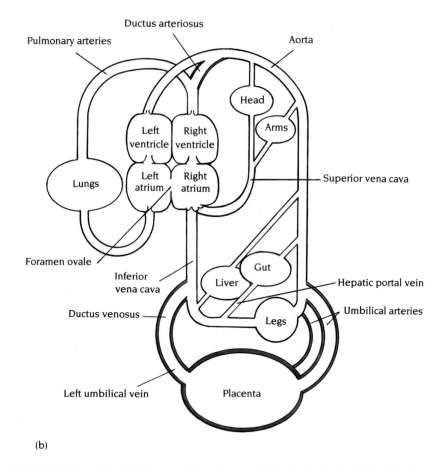

(b)

FIGURE 7.6 (*contd*)   (b) Corresponding diagram of circulation before birth. The features that are present before, but not after, birth are shown in red.

arteriosus (see Chapter 21). The pulmonary arteries carry very little blood, as they are constricted by the fluid-filled lungs.

At birth the fetal circulation must be rapidly converted to a neonatal form, which develops into the adult form over the next few months. As the first breath is taken the pulmonary arteries begin to carry more blood and the pressure in the aorta drops. This results in the ductus arteriosus beginning to contract, a process that takes a number of hours to complete (see p. 291). The umbilical arteries also contract, but much more rapidly, shutting off the blood supply to the placenta: this may be mediated by the release of hormones into the blood. The left umbilical vein constricts more slowly than the umbilical artery, allowing blood to continue to leave the placenta. The ductus venosus also begins to shut down and pressure changes lead to closure of the foramen ovale (Chapter 21).

Those vessels closed off during the neonatal period gradually become fibrous cords. The umbilical arteries form the median umbilical ligaments, the left umbilical vein becomes the ligamentum teres hepatus, the ductus venosus becomes the ligamentum venosum and the ductus arteriosus develops into the ligamentum arteriosum.

Further reading

Clark E.R. and Clark E.L. (1939). Microscopic observations on the growth of blood capillaries in the living mammal. *Am. J. Anat.*, **64**, 251–301

Goldwasser E. (1975). Erythropoietin and the differentiation of red blood cells. *Fed. Proc.*, **34**, 2285–92

Hopper A.F. and Hart N.H. (1980). *Foundations of Animal Development*. Oxford: Oxford University Press

Hughes A.F.W. (1935). The first differentiation of the vitelline artery. *J. Anat.*, **70**, 76–122

Metcalf D. (1985). The granulocyte–macrophage colony stimulating factors. *Science*, **229**, 16–22

Perera P., Kurban A.K. and Ryan T.J. (1970). The development of the cutaneous microvascular system in the newborn. *Br. J. Dermatol.*, **80**, 86

Sabin F.R. (1917). Origin and development of the primitive vessels of the pig and of the chick. *Carnegie Contributions to Embryology*, **6**, 61–124

Sabin F.R. (1920). Studies on the origin of blood vessels and of red blood corpuscles as seen in the living blastoderm of the chick during the second day of incubation. *Carnegie Contributions to Embryology*, **9**, 213–64

van der Putte S.C.J. (1975). The development of the lymphatic system in man. *Adv. Anat. Embryol. Cell Biol.*, **51**, 1–60

Wilson D. (1983). The origin of the endothelium in the developing marginal vein of the chick wing bud. *Cell Diff.*, **13**, 63–7

8

The musculature

There are three kinds of muscle: skeletal, smooth and cardiac. Cardiac and skeletal muscle both exhibit regularly spaced transverse bands and are described as **striated muscle**. Much striated skeletal muscle is under voluntary control. **Smooth muscle** does not have striations: it is particularly well suited to prolonged contractions such as those that control gut movements.

In general, muscle cells arise from the mesoderm, though there are exceptions: the smooth muscle of the iris is believed to derive from neurectodermal cells, and the smooth muscle associated with sweat, salivary and mammary glands is believed to originate from surface ectoderm.

Striated muscles

Skeletal muscle

The exact origin of skeletal muscle cells in higher vertebrates has long been controversial but it is now clear that skeletal muscle cells arise in the somites (Box 8.1) from where they migrate to form the skeletal musculature throughout the body. This migration can occur either by lateral extension of the somites themselves or as a result of the detachment of single cells from the lateral edge of the

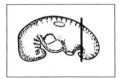

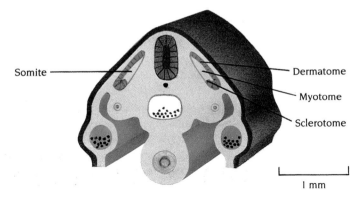

Somite

Dermatome

Myotome

Sclerotome

1 mm

FIGURE 8.1   Somite development during week 4.

somite known as the dermomyotome (Figure 8.1). The part of the somite known as the myotome contributes to the axial muscles.

The migratory single cells (myoblasts or premyoblasts) invade the surrounding mesoderm and condense in regions where muscles are to form. The mechanism underlying this is not clear, but it seems likely that it reflects a prepattern of muscle connective tissue. If somites are removed to prevent migration of muscle cells, then a 'ghost' pattern of connective tissue can be observed to form briefly before degenerating. The connective tissue prepattern may arise in direct response to some form of positional signalling (see Chapter 5). Similarly, the lateral extensions of the somites split into individual muscles and muscle sheets, also probably under the influence of the cells that will form the connective tissue.

Within the condensing premuscle masses individual myoblasts cease to divide and then begin to fuse together to form elongated tubes, which later develop visible striations. A proportion of the myoblasts remains capable of division to expand the muscle population during growth (see regeneration of skeletal muscle below). For myoblast populations the decision to divide or to differentiate seems to be mediated by growth factors (see Box 8.1).

Box 8.1   Experimental analysis of muscle development

The origin of skeletal muscle cells was unknown for many years. It was clear that in lower vertebrates somites give rise to most, if not all, of the skeletal muscles by the extension of long processes, but in higher vertebrates the muscles of the limbs and face appear without the intervention of processes of this kind, leading to the belief that they differentiated directly from the local mesoderm.

This is now known not to be the case, as was discovered by exploiting recognizable differences in individual cells from different species of birds. Quail cells possess a distinct nuclear marker that distinguishes them from cells of the domestic chick. Short lengths of somitic mesoderm were removed from early chick embryos, and replaced with equivalent lengths of quail somitic tissue (Figure 1). The grafted chick embryos were incubated until the time at which muscle cells were detectable in the limbs, and were then analysed. The striated muscle cells of the limb were indeed quail in origin: they had migrated into the limb from the somites. All the connective tissue cells of the muscles and their tendons were derived from the host chick, showing that they had differentiated in the limb itself.

There are minor differences between chick and quail embryos in terms of their muscle mass splitting timetable. In grafted chick hosts the

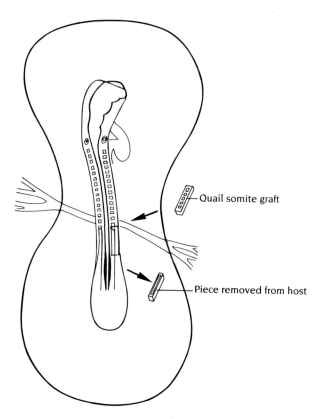

Quail somite graft

Piece removed from host

FIGURE 1   Replacement of chick somites by quail somites leads to the formation of chick muscles in which all the striated muscle cell are quail, showing that these cells arise only from somites.

Box 8.1 Experimental analysis of muscle development • 119

muscles behaved in a manner characteristic of the chick, even though the actual muscle cells were quail, indicating that the connective tissue controls the morphology and splitting timetable of the muscles.

Although for technical reasons such experiments are difficult to carry out in mammals, there are no grounds for believing that the situation is any different in the higher vertebrates.

Once cells have become muscle they can either proliferate or commence differentiation but once they have begun to differentiate proliferation is no longer possible: in the fused muscle fibres the nuclei are inactivated. Muscle growth in response to exercise therefore takes place by splitting of fibres rather than by cell division.

The decision to proliferate or differentiate appears to be modulated by growth factors. In the presence of fibroblast growth factor (FGF), myoblasts remain in division. If FGF is withdrawn, even in the presence of other factors that allow cell division, myoblasts enter the differentiation pathway. FGF is present in the embryo during development, and so it is a plausible candidate as a control molecule. Moreover, FGF is a mesoderm-inducing factor (see Box 2.1, p. 35–9). This hints at an elegant mechanism in which the appearance of FGF in the embryo commits cells to muscle differentiation but keeps them proliferating without differentiating; its withdrawal acts as the signal for differentiation.

Limb muscles

The migratory cells enter the limb bud and collect in dorsal and ventral muscle masses (Figure 8.2), which correspond to the extensor and flexor compartments respectively of the adult musculature. These masses then split in a binary fashion until the definitive muscle pattern is established. The mechanism underlying muscle splitting is not yet known: several explanations such as differential contraction under the influence of the ingrowing nerves or mechanical stresses caused by elongation of the limb have been ruled out by experiment, but it is likely that the connective tissues are involved in some way.

Trunk muscles

The somites extend down the flanks during the embryonic period (Figure 8.3), their segmental nature becoming less clear with time. In the abdominal region the segmentation is lost and the muscles form a continuous sheet but in the thorax the development of the ribs reimposes patent segmentation.

Two distinct dorsoventral divisions can be recognized in the trunk myotomes at about week 5 (Figure 8.3): the dorsal division, the **epimere**, will give rise to the extensor muscles of the spine and to the intervertebral muscles; the ventral division, the **hypomere**, extends laterally and ventrally and produces

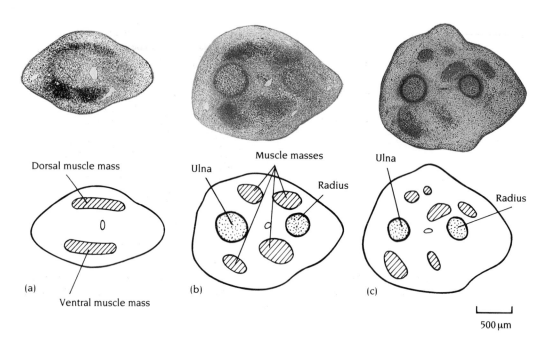

FIGURE 8.2 Dorsal and ventral muscle masses in the forelimb of the chick embryo, at mid-radius/ulna level. (a) Equivalent to approximately 5 weeks after fertilization in humans; (b) 6 weeks; (c) 7 weeks.

the layered muscles of the abdomen and thorax. The hypomere develops into three layers corresponding to the external, internal and innermost intercostal muscles in the thorax, and to the external oblique, internal oblique and transversus abdominus in the abdomen. This delamination is thought to be controlled by muscle connective tissue. The most ventral part of the hypomere becomes the infrahyoid musculature in the cervical region, the sternalis muscle (where present) in the thoracic region and the rectus abdominis muscle in the abdominal region.

As the epimere and hypomere form from the myotome posterior primary division, the corresponding spinal nerve supplies the epimere and an anterior primary division supplies the hypomere.

Head and neck muscles

Differentiated somites do not form in the head region. However, in many vertebrate embryos it is possible to see faint segmental condensations running cranially from the first distinct somite. These are referred to as **somitomeres**. Grafting experiments, such as those described in Chapter 5, reveal that the somitomeres also give rise to migratory premuscle cells that populate the head and neck. These are described more fully in Chapter 14.

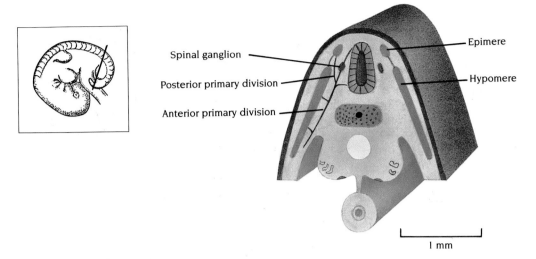

Spinal ganglion

Posterior primary division

Anterior primary division

Epimere

Hypomere

1 mm

FIGURE 8.3 The somitic myotome divides into the epimere and hypomere. The segmental nature of the myotome becomes less obvious over much of the trunk. The spinal nerve branches to supply both divisions of the myotome.

Fast and slow muscle fibres

There are two main types of striated skeletal muscle fibre: 'slow' fibres are well suited to prolonged and/or repetitive contraction as required in maintenance of posture whereas 'fast' fibres are adapted for the rapid contraction required during movement. A particular muscle may contain both types in proportions, depending on its function. Though these fibres are different in appearance and biochemical properties, they arise from identical embryonic skeletal muscles; the differences are induced by particular patterns of nerve firing in the innervating muscles. This can be shown by diverting the nerves that usually supply fast muscles to muscles that are usually slow. The muscle then develops as a fast muscle: in other words, the fibres develop in accordance with their innervation. Frequency of neural activity appears to be the active determinant: the more frequent the neural activity, the greater the disposition to form fast muscle fibres.

Regeneration of skeletal muscle

Once muscle fibres have formed, the nuclei lose their ability to replicate. Subsequent muscle growth in response to exercise is due to hypertrophy and extension of the fibres. However, damaged muscle can regenerate since muscle stem cells ('satellite cells') remain in a myoblastic state, and can divide to produce new muscle when signalled to do so by trauma.

Cardiac muscle

Cardiac muscle is derived from the splanchnic mesoderm at the cranial end of the embryonic disc, perhaps under the influence of the endoderm. If this mesoderm is isolated, and the tissue dissociated to single cells, each of these cells begins to contract spontaneously, showing that contractility is an intrinsic property of the differentiating cells. At first, when the cells are widely dispersed, the cells all contract at different rates but later, as they multiply, they come into contact with each other. At this point their rates of beating entrain on to the fastest cells and a mass of tissue is formed with all the cells beating in synchrony.

The development of the heart is discussed in Chapter 21.

Smooth muscle

It is believed that most smooth muscle cells arise in the splanchnopleural mesoderm, although their lineage has not been traced in as much detail as that of the skeletal muscle cells. It is also possible that some smooth muscle develops from the intermediate mesoderm. The smooth muscle of the iris is, very unusually, derived from neurectoderm (Chapter 17). Smooth muscle cells, like striated muscle cells, fuse to form fibres, but these are often in the form of 'straps' or fascicles and may be interwoven in different orientations to give a sheet of muscle that can contract in more than one direction.

Further reading

Bardeen C.R. and Lewis W.H. (1901). Development of the limbs, body wall and back in man. *Am. J. Anat.*, **1**, 1–36

Buller A.J., Eccles J.C. and Eccles R.M. (1960). Interactions between motoneurones and muscles in respect of the characteristic speeds of their responses. *J. Physiol.*, **150**, 417–39

Burnstock G. (1970). Structure of smooth muscle and its innervation. In *Smooth Muscle*. (Bulbring, E., Brading, A.F., Jones, A.W. and Tomita, T., eds.), pp. 1–69. London: Edward Arnold

Christ B. and Cihak R. (1986). *Development and Regeneration of Skeletal Muscle*. Basel: Karger

Haan R.L. (1967). Regulation of spontaneous activity and growth of embryonic chick heart cells in tissue culture. *Dev. Biol.*, **16**, 216–49

Kollman J. (1907) *Handatlas der Entwicklungsgeschichte des Menschen*. Vol. 1. Jena: Gustav Fischer

Lipton B.H. and Schultz E. (1979). Developmental fate of skeletal muscle satellite cells. *Science*, **205**, 1292–4

McLachlan J.C. and Wolpert L. (1980). The spatial pattern of muscle development in chick limb. In *Development and Specialisation of Skeletal Muscle* (Goldspink D.F., ed.), pp. 1–17. Cambridge: Cambridge University Press

Noden D.M. (1984). Craniofacial development: new views on old problems. *Anat. Rec.*, **208**, 1–13

Noden D.M. (1988). Interactions and fate of avian craniofacial mesenchyme. *Development*, **103**, 121–40

Reznik M. (1976). Origin of the myogenic cell in the adult striated muscle of mammals. A review and a hypothesis. *Differentiation*, **7**, 65–73

Shafiq S.A. *et al.* (1967). An electron microscopic study of regeneration and satellite cells in human muscle. *Neurology*, **17**, 567–74

Tandler B. (1972). Microstructure of salivary glands. In *Proceedings of Symposium on Salivary Glands and their Secretions* (Rowe, N.H. ed.), pp. 8–21. Ann Arbor: University of Michigan

Vrbova G. (1980) Innervation and differentiation of muscle fibres. In *Development and Specialisation of Skeletal Muscle* (Goldspink, D.F., ed.), pp. 37–50. Cambridge: Cambridge University Press

Wachtler F. and Jacob M. (1986). Origin and development of the cranial skeletal muscles. *Bibl. Anat.*, **29**, 24–46

Box 8.1

Christ B., Jacob H.J. and Jacob, M. (1979). Differentiating abilities of avian somatopleural mesoderm. *Experientia*, **35**, 1376–8

Linkhart T.A., Clegg C.H. and Hauschka S. (1980). Control of mouse myoblast commitment to differentiation by mitogens. *J. Supramol. Struct.*, **14**, 483–98

Mauger A., Kient M., Hedayat I. and Goetick P.F. (1983). Tissue interactions in the organization and maintenance of the muscle pattern in the avian limb. *J. Embryol. Exp. Morph.*, **76**, 199–215

Shellswell G.B. (1980). Cellular events in the early development of skeletal muscles. In *Development in Mammals 4* (Johnson M.H., ed.), pp. 137–59. Amsterdam: Elsevier/North Holland Biomedical Press

9

The skeleton

The strength of structures formed by direct cell-to-cell adhesion is rather low, being limited by the strength of the cell membrane. Mechanical strength is instead gained by secretion of extracellular materials by cells. The enamel of the teeth is the hardest material thus formed; bone is next in hardness but is rather stiff and is frequently partnered by cartilage, which is more flexible.

Cartilage

Cartilage is a largely avascular tissue, in which cells (**chondrocytes**) are embedded in a tough fibrous matrix with a large collagen component. In the adult, variations in the composition of the ground substance lead to different types such as hyaline cartilage, elastic cartilage and fibrocartilage. Cartilage is an ancient tissue in evolutionary terms, probably predating bone. It forms directly from mesoderm, both somatic and somitic. In the embryo most of the bony elements are prefigured by cartilage models, which begin to ossify during the embryonic period. This process continues throughout the fetal period and early life until adulthood, when cartilage remains mainly at the joints.

Cartilage models of bones are initially indistinct in form, but by the end of the embryonic period they have developed into recognizable, if simplified, miniatures of the adult structure. The cartilage and the developing bone can be extensively modified by mechanical forces.

Cartilage grows by cell division, by cell enlargement (often just before the death of the chondrocyte) and by increased secretion of extracellular materials by the chondrocytes.

Bone

Bone is a vascular tissue in which the cells (**osteocytes**) are dispersed in a protein matrix with a large collagen component and calcium phosphate salts crystallized throughout. Bone forms in one of two ways, either as **endochondral** or **intramembranous bone**.

Endochondral (replacement) bone formation

Most bones in the body are formed by this process, which is seen most clearly in the long bones. An avascular cartilage model develops first, as described earlier, and is gradually refined into the general shape of the adult bone. After the cartilage element is formed it continues to grow, mainly at the ends, but also radially. The individual chondrocytes show a distinct ageing process that culminates in hypertrophy and death, initially at the midpoint of the cartilage element. As the chondrocytes die blood vessels begin to enter the previously avascular cartilage, carrying cells known as **chondroclasts**, which remove the dead chondrocytes and another blood-borne family of cells, known as **osteoblasts**, lay down bone in their place. A race commences between the growth of cartilage and the process of ossification: when ossification finally catches up, the bone ceases to grow.

Intramembranous bone formation

The rather unfortunate name of this bone should not be taken to imply that it forms in membranes. Mesoderm cells start to proliferate and blood vessels form in the resulting dense tissue. Cells in the mesoderm (either mesodermal in origin or originating from the neural crest) then secrete strands of bone, so that osteoblasts appear directly from the mesoderm.

The process begins in discrete centres, which may then grow to meet each other. As in a number of other tissue types, dermal bone cells respond to mechanical stress by commencing (or remaining in) division, which enables them to respond to physical forces both before and after birth. Bones formed, at least in part, by intramembranous ossification include the vault of the skull, some of the facial bones and the clavicle.

Turnover of bone

There is a fairly rapid turnover even of mature bone, with osteoclasts eating away old bone and osteoblasts laying it down anew. Coupled with the ability of bone cells to respond to physical forces by proliferating this means that bones have a considerable capacity for responding to mechanical stresses by remodelling. In some eastern and ancient American cultures this capacity has been exploited to produce particular skull shapes: wooden boards bound tightly to either side of the skull to produce marked elongation, for example. This property is also exploited in the treatment of congenital or traumatic malformation: artificial stresses are imposed on the skull and jaw by use of wires and braces causing extensive shape changes.

Particular skeletal elements

Perhaps the most interesting and complex bony structure is the skull, which is discussed in Chapter 13. The limb skeleton is described in Chapter 18.

The vertebral column

Each somite differentiates into three separate zones (see Figure 8.1). The dermatome lies most dorsolaterally: underneath this, separated from it by a small lumen, is the myotome and medial and ventral to the myotome are the loose cells collectively described as the sclerotome. The sclerotome cells will give rise to the vertebrae (Figure 9.1). At first they move ventrally and surround the notochord preserving their original segmental arrangement; they are therefore still in register with the segmental myotomes or muscle blocks of the somites. Later, however, the developing vertebrae are shifted half a segment with respect to the myotomes (Figure 9.2). The cellular mechanism underlying this important process is still rather unclear. The cranial and caudal halves of each segment are known to differ from each other in a number of properties and to express different molecules. The caudal cells of each original somitic segment are more densely packed than the cranial cells. They come to lie opposite the midpoint of the next cranial myotome and later contribute to the intervertebral disc as well as the cranial portion of the vertebra caudal to this disc. The vertebra is also thought to receive a contribution from the loose cells from the cranial half of the next segment down the body axis: each vertebra would then comprise the caudal part of one original segment and the cranial part of the next most caudal segment.

The reason for this complicated process is not entirely clear. Perhaps, by offsetting the vertebrae and the vertebral muscles, it enables the muscles to act on the joints to flex the vertebral column. The notochord will eventually degenerate, except at the level of the intervertebral disc, where it forms the central **nucleus pulposus**.

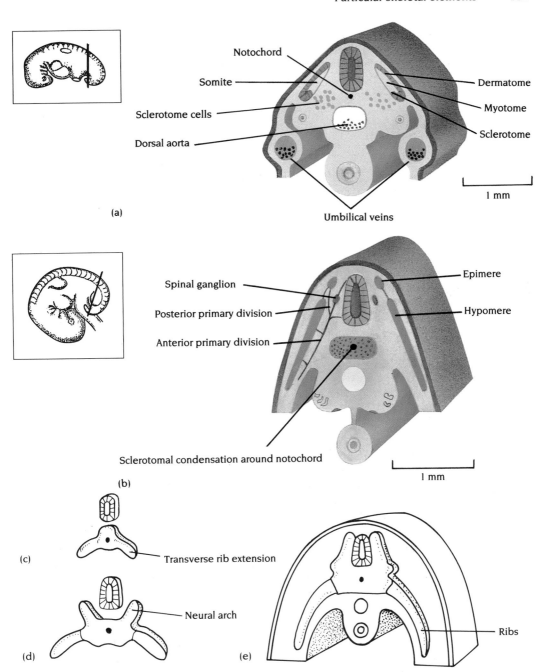

FIGURE 9.1 Formation of vertebrae during the embryonic period. (a) The sclerotome cells migrate to cluster round the notochord. (b) Gradually a distinct condensation – the basal body – is formed between the neural tube and dorsal aorta. (c) The thoracic vertebrae extend processes that will become ribs. (d) The basal condensations extend processes dorsally – the neural arches – that grow round the neural tube. (e) Eventually the neural tube lies in a trough of neural arches, and the ribs are beginning to approach one another in the ventral midline.

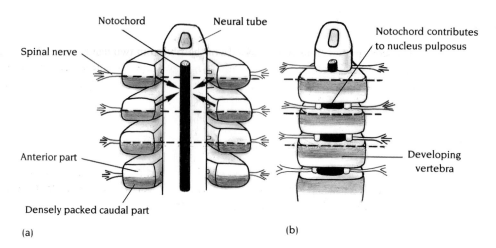

Notochord   Neural tube

Notochord contributes to nucleus pulposus

Spinal nerve

Anterior part

Densely packed caudal part

Developing vertebra

(a)

(b)

FIGURE 9.2 (a) Arrangement of somites. (b) Arrangement of vertebrae. The cells of the caudal half of each somitic segment are more densely packed than the cranial cells. As they migrate to form the vertebral basal bodies a segment shift occurs. The spinal nerves which ran through the original somites now therefore run between vertebrae. The odd cranial half-segment fuses to the base of the developing skull.

During this period, scelerotome cells have made their way ventrally between the myotomes and the spinal ganglia, so that the neural tube lies in a shallow sclerotome 'conduit'. Eventually the sides of this conduit grow dorso-medially to enclose the neural tube.

Up to the sixth week the sclerotome is composed of loose cells, but after this centres of cartilage formation begin to appear. The extension of these centres results in the transverse and spinous processes.

Ribs

While the sclerotome cells are forming the segmental mass around the notochord, the ribs begin to develop. Dense masses of cells extend laterally and ventrally between the myotome muscle sheets from the thoracic vertebrae, until they start to converge on the ventral midline. The cartilaginous extensions of the seven most cranial ribs fuse with the developing sternum (see below). The remaining three ribs form cartilaginous fusions with the rib lying cranial to them. Initially the extending rib process in the thoracic region is continuous with the sclerotome mass but a narrow band of tissue close to what will be the body of the vertebra fails to chondrify and in time develops into a joint.

Occasionally ribs develop on the lumbar or cervical vertebrae adjacent to the thoracic vertebrae. The latter are more significant clinically: persistent cervical ribs on the eighth cervical vertebra may compress the nerves or blood vessels between this and the first thoracic vertebra.

Sternum

The sternum develops independently of the ribs from two bands of cartilage running in the craniocaudal axis (Figure 9.3), which move towards each other as the body cavity closes and finally fuse. The structure later develops surface features corresponding to the divisions of the sternum.

Clavicle

The clavicle develops in the main as a dermal bone, with cartilaginous ends. It commences ossification between the sixth and seventh weeks after fertilization, making it the earliest bone to ossify in the body.

Sacrum

The sacrum is derived from the upper two or three sacral vertebrae, by projections similar to those which give rise to the ribs in the thoracic vertebrae. These extend, flatten, and fuse to form the lateral mass of the sacrum (Figure 9.4).

Tail

Human embryos possess a distinct tail, which regresses as a result of cell death during the fetal period; the derivatives of the most caudal somites vanish, and the last few vertebrae now present fuse together to form the coccyx. Rarely the tail may persist, presumably due to failure of this process.

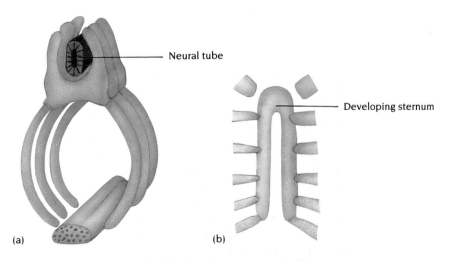

(a)   (b)

FIGURE 9.3   Relationship of the forming sternum to the ribs.

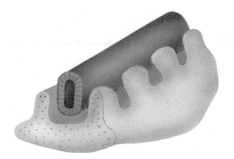

FIGURE 9.4   A flattened fused extension of the vertebrae in the tail region forms the sacrum.

Ossification centres

As mentioned above, the clavicle begins to ossify first. In the sixth week, it is followed by the scapula, mandible and maxilla, the frontal bone and narrow collars of bone surrounding the middle of the femur and humerus. During the next week the radius and ulna and tibia and fibia commence ossification, and the ribs and cranial vault bones become evident. By the eighth week, ossification has commenced in the long bones of the hands and feet. Complete guides to ossification in the human embryo are obtainable.

Defects in skeletogenesis

Because both cartilage and bone rely on collagen for their ground substance any genetic defect in collagen formation – failure of the subunit molecules to unite properly, for instance – will lead to skeletal abnormalities.

Achondroplasia   In achondroplasia endochondral ossification is particularly affected, and afflicted individuals have shortened limbs and trunk although the head is relatively normal in size.

Further reading

Dalgleish A.E. (1985). A study of the development of thoracic vertebrae in the mouse assisted by autoradiography. *Acta Anat.*, **122**, 91–8

Fallon J.F. and Simandl B.K. (1978). Evidence of a role for cell death in the disappearance of the embryonic human tail. *Am. J. Anat.*, **152**, 111–30

Gasser R.F. (1982). *Atlas of Human Embryos*. Hagerstown: Harper & Row.

Norris W.E., Stern C.D., and Keynes R.J. (1989). Molecular differences between the rostral and caudal halves of the sclerotome in the chick embryo. *Development*, **105**, 541–8

O'Rahilly R., Muller F. and Meyer D.B. (1980). The human vertebral column at the end of the embryonic period proper. I. The column as a whole. *J. Anat.*, **131**, 567–75

O'Rahilly R., Muller F. and Meyer D.B. (1983). The human vertebral column at the end of the embryonic period proper. I. The occipitocervical region. *J. Anat.*, **136**, 181–95

Ranscht B. and Bronner-Fraser M. (1991). T-cadherin expression alternates with migrating neural crest cells in the trunk of the avian embryo. *Development*, **111**, 15–22

Stern C.D. and Keynes R.J. (1987). Interactions between somite cells: the formation and maintenance of segment boundaries in the chick embryo. *Development*, **99**, 261–72

10

Skin and its derivatives

In the early embryo the mesoderm is overlaid by a single layer of ectoderm, from which it is separated by an acellular basal membrane (Figure 10.1(a)). Together, ectoderm and mesoderm will give rise to the skin but also to a number of repetitive structures that at first glance seem quite dissimilar to each other: teeth, hair, sweat glands, salivary glands, mammary glands. Each of these, however, develops in a basically similar way, as will be seen below, and the development of these diverse structures found in various parts of the body is grouped together in this chapter.

Skin

Skin consists of an epidermal layer and a dermal layer, derived from ectoderm and mesoderm respectively (Figure 10.1(b)). The embryonic ectoderm remains as a single layer until about the beginning of the fetal period, at which time the ectodermal cells next to the basal layer begin multiplying (functioning as a germinative layer) and these underlying cells produce a superficial layer known as the **periderm**. This may help to protect the fetus from the effects of immersion in amniotic fluid. Gradually, over the remainder of the fetal period, the epidermis differentiates into different strata, corresponding to various stages in the dif-

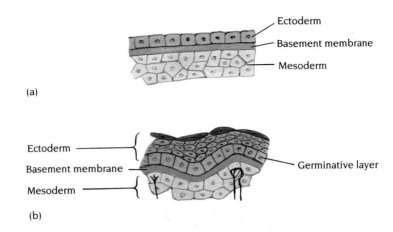

FIGURE 10.1   (a) Early embryonic skin; (b) early fetal skin.

ferentiative process, from the stem cells of the germinative layer to the skin flakes that are finally shed from the surface. By the sixth month of pregnancy, the shed peridermal cells and debris and the oily secretions of the sebaceous glands have together formed a whitish coating – the **vernix caseosa** – which continues the protective role of the periderm.

Fingerprints

Fingerprints are formed as folds of the epidermal layers during the early fetal period. Epidermal cells in culture form ridges and whorls

Pigment cells

During the third month after fertilization, neural crest cells invade the epidermis and differentiate to form pigment cells (melanocytes). Melanin may be produced in the fetal period in races with dark skin, though in other racial groups this ability remains latent until stimulated by sunlight after birth. Melanocytes can also transfer melanin to neighbouring cells and to hair shafts.

Dermis

The dermis arises from the mesoderm: in particular, from the dorsal component (dermomyotome) of the somites. At first the interface between dermis and epidermis is smooth but during fetal life the dermis begins to form papillae, or indentations projecting into the epidermal layer. The papillae contain nerves and blood vessels, which the epidermis lacks.

Derivatives of skin

Although the structures formed by the skin are very diverse, a common developmental pathway underlies many of them. Essentially this takes the form of an invasion of the epidermal component into the underlying mesoderm, followed by the formation of complex epidermal morphology – branching or coiling. In the second stage the epidermal part begins to hollow out while the mesoderm condenses around the structure. In the final phase the hollowed-out glands begin to secrete extracellular product and, if they have lost their communication with the surface entirely during the invasion phase, they now redevelop it.

Often these structures are arranged in regular arrays gathered in particular parts of the body and positioned accurately with respect to each other. The position in which each element forms, and the precise nature of the structure formed, relies on information conveyed to the ectoderm by the mesoderm (see Box 10.1).

Box 10.1 Experimental analysis of integument development

Structures developing in the integument commonly form ordered arrays, which are confined to particular parts of the body: teeth, hair and sweat glands, for example, all have particular regional distributions on the body surface. How does this come about? Experiments in which the ectodermal and mesodermal components of skin are separated and recombined in various ways reveal much about the nature of this process.

For practical reasons, chick embryos are often used for such experiments, but there are strong grounds for believing that the results observed are generally applicable within the vertebrates, including mammals. Feather formation is often chosen for study because the rudiments of feathers are distinctly recognizable, and form a regular array from early in development.

The first hint of feather formation is the appearance of condensations in the mesoderm, associated with corresponding thickenings in the overlying ectoderm. The ectoderm then forms a distinct bud, or germ, with a mesodermal core. These buds have regional differences, and experiments show that the differences depend only on the mesoderm.

If mesoderm in which the first condensations have developed is combined with ectoderm that has not started to show any signs of differentiation, feather germs will form in the ectoderm to correspond with the condensations in the mesoderm; older mesoderm loses this ability. In other words, the capacity of the mesoderm to induce the ectoderm is transient.

If ectoderm in which thickenings have begun to appear is combined with early mesoderm that lacks condensations it induces corresponding

Box 10.1 Experimental analysis of integument development • **135**

thickenings in the mesoderm. This shows that, although the mesoderm may initiate the formation of the integumentary structure, there is reciprocal interaction between the ectoderm and mesoderm.

Generally similar results have been seen in studies of mammary gland formation and tooth development in mammals.

In summary, the mesoderm induces the ectoderm to respond but the interaction then becomes reciprocal. A similar interaction between mesoderm and endoderm will be seen later.

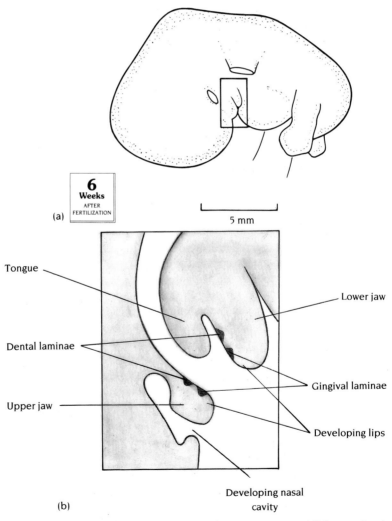

FIGURE 10.2 Two extended ectodermal thickenings run parallel to each other just inside the upper and lower jaw. The gingival laminae will hollow out to mark the formation of the lips and the dental laminae mark where the gums will form.

Teeth

Teeth have an extended evolutionary history. It seems likely that they were originally armour scales on the surface of the head and subsequently became associated with jaws. This is by no means a rule; in many animals, tooth-like structures can be found in the skin of the head, on the palate or elsewhere. The extracellular material **enamel** is secreted to form the biting surface. This is the hardest material in the body.

The gums form as twin U-shaped structures in the floor and roof of the mouth (Figure 10.2), defined by the formation of a **lip furrow band**. As this occurs the ectoderm along the crest of the developing gums begins to thicken and then to invade the mesoderm, forming the continuous **dental laminae**. From each of these, ten further individual processes or buds will form in humans, representing the first or milk teeth (Figure 10.3(a,b)), and will begin to spread out, forming a structure like an inverted cup or a cap. Inside this cup the mesoderm is shaped into a **papilla** (Figure 10.3(c)). All of these events correspond to the invasive phase of tooth development, often divided into the **bud** and **cap** stages in accordance with the appearance of the rudiment. In the next phase the ectoderm of the cap begins to develop a fluid-filled lumen, which also contains extracellular matrix molecules and a network of scattered cells and processes described as the **stellate reticulum** (Figure 10.3(d)).

At these stages the rudiment of the definitive tooth can be seen developing from the thread of ectoderm connecting the developing primary tooth to the surface (Figure 10.3(d,e)).

Meanwhile, the mesoderm is condensing round the developing tooth to form a capsule, while nerves and blood vessels will come to lie inside the dermal papilla at the core of the tooth.

As we will see in more detail later the jaw bones – the maxilla and the mandible – are forming in the mesoderm parallel to, but deeper under the surface than, the dental laminae. The capsular regions surrounding each tooth impinge on the bone, leading to sockets in which the teeth will lie (Figure 10.4). The capsular condensation will eventually form the **cementoblasts** and **periodontal ligaments** hold the tooth in place.

In the secretory phase of tooth development the ectodermal component next to the mesoderm begins to secrete enamel and the mesoderm begins to secrete

FIGURE 10.3 *(opposite)* Ectodermal buds from the dental lamina (a) begin to invade the underlying mesoderm (b). As the ectoderm begins to spread (c), mesoderm condenses in the cavity. A mesodermal capsule forms round the entire tooth (d). This mesodermal condensation is invaded by blood vessels and nerves. The 'stellate reticulum' forms between the delaminating layers of ectoderm. A secondary tooth bud becomes apparent (d,e). Later still, enamel and dentine are secreted at the interface between ectoderm and mesoderm (f). The ectodermal cells (ameloblasts) secrete the enamel and odontoblasts (derived from the neural crest) secrete the dentine. The teeth erupt during the second year (g) to expose the enamel surface.

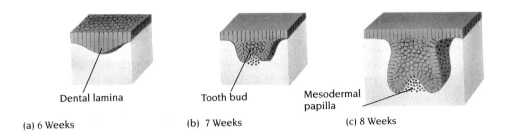

Dental lamina

(a) 6 Weeks

Tooth bud

(b) 7 Weeks

Mesodermal papilla

(c) 8 Weeks

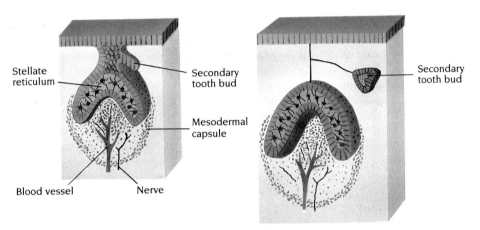

Stellate reticulum

Secondary tooth bud

Mesodermal capsule

Blood vessel

Nerve

(d) 9 Weeks

Secondary tooth bud

(e) 12 Weeks

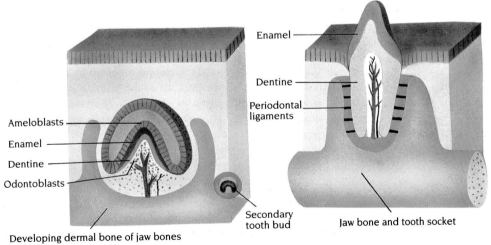

Ameloblasts

Enamel

Dentine

Odontoblasts

Developing dermal bone of jaw bones

(f) 28 Weeks

Enamel

Dentine

Periodontal ligaments

Secondary tooth bud

Jaw bone and tooth socket

(g) Birth plus 18 months

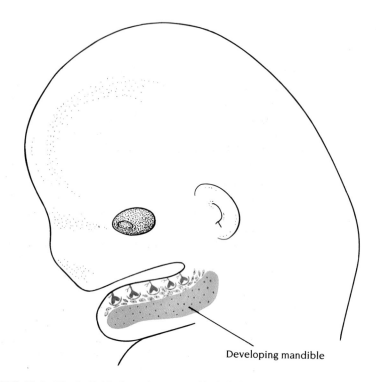

FIGURE 10.4 The individual tooth germs with their forming capsules lie close to the developing jaw bones. As these structures grow they fuse.

dentine (Figure 10.3(f)). This is known as the **bell** stage, on the basis of the appearance of the tooth rudiment. Generally, the teeth erupt through the surface of the gum 6–24 months after birth (although teeth are occasionally present at birth) in a process that can cause considerable inflammation and pain.

In humans the primary or milk teeth are replaced by the secondary teeth from the age of 6 years onwards: the root of the primary tooth is resorbed and the remainder is pushed out by the secondary tooth. Humans are rather limited in their tooth-forming capacity: some non-mammalian animals can replace missing teeth many times.

Humans possess 32 permanent teeth, 20 of which arise in association with the primary tooth buds as described above. The other 12, three from each half-jaw element, arise directly from an extension of the dental lamina.

The human jaw has decreased in size in recent evolutionary history and, as a result, the molars that lie furthest back and do not develop until early adulthood (hence their slightly inappropriate name 'wisdom teeth') are restricted for space. This may cause quite severe dental problems.

Hair

Hair is thought to have evolved from sensory structures. Hair development begins in a manner reminiscent of tooth development. A **hair bud** grows from the ectoderm into the underlying mesoderm (Figure 10.5) and extends out to enclose a dermal **hair papilla**. A secondary growth from the connecting stalk begins to form during the fifth month after fertilization: this will develop into the sebaceous gland associated with each hair. The adjacent mesoderm begins to condense around the hair follicle to form the root capsule. Nearby mesoderm cells align themselves to form the erector pili muscles associated with each hair which, when they contract in the adult or child, are responsible for the phenomenon of 'goose-bumps' or 'goose-pimples'.

A lumen develops in the ectodermal component of the hair bud and keratin is secreted, which forms the developing hair shaft. This will erupt during the fetal period, so that the fetus is covered with a coating of fine hair – the **lanugo**. It may persist to birth, but is generally lost within the first few weeks.

Eyelashes and eyebrows develop in the same way as hair. In other animals, hairs may form large sensitive whiskers as sensory organs or substantial structures formed from fused hair as in rhinoceros horn.

Hair follicles undergo regular cycles of activity and quiescence, so each hair grows in bursts. In male-pattern baldness, follicle recovery becomes poorer after each quiescent period. Hair follicles have considerable regenerative powers and can reform from the upper portion only.

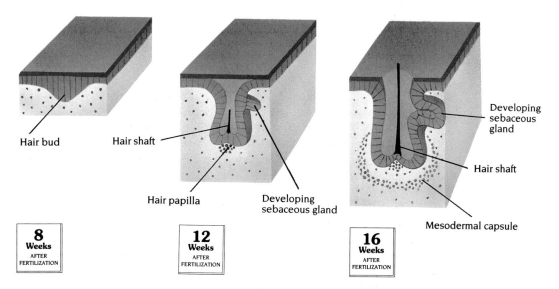

FIGURE 10.5 Hair buds begin to form in a manner reminiscent of tooth buds. Hair develops first on the upper lip, chin, eyebrows and eyelids. Gradually it will spread over the whole body. Sebaceous glands mostly develop in association with hair, but in the glans penis and labia minora they develop independently. The sebaceous glands will branch.

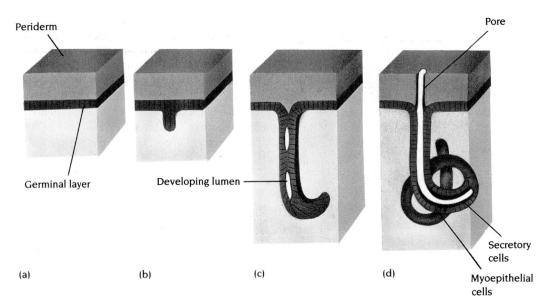

Periderm

Pore

Germinal layer

Developing lumen

Secretory cells

(a)   (b)   (c)   (d)

Myoepithelial cells

FIGURE 10.6 Sweat glands begin to develop relatively late, four to five months, so the skin has already formed a distinct germinal layer (a). This forms the bud (b), which goes on to coil and to form a lumen (c). The germinal layer grows a smooth muscle myoepithelium on the outer surface and a layer of secretory inner cells (d). Apocrine sweat glands are present over the body during early fetal development but at birth are only found in the armpits and around the sexual organs. They become active at puberty.

Sweat glands

Sweat glands form at about 4–5 months after fertilization. They grow down into the underlying mesoderm, but instead of branching will coil before forming a central lumen (Figure 10.6). The outer cells of the ectodermal component are believed to form the smooth-muscle myoepithelium coating the gland.

Salivary glands

The salivary glands develop from the epithelium of the mouth during the third month after fertilization. The submandibular glands appear first as a pair of extended epithelial thickenings in the floor of the mouth running parallel with and lateral to the tongue. These thickenings detach from the surface at the end nearest the mouth, becoming solid epithelial cords attached to the surface only at their posterior end. The cords branch and develop lumina, while the mesoderm condenses around the developing gland to form a capsule.

The parotid gland forms in a rather similar way, behind the angle of the jaw. During the branching of the gland, nearby nerves and blood vessels are engulfed by the gland structures. Again, a mesodermal capsule will develop. Pain will result if the gland becomes inflamed, as in parotiditis or mumps, and presses the nerves and lymphatics against this capsule. The sublingual glands develop lateral to the submandibular glands.

Mammary glands

Mammary glands are the structures that distinguish the class Mammalia. In evolutionary terms they are modified sweat glands, as can be seen clearly in very primitive mammals such as the duck-billed platypus. In mammals in general, a **mammary ridge** forms on which the glands develop (Figure 10.7). The number of pairs of teats formed is related to litter size.

The ectoderm invades, branches and forms a lumen, while the mesoderm forms a surrounding capsule (Figure 10.8). Initially, mammary glands are identical in males and females but at puberty fat and connective tissue are deposited in the mesoderm of the gland of females under hormonal influence. In pregnancy the mammary ducts lengthen, branch and form alveoli, replacing fat, although the overall size of the gland also increases. The requirement for proliferation at a relatively late stage in life has important consequences in pathological terms. Cell division in the mammary gland is held in check by the presence of a growth inhibitor, TGF-β. This in turn is suppressed by high levels of oestrogen. In consequence, high oestrogen levels, as were employed in early versions of the con-

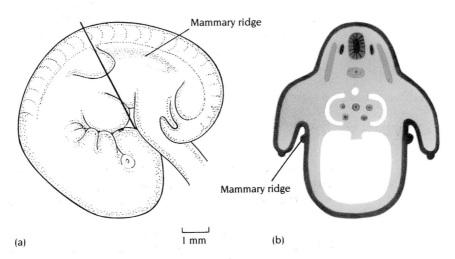

(a)   1 mm   (b)

FIGURE 10.7   The mammary ridge.

Mammary ridge

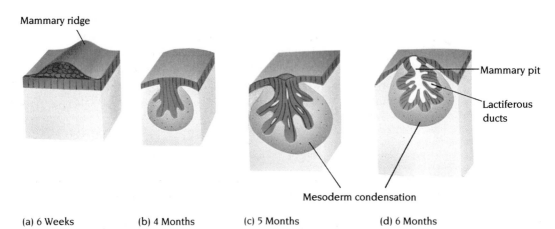

Mammary pit

Lactiferous ducts

Mesoderm condensation

(a) 6 Weeks   (b) 4 Months   (c) 5 Months   (d) 6 Months

FIGURE 10.8   Development of the mammary gland. From the mammary ridge (a) a primary bud invades into the mesoderm and begins to branch (b). Lumina gradually form within the buds to give a branching structure (c,d).

traceptive pill, or as occur naturally in some women, increase the chances of breast cells escaping from normal cell division controls and becoming cancerous. Some women are overly sensitive to their natural levels of oestrogen, or insensitive to the natural TGF-β. This increases their chances of developing breast cancer.

Extra breasts or nipples often develop along the line of the mammary ridge, and occasionally elsewhere. These may be present in about 1% of all females, but are often mistaken for a mole. The hormones of pregnancy may cause these structures to enlarge and even to commence lactation.

Nails

A thickening known as the **nail field** is evident on the dorsal surface of the digit at about 12 weeks after fertilization. This becomes emphasized by **lateral nail folds** on either side, which sweep round to join the **proximal nail fold** (Figure 10.9). The nail field extends laterally under the lateral nail folds and proximally under the proximal nail fold to form the **nail root**. The true nail grows forward from the root to reach the tip of the digit shortly before birth.

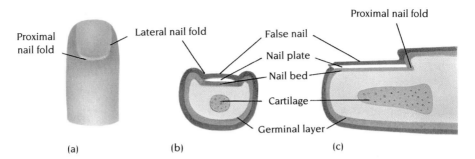

FIGURE 10.9 Development of the nail. At week 12 a thickening of the dorsal surface of the finger is bordered by two lateral folds and one proximal fold (a). Sections through the tip of the digit, (b) transverse and (c) sagittal to the long axis of the finger, reveal the definitive nail will grow from the proximal nail fold, underlying surface layers of epidermis which form the false nail.

Further reading

Dawber R.P.R. (1988). The embryology and development of human scalp hair. In *Clinics in Dermatology: Androgenetic Alopecia – from Empiricism to Knowledge* (De Villez R.L., Griggs L.M.P. and Freeman B., eds), pp. 1–6. Philadelphia: Lippincott

De Weert J. (1989). Embryogenesis of the hair follicle and hair cycle. In *Trends in Human Hair Growth and Alopecia Research* (Van Neste D., Lachapelle J.M. and Antoine J.L., eds), pp. 3–10. Lancaster: Kluwer Academic Publishers

Hashimoto K. (1988) The structure of human hair. In *Clinics in Dermatology: Androgenetic Alopecia – from Empiricism to Knowledge* (De Villez R.L., Griggs L.M.P. and Freeman B., eds), pp. 7–25. Philadelphia: Lippincott

Holbrook K.A., Fisher C., Dale B.A. and Hartley R. (1989). Morphogenesis of the hair follicle during the ontogeny of human skin. In *The Biology of Wool and Hair* (Rogers G.E., Reis P.J., Ward K.A. and Marshall R.C., eds), pp. 15–36. London: Chapman & Hall

Ito M. (1986). The innermost cell layer of the outer root sheath in human anagen hair follicle. Light and electron microscopy study. *Arch. Dermatol. Res.*, **279**, 112–19

Kollar E.J. (1981). Tooth development and dental patterning. In *Morphogenesis and Pattern Formation* (Connely T.G., ed.) New York: Raven Press

Lumsden A.G.S. (1988). Spatial organisation of the epithelium and the role of the neural crest cells in the initiation of the mammalian tooth germ. *Development*, **103**, 155s–69s

Maderson P.F.A. (1972). When, why and how? Some speculations on the evolution of the vertebrate integument. *Am. Zool.*, **12**, 159–71

Mayor G.H. and Griggs L. (1988). Commentary. In *Clinics in Dermatology: Androgenetic Alopecia – from Empiricism to Knowledge* (De Villez R.L., Griggs L.M.P. and Freeman B., eds), pp. XI–XIII. Philadelphia: Lippincott

Ruch J.V. (1984). Tooth morphogenesis and differentiation. In *Dentin and Dentinogenesis* (Lind A., ed.), pp. 47–80. Boca Raton: CRC Press

Vermorken A.J. (1989). Foreword. In *Trends in Human Hair Growth and Alopecia Research* (Van Neste D., Lachapelle J.M. and Antoine J.L., eds), pp. IX–X. Lancaster: Kluwer Academic Publishers

Worst P.K.M., Mackenzie I.C. and Fusenig N.E. (1982). Reformation of organised epidermal structure by transplantation of suspensions and cultures of epidermal and dermal cells. *Cell Tissue Res.*, **225**, 65–7

Box 10.1

Kollar E.J. and Fisher C. (1980). Tooth induction in chick epithelium: expression of quiescent genes for enamel synthesis. *Science*, **207**, 993–5.

Saunders J.W. Jr. (1980). *Developmental Biology*. New York: Macmillan

Sengel P. (1986). Epidermal–dermal interactions. In *Biology of the Integument II: Vertebrates* (Bereiter-Hahn J., Maltoltsy A.G. and Richards K., eds), pp. 374–408. Berlin: Springer-Verlag

11

Neural crest cells

Neural crest cells disperse throughout the body from their sites of origin in the neural tube to give rise to a bewildering array of derivatives. The study of their migration and differentiation poses a number of fascinating problems.

The embryological origin of neural crest cells

Neural crest cells originate in the dorsal and lateral neural tube (Figure 11.1). Initially they may be considered as part of the neural tube itself. The adhesive bonds holding them in place must therefore loosen before they are able to disperse.

Neural crest cells first appear in the mesencephalon, before the neural tube has fused; later they are found in more cranial brain regions, and caudally down the neural tube. Migration occurs in a craniocaudal sequence, beginning at the start of the fourth week.

Three major pathways are followed by the migrating cells (Figure 11.2):

(1) The first of these leads cells to migrate between the surface ectoderm and the somites. These cells become pigment cells.

(2) Cells opposite the cranial half of each somite migrate through it, to produce the dorsal root ganglia, and some of these cells continue ventrally, forming

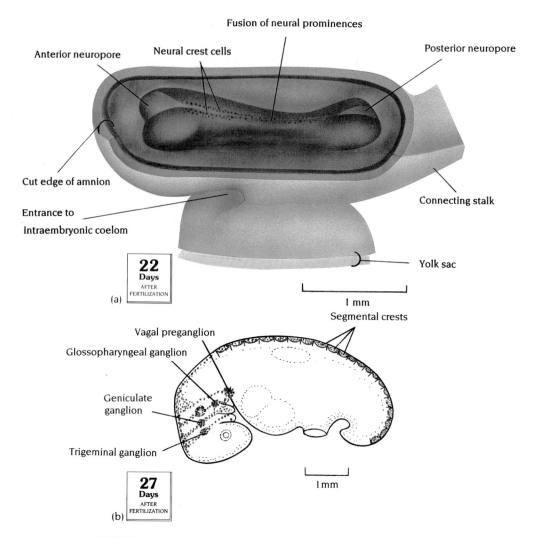

FIGURE 11.1 Successive stages in the origin and migration of neural crest cells (shown in red) at the 22nd (a) and 27th (b) days after fertilization.

the sympathetic ganglia and a plexus around the aorta. At the appropriate level, cells in the last group contribute to the adrenal glands.

Deep migrating cells divide into three further streams that migrate between the somites and the neural tube, between the somites to the aorta and ventrally to the spinal cord to form dorsal root ganglia.

(3) The third pathway is for cells opposite the caudal half of each somite, which migrate cranially *and* caudally along the neural tube, to contribute to the nearest dorsal root ganglion.

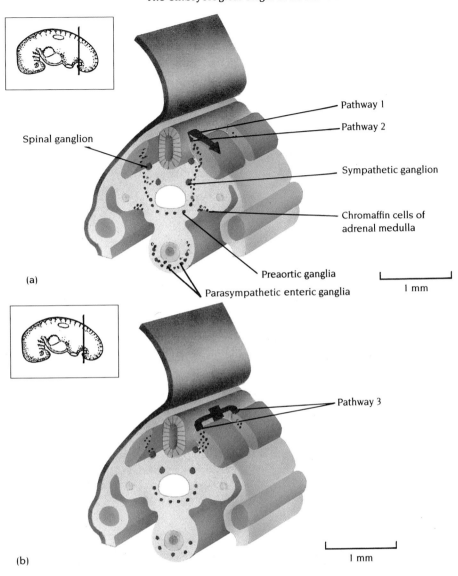

Spinal ganglion

Pathway 1
Pathway 2

Sympathetic ganglion

Chromaffin cells of adrenal medulla

(a)

Preaortic ganglia
Parasympathetic enteric ganglia

1 mm

Pathway 3

(b)

1 mm

FIGURE 11.2 Pathways of neural crest cells in a section through the trunk. (a) Pathway 1 runs between the somite and the ectoderm, and in the trunk these cells give rise to the pigment cells. Pathway 2 runs through the somite initially. Some of these cells contribute to the sensory dorsal root ganglia (perhaps because their migration is interrupted by the developing sclerotome). Others continue ventrally to form the sympathetic ganglia and, in the trunk region, the chromaffin cells of the adrenal medulla. The parasympathetic enteric ganglia arise from this migration pathway in the first seven crests and from the sacral region crests. The cranial neural crest cells (derived from the 'vagal' region) then migrate caudally along the gut, forming the enteric ganglia. The third pathway begins opposite the caudal half of each somite (b). Neural crest cells cannot enter this, so they migrate cranially and caudally to join pathway 2, whence they contribute to the dorsal root ganglia.

Tracing neural crest cells

The derivatives of these cells, and the routes they take, can be identified by two methods.

Ablation

In ablation experiments regions of neural crest are removed from the embryo before migration begins and the resulting embryo examined to see which structures are abnormal or missing.

Marking

In marking experiments regions of the neural crest are 'identified' in some way so that the cells may be traced throughout development. The region may be marked in a number of ways; for example transplants can be carried out between equivalent embryos whose cells can be distinguished from each other in some way (see Chapter 8). The distinguishing feature could be possession of different pigmentation or nuclear structure, or result from previous labelling of the embryo. It is now also possible to inject single cells with a marker dye. A list of neural crest derivatives is shown in Table 11.1.

Sensory nervous system

Neural crest cells give rise in whole or in part to the trigeminal ganglion, the facial root ganglion, the glossopharyngeal ganglion and the vagal ganglion. Caudally, the ganglion crest forms a scalloped structure that produces the individual spinal ganglia.

Autonomic nervous system

Ganglia of the parasympathetic system (including the ciliary, ethmoidal, sphenopalatine and submandibular ganglia, and the visceral and enteric ganglia) also arise from the neural crest.

Neural crest cells also form the chain ganglia of the sympathetic nervous system, migrating laterally at each body level.

Supporting cells of the nervous system

In addition to neurons a variety of cells associated with the nervous system originate from the neural crest, in a range of support roles. The Schwann cells, which wrap around the nerve axons and increase the speed of conduction, are derived from the neural crest, as are a variety of glial cells. The neural crest is also thought to contribute to the arachnoid and pia mater surrounding the brain and spinal cord.

TABLE 11.1 Derivatives of the neural crest.

Pigment cells

Sensory nervous system
  Spinal ganglia
  Trigeminal ganglion
  Facial root ganglion
  Glossopharyngeal ganglion
  Vagal ganglion

Autonomic nervous system
  Sympathetic ganglia
    Superior cervical ganglia
    Prevertebral ganglia
    Paravertebral ganglia
    Adrenal medulla
  Parasympathetic ganglia
    Remak's
    Pelvic plexus
    Visceral and enteric ganglia
    Ciliary
    Ethmoidal
    Sphenopalatine
    Submandibular
    Intrinsic ganglia of viscera

Supporting cells of the nervous system
  Glial cells
  Schwann cells
  Meningeal cells of pia and arachnoid mater

Mesoderm-like cells (ectomesenchyme)
  Connective tissue of parathyroid
  Smooth muscle walls of aortic arches
  Cartilage and membrane bone components of the skull
  Odontoblasts

Endocrine cells
  Adrenal medulla
  C cells (calcitonin-secreting cells of superior parathyroid derived from ultimobranchial body)
  Type 1 cells of the carotid body
  Parafollicular cells of the thyroid

Pigment cells

It may not be surprising that the neural crest produces cells associated with the nervous system, because it is derived originally from the neural tube. Much less expected is that melanocytes, the pigment cells that establish skin, hair and eye coloration, also come from the neural crest.

Mesoderm-like cells (ectomesenchyme)

Some structures taken to be characteristic of mesoderm derivatives in fact originate from neural crest: many cartilage and bony elements of the skull, the smooth muscle walls of the aortic arches, the connective tissue cells of the parathyroid glands and the dentine-secreting odontoblasts in tooth formation.

Endocrine cells

The adrenaline-secreting cells of the adrenal medulla (see Chapter 24), the calcitonin-secreting cells (C cells) of the superior parathyroid (Chapter 15), Type 1 cells of the carotid body (which measures the pH and oxygenation of the blood) and the parafollicular cells of the thyroid are all also derived from the neural crest.

Movement and differentiation

Two key questions related to neural crest cells are: what controls their movement and what controls their differentiation?

Movement

Initially neural crest cells are closely adherent to other cells of the developing neural tube. Before migration can begin this mutual adhesion must lessen.

Cell adhesion in the neural system is mediated by a class of molecules known as neural cell adhesion molecules (N-CAMs). Concentrations of these decrease at the time of onset of migration, so that cell–cell adhesion is reduced.

Migration is promoted by the expression of plasminogen activator, which helps cells to penetrate between other cells.

A third component in initiating migration is an increase in the production of hyaluronic acid. This molecule expands rapidly when hydrated and is believed to be important in opening up spaces between cells into which neural crest cells can migrate. Conversely, at the time when migration ceases, hyaluronidase is produced, which breaks up the hyaluronic acid matrix and causes gaps between cells to close rapidly.

In these ways, differential patterns of production of particular molecules lead to corresponding changes in cell behaviour. The changing patterns of expression of these molecules can be related to molecular biology, and a way is open in principle to provide a complete explanation from the gene, via the molecule and its effect on cell behaviour, to the morphology and development of the tissue involved.

Direction of movement

Onset and cessation of migration are only part of the problem: neural crest cells also need to know *where* to go. Again, patterns of expression of particular 'behavioural' molecules seem to be important. Neural crest cells migrating through the segmental sclerotome avoid the caudal half of each segment, preferring the cranial

Box 11.1 Experimental analysis of neural crest development • 151

half. This creates a segmental pattern of outgrowth. If the segmental arrangement of the sclerotomes is altered, by, for example, surgically creating double cranial or double caudal segments, then the neural crest cells respond appropriately. Neural crest cells form a broad double-width stream when faced with a double cranial segment, but are inhibited in outgrowth by double caudal segments.

The difference between cranial and caudal half-segments is of vital importance. This has not yet been completely elucidated at the molecular level, although the migration-inhibitory molecule T-cadherin is present at higher levels in the caudal half of each segment than in the cranial half.

Neural crest cells are capable in vitro of following artificial trackways of cell adhesion molecules, fibronectin in particular. Fibronectin pathways are present in the embryo, and may play a role in determining migration pathways of neural crest cells. However, it is unlikely that the distribution of one single molecule determines the migration of neural crest cells. It is more likely that a variety of molecules present in the extracellular matrix are involved, and there may be redundancy in path specification.

Differentiation

Once neural crest cells have reached their destination they develop cell types appropriate to that locality. The study of this phenomenon is even more difficult than that of controls of cell movement but certain general principles seem to be emerging (see Box 11.1).

The type of cell formed bears a strong relationship to the level at which the cells arise on the craniocaudal axis of the neural tube. For example, the most cranial neural crest cells will produce skeletal structures: those from more caudal levels do not usually appear to do so. This could reflect differences in the neural crest cells present at each level or the different environments through which the cells migrate. Experimentation (see Box 11.1) has shown that individual neural crest cells begin with a wide range of possible differentiation outcomes, which progressively narrows as their migration continues. This is likely to be due to influences from the tissues that line their route.

Box 11.1 Experimental analysis of neural crest development

The mechanisms of neural crest cell movement may well prove to be of major clinical relevance but it does not follow that the mechanisms are best studied using systems that are themselves of clinical interest. On the contrary, other systems may be technically much easier to study and may provide information that is applicable to the clinical situation.

Melanocytes are the easiest product of the neural crest to investigate because their pigment renders them readily identifiable.

The strain of chicken known as Barred has black and white stripes on its wing. How these arise may be investigated by transferring small regions of the dorsal neural tube of Barred chick embryos to the all-white White Leghorn chick embryo before migration has begun.

The result of such a graft is that the host develops stripes in its wing, instead of being all white. In the white stripe regions melanocytes are present, but they are not expressing any melanin, indicating that the expression of the differentiated products of neural crest cells is not modulated by their presence or absence but by the control of expression of their genes. It also demonstrates that the cells respond in a manner appropriate to their position, even in the 'wrong' species (see Chapter 5).

In a mouse mutant called White the heterozygote has a white patch on its belly. This is believed to be because the melanocytes have not migrated all the way ventrally before being instructed to stop. The homozygote is all white except for the eyes, which are black (due to the pigmented layer of the retina). This shows that the mouse is not an albino, where melanin cannot be expressed, but that it is the movement of melanocytes that is affected.

Differentiation

Cervical neural crest cells contribute to parasympathetic nerves, which make acetylcholine as their neurotransmitter. Thoracic neural crest cells contribute to the sympathetic system, in which noradrenaline is the neurotransmitter. This provides a convenient biochemical marker for the cell type that has been formed.

Marked regions of neural crest can be swapped from one region to another and their offspring followed. As a result of this experiment, cells derived from the cervical region were found to give rise to noradrenaline-secreting cells when grafted to the thoracic level. Cells from the thoracic area can be led to express acetylcholine when grafted to the cervical region and those studied before migration commences can be seen to express both neurotransmitters. This implies that the cells begin by making either neurotransmitter, but that something they encounter *en route* selects one particular phenotype.

What could this 'something' be? Cranial neural crest cells cultured in medium that normally permits cartilage and bone differentiation express neither of these differentiation types when no other tissues are present. However, if head ectoderm, which is passed on the way to their final site, is added to the culture medium then cartilage is formed by the neural crest cells. Such experiments support the above hypothesis.

This is unlikely to be the complete story: several levels of decision may well be involved, of which this is only one. However, it does indicate how neighbour tissue relationships established at an earlier stage generate new interactions and differentiation later.

Defects arising from neural crest abnormalities

A system of such complexity must sometimes go wrong but it can be rather difficult to prove that the resulting defect was due to a fault with the neural crest itself.

Colon agangliosis (or Hirschprung's disease) In this condition the submucosal and myenteric ganglion cells are absent, probably from a failure of neural crest cell migration to the hindgut region. In consequence the colon is greatly enlarged since there is no peristaltic movement in the colon. This condition is alleviated by removal of the affected section of colon.

Effects of retinoic acid Cranial neural crest cell proliferation and migration are specifically inhibited by the vitamin A analogue, retinoic acid, which is often prescribed for severe cases of acne. Although it is recommended that pregnant women avoid this medication, in a number of cases women have become pregnant during the course of treatment and children have been born with abnormalities including defects of the ears and jaws, thymus, nervous system and aortic arches.

DiGeorge syndrome Various kinds of craniofacial defects are related to neural crest abnormalities. In DiGeorge syndrome the parathyroid glands and the thymus are missing or reduced. Affected children are prone to infections, and the absence of parathyroid hormones has a variety of deleterious effects. Fetal thymus transplant and hormone replacement therapy can alleviate the symptoms.

Special Topic 5 Formation of functional structures

Even simple body structures take a lot of describing. In the adult arm, for instance, blood vessels, nerves, muscles and tendons are present in bewildering complexity. As a result, merely to describe the body fully would take millions of bits of information. Does the embryo therefore contain a full description of all this complexity? It scarcely seems possible. Although the information-carrying capability of the genome is perhaps large enough, the information it carries, sequences of peptides, is not easily converted into spatial and temporal arrangements of tissues: in fact it is likely that even if the human genome were completely sequenced it would still not be clear how development occurs.

Further, if all the tissues of the body were specified separately there would be many opportunities for fatal errors to occur. Given the ways in which tissues need each other to function properly, almost any error would render whole regions of the body non-functional. Fortunately, there is evidence that the tissues of the body are not all specified independently but that they interact in ways which lead to their correct relative deployment.

By the end of the pre-embryonic period the major tissue lineages have been established but are not in their final relationships. They are established in a rather simple segmental pattern, which is essentially identical for all the higher vertebrates. How will this become the complex network of structures we recognize as the adult? It is useful to think of the tissues as being placed like chess pieces at the start of a game. A complex, interactive set of rules will operate the pieces to generate a complex outcome. In development one set of moves gives a chicken, a different set gives a mouse but the rules are the same for the two organisms. The 'moves' for individuals of each species (e.g. two mice) are similar, but perhaps not identical.

Each tissue blindly follows certain interactive rules: it does not know what the overall outcome will be, merely that it must interact in certain ways with its environment. Tissues in culture will continue to follow these rules to the best of their ability.

It is possible to study these rules in detail, using several tissues as examples. As will be explained in Chapter 18, the embryonic limb bud is a convenient model system for studying such interactions and many experiments are carried out using limb buds. They are, however, of general applicability.

Interactions between motor nerves and voluntary muscles

Motor nerves originate in the ventral neural tube (Chapter 6). Striated skeletal muscle cells originate in the somites (Chapter 8). Both migrate into the body, where each forms a complex pattern: these patterns stand in a clear relationship to each other. How this is achieved can be deduced from a small number of critical experiments.

Nerve outgrowth is initially not patterned

If a chick embryo limb bud is removed before motor nerves have grown into it and is grafted to the head it becomes invaded by cranial nerves. However, the deployment of these 'cranial' nerves within the limb is exactly the same as those in an undisturbed limb: in other words the 'wrong' nerves have reached the 'right' target. The cranial nerves do not appear to know where they 'ought' to be going, but are organized in some way by the limb. In culture, it can easily be demonstrated that nerves will follow pathways of extracellular molecules such as laminin: perhaps such pathways are present in the limb connective tissue.

This lack of specificity is the case for **major** mismatches between muscle and nerve. If the mismatch occurs over a short distance in the craniocaudal axis of the embryo there is evidence of nerve specificity: given a choice between its 'normal' muscle and a near neighbour, nerves often prefer their usual partner. This may reflect an ability of nerves to detect the craniocaudal level of muscles and for more 'cranial' nerves to prefer more 'cranial' muscles. As this might predict, rotation of a limb so that it is upside down (and there is no craniocaudal displacement) causes the muscles now lying dorsally to be innervated by the nerves that usually supply the dorsal muscles, while the original dorsal muscles are now supplied by ventral nerves. It is to be expected that multiple mechanisms, mutually reinforcing, will underlie a process as important as nerve development.

Muscle outgrowth is initially not patterned

Experiments involving limbs into which muscle cells have not yet penetrated indicate that muscle pattern is not specified by the somites: a leg bud placed next to neck somites is invaded by muscle cells, which then form muscles characteristic of the leg, not the neck. Again, the limb seems to organize the muscle cells in some way.

A chick mutant in which muscles are highly disorganized provides a clue to the underlying mechanism. Combining 'mutant' somites with normal limbs gives normal muscles but the combination of mutant limbs with normal somites produces abnormal muscles.

Because muscle connective tissue is derived not from the somites but from the lateral mesoderm, it seems a plausible candidate as the organizing tissue. It is thought to receive its initial pattern information from positional information signals (see Chapter 5).

Muscles send local signals to nerves

If a length of somites is killed in place (by radiation, for example) no muscle cells can grow out and a muscle-less region is created lateral to the irradiated zone. Nerves are able to grow across this zone without difficulty and a muscle-less limb can be created, which is still supplied with nerves. In such limbs the pattern of main nerve tracts is exactly like that in a normal limb, but the small local branches to individual muscles are lacking. This suggests that the limb organizes the nerves into main pathways but that the fine detail that establishes innervation is controlled by local signals.

Developing muscle in culture secretes a protein factor that stimulates nerve outgrowth. This 56-kDa motor neuron growth factor may be the initiator of local branching of nerves as they pass the muscle on the main nerve trunk.

An excess of nerves grow into the limb

The nerve supply of the embryonic limb is about twice as rich as that of the adult. This is brought about by nerves having to compete for limited binding sites on the muscle as the muscle matures. Nerves that do not form the proper connections die. Targets of sensory nerves may manufacture 'nerve survival substances' in the form of growth factors such as nerve growth factor and brain-derived neurotrophic factor to support the survival of the appropriate proportion of nerves.

This competition for nerves gives great flexibility to the system. If by some combination of circumstances one nerve tract fails to form, other nerves which would have died will supply its targets instead, and some kind of functional relationship will be formed.

Muscles without nerves die

As muscle matures it requires nerves: or it will atrophy and die (as happens with nerve damage in the adult). More positively, the pattern of nerve firing can determine whether the muscle differentiates as 'fast' or 'slow' muscle (see Chapter 8).

By this combination of programming and interaction a functional neuromuscular pattern is established. Generally, the pattern varies little between individuals, but clinically significant variations can occur.

Interactions between blood vessels and their targets

After the initial blood vessel network has formed new blood vessels grow out from these by the formation of solid cords, which eventually hollow out (see Chapter 7). A relationship has to be developed between the vascular system and the tissues in the body that require a blood supply. Much study still has to be done on how this is controlled in the embryo, but valuable clues have come from cancer studies.

Tumours secrete factors that attract blood vessels

The growth of tumour cells is so rapid that they soon exhaust the local supply of nutrients, at which point they stop dividing. It is common to find that tumours consist of a ball of cells with a core of dead cells, where nutrient levels are low. In this condition, the tumours may be relatively harmless; however, a number of tumours are able to attract blood vessels from the vascular network. When the blood vessels reach the tumour it can grow rapidly, and the chances of metastasis become very much greater as tumour cells enter the blood supply and pass rapidly round the body. This process of tumour vascularization is therefore of major clinical importance. If it could be prevented, it might be possible to avoid the growth of secondary tumours after the primary is removed.

Experiments revealed that tumours produce a protein (named as tumour angiogenic factor). This was eventually found to belong to a class of growth factors known as the endothelial cell growth factors, which stimulate the endothelial cells of the blood vessel walls to divide, and by doing so provoke the local outgrowth of the cords that will become new blood vessels. These growth factors are actively expressed in embryos. It is possible to speculate that a developing muscle in the embryo secures its vascularization by producing endothelial cell growth factors, in the same way that it secures its innervation by producing motor neuron growth factors.

Factors in the embryo inhibit vascularization

Developing cartilage regions are essentially avascular. In experiments using tumours, this was found to be due to the production of anti-angiogenic factors by the developing cartilage. This is of major clinical interest in that it offers the hope of discovering factors that inhibit tumour vascularization. In addition, it offers another clue to the development of blood vessel patterns in the embryo: blood vessels may be actively attracted towards particular regions and repelled from others.

Interactions between muscles and tendons

Muscles also need tendons to exert their function. Tendon cells appear to belong to the same lineage as cartilage cells, and are therefore derived from the somatopleural mesoderm. Tendons will begin to condense from the mesoderm in the correct general area, even in the absence of muscle, but will regress if they do not make contact with a muscle. If tendons are displaced during development they will join up with a muscle, any muscle, even if it is some distance away. It almost appears as if they have a 'seek-and-join' rule. In the absence of a connection to a tendon, the muscle will also die.

The tendon cells form a sharp boundary with muscle cells, which contains many interdigitations in order to increase the area of 'grip'. At its cartilage end the tendon and cartilage elements merge imperceptibly, implying that the tendon cells are of a different type from muscle cells, but of the same type as cartilage.

By such mechanisms functional structures are formed with a great deal of flexibility. Many abnormalities will be smoothed out and extraneous tissues disappear. Inevitably there will be a degree of variability from individual to individual, although in general the various arrangements all work in rather similar ways.

Mechanisms such as those described above persist in the adult, though they tend to work rather more slowly. If ways could be found of enhancing revascularization in ulcers, or reinnervation following accidents such as spinal cord damage, then understanding of the developmental mechanisms might prove of very great clinical relevance, quite apart from their implications for cancer treatment.

Further reading

Davies A.M. and Lumsden A. (1990). Ontogeny of the somatosensory system: origins and early development of the primary sensory neurons. *Annu. Rev. Neurosci.*, **13**, 61–73

Erickson C.A. (1988). Control of pathfinding by the avian neural crest. *Development*, **103** (suppl.), 63–80

Klottmeier P.K. and Clattworthy H.W. Jr. (1965). Aganglionic and functional megacolon in children. *Pediatrics*, **36**, 572

Lammer E.J. *et al.* (1985). Retinoic acid embryopathy. *New Engl. J. Med.*, **313**, 837–41

Lofberg J., Ahlfors K. and Fallstrom C. (1980). Neural crest cells migration in relation to extracellular matrix secretion in the embryonic axolotl trunk. *Dev. Biol.*, **75**, 148–67

Ranscht B. and Bronner-Fraser M. (1991). T-cadherin expression alternates with migrating neural crest cells in the trunk of the avian embryo. *Development*, **111**, 15–22

Swenson O. (1989). My early experience with Hirschprung's disease. *J. Ped. Surg.*, **24**, 839–46

Tucker G.C., Duband J.-L., Dufour S. and Thiery J.P. (1988). Cell adhesion and substrate-adhesion molecules: their instructive roles in neural crest cell migration. *Development*, **103** (suppl.), 82–94

Weston J.A. (1970). The migration and differentiation of neural crest cells. *Adv. Morph.*, **8**, 41–114

Box 11.1

Bee J.A. and Thorogood, P.V. (1980). The role of tissue interactions in the skeletogenic differentiation of avian neural crest cells. *Dev. Biol.*, **78**, 47–62

Le Douarin N.M., Renaud D., Teillet M.-A., and Le Douarin G.H. (1975). Cholinergic differentiation of presumptive adrenergic neuroblasts in interspecific chimeras after heterotopic transplantation. *Proc. Natl Acad. Sci. USA*, **72**, 728–32

Weston J. (1963) A radiographic analysis of the migration and localisation of trunk neural crest cells in the chick. *Dev. Biol.*, **6**, 274–310

Willier B.H. (1952). Cells, feathers and colors. *Bios*, **23**, 109–25

Special Topic 5

Beresford B. (1983). Brachial somites in the chick embryo: the fate of individual somites. *J. Embryol. Exp. Morph.*, **77**, 99–116

Berg D.K. (1984). New neuronal growth factors. *Annu. Rev. Neurosci.* **7**, 149–70

Bonner P.H. (1980). Differentiation of chick embryo myoblasts is transiently sensitive to functional innervation. *Dev. Biol.*, **76**, 79–86

Bonner P.H. and Adams T.R. (1983). The involvement of nerves in chick myoblast differentiation. In *Progress in Clinical and Biological Research Vol. 110B. Limb Development and Regeneration* (Kelly R.O., Goetinck P.F. and MacCabe J.A., eds), pp 359–68. New York: Alan Liss

Chevallier A. and Kieny M. (1982). On the role of the connective tissue in the patterning of the chick limb musculature. *Wilhelm Roux's Arch.*, **191**, 277–80

Chevallier A., Kieny M., Mauger A. and Sengel P. (1977). Developmental fate of the somitic mesoderm in the chick embryo. In *Vertebrate Limb and Somite Morphogenesis* (Ede D.A., Hinchliffe J.R. and Balls M., eds), pp. 421–32. Cambridge: Cambridge University Press

Christ B. Jacob H.J. and Jacob M. (1979). Differentiating abilities of avian somatopleural mesoderm. *Experientia*, **35**, 1376–8

Crum R., Szabo S. and Folkman J. (1985). A new class of steroids inhibits angiogenesis in the presence of heparin as a heparin fragment. *Science*, **230**, 1375–8

Davies A.M. and Lumsden A. (1990). Ontogeny of the somatosensory system: origins and early development of primary sensory neurons. *Annu. Rev. Neurosci.*, **13**, 61–73

Diwan F.H. and Milburn A. (1986). The effects of temporary ischaemia on rat muscle spindles. *J. Embryol. Exp. Morph.*, **92**, 223–54

Eastlick H.L. (1943). Studies on transplanted embryonic limbs of the chick. I. The development of muscle in nerveless and in innervated grafts. *J. Exp. Zool.*, **93**, 27–45

Eastlick H.L. and Wortham R.A. (1947). Studies on transplanted embryonic limbs of the chick. III. The replacement of muscle by adipose tissue. *J. Morphol.*, **80**, 369–85

Folkman J. (1985). Towards an understanding of angiogenesis: search and discovery. *Perspect. Biol. Med.*, **29**, 10–36

Folkman J. (1985). Tumour angiogenesis. *Adv. Cancer Res.*, **43**, 175–203

Goldspink G. (1980). Growth of muscle. In *Development and specialisation of skeletal muscle* (Goldspink D.F., ed.), pp. 19–35. Cambridge: Cambridge University Press

Gurney M.E. (1984). Suppression of sprouting at the neuromuscular junction by immune sera. *Nature*, **307**, 546–8

Haines R.W. (1932). Laws of muscle and tendon growth. *J. Anat.*, **66**, 578–85

Henderson C.E., Hachet M. and Changeux J.P. (1981). Neurite outgrowth from embryonic chicken spinal neurons is promoted by media conditioned by muscle cells. *Proc. Natl Acad. Sci. USA*, **78**, 2625–9

Hsu L., Natyzak D. and Trupin G.L. (1982). Neurotrophic effects of skeletal muscle fractions on spinal cord differentiation. *J. Embryol. Exp. Morph.*, **71**, 83–95

Kieny M. and Chevallier A. (1979). Autonomy of tendon development in the embryonic chick wing. *J. Embryol. Exp. Morph.*, **49**, 153–65

Lewis J., Chevallier A., Kieny M. and Wolpert L. (1981). Muscle nerve branches do not develop in chick wings devoid of muscles. *J. Embryol. Exp. Morph.*, **64**, 211–32

Pittman R. and Oppenheim R.W. (1979). Cell death of motoneurones in the chick embryo spinal cord. 4: Evidence that a functional neuromuscular interaction is involved in the regulation of naturally occurring cell death and the stabilisation of synapses. *J. Comp. Neurol.*, **187**, 425–36

Shing Y., Folkman J., Sullivan J. Butterfield C., Murray J. and Klagsbrun M. (1984). Heparin affinity and purification of a tumour derived capillary endothelial cell growth factor. *Science*, **223**, 1296–9

Sorgente N., Kuettner K.E., Soble L.W. and Eisenstein R. (1975). The resistance of certain tissues to invasion. II. Evidence for an extracellular factor in cartilage which inhibits invasion by vascularised mesenchyme. *Lab. Invest.*, **32**, 217–22

Swanson G. and Lewis J. (1982). The timetable of innervation and its control in the embryonic chick wing bud. *J. Embryol. Exp. Morph.*, **71**, 121–37

Wilson D. (1983). The origin of the endothelium in the developing marginal vein of the chick wing bud. *Cell Diff.*, **13**, 63–7

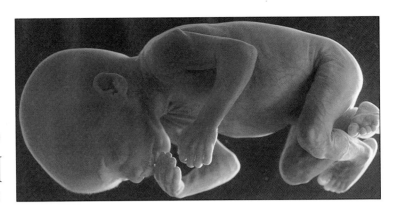

PART III

Regional embryology

Abdomen and pelvis

HEAD AND NECK

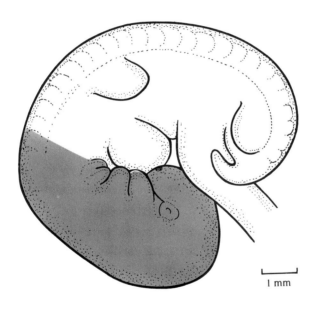

1 mm

12

The brain

EVOLUTION

Most of what is visible of the adult human brain is of comparatively recent evolutionary origin. The early vertebrate brain was a simple tube in which motor functions were carried out in the ventral regions and sensory functions in the dorsal regions. Sensory and motor regions were approximately equal in size. During evolutionary history sensory functions, and regions of the brain involved with associations between sensory inputs, became more important. In particular the optic lobes, concerned with visual input, and the olfactory lobes, concerned with chemical detection, increased markedly in size and finally the forebrain began to play an increasing role in coordinating neural activities. In humans the forebrain has grown dorsally and caudally until it completely covers the primitive brain stem. The embryonic development of the human brain is reminiscent of this evolutionary process in a number of ways.

Very primitive brains were segmental in structure over at least part of their length, and students of mammalian embryo morphology have disagreed for decades as to the nature of this segmentation during development. In the most unexpected way this debate has recently been elucidated by the discovery of segmental patterns of gene expression in the hindbrain (see Special Topic 6, pp. 174–7). These segments are associated with outgrowth of the cranial nerves.

Regionalization of the brain

The primordia of the brain are visible even before the neural tube begins to fuse (Chapter 3). When fusion commences the brain represents a much larger proportion of the neural tube in the early embryo than it does in the adult (about half the length of the neural tube present will contribute to the brain). Throughout the embryonic period the overall growth of the brain is rapid and small differences in regional growth rates to lead to marked changes in form. (The constant-scale illustrations in Chapter 15 indicate the nature of this growth.)

The brain at the beginning of the fourth week possesses three distinct regions: the **forebrain**, **midbrain** and **hindbrain** (also known as the prosencephalon, mesencephalon and rhombencephalon, respectively) (Figure 12.1). The early brain shows signs of being further divided into rather indistinct segments, known as **neuromeres**. These can be observed most clearly in the hindbrain, where they are known as **rhombomeres** (see Figure 12.3 for a later view). As described in Special Topic 6 (pp. 174–7), these are now known to reflect underlying gene expression patterns.

During the fourth week, the neural tube closes cranially and caudally and the three primary divisions give rise to a number of subsidiary structures. Even before the neural folds in the forebrain region fuse, lateral outpushings known as the **optic sulci** have formed (Figure 12.2). After fusion these form the **optic vesicles**, which will give rise to the retina and optic nerve (Chapter 17).

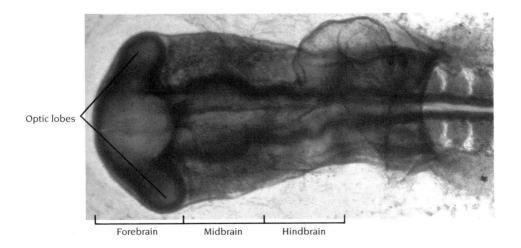

Optic lobes

Forebrain   Midbrain   Hindbrain

FIGURE 12.1 The early brain.

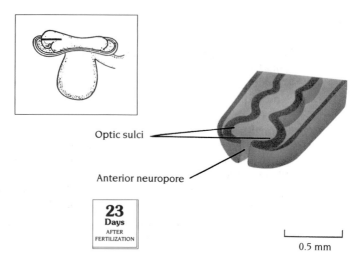

Optic sulci

Anterior neuropore

23
Days
AFTER
FERTILIZATION

└──────────┘
0.5 mm

FIGURE 12.2 The optic sulci of the forebrain. The mesoderm intervening between brain and ectoderm is not shown.

Division of forebrain

The forebrain (or prosencephalon) divides into the **telencephalon** cranial to the optic vesicles and the **diencephalon**, which extends back to the mesencephalon (Figure 12.3). The boundaries of these regions are not always clear, but the names may help to simplify the complex task of describing the developing brain.

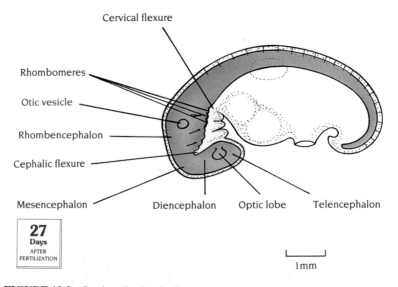

Cervical flexure

Rhombomeres

Otic vesicle

Rhombencephalon

Cephalic flexure

Mesencephalon   Diencephalon   Optic lobe   Telencephalon

27
Days
AFTER
FERTILIZATION

└──────┘
1mm

FIGURE 12.3   Regionalization in the neural tube.

Midbrain

The midbrain remains undivided, and is given the definitive name of **mesencephalon**.

Hindbrain

The hindbrain (or rhombencephalon) gives rise to the **metencephalon** and the **myelencephalon** (Figure 12.4(a)). The roof of the hindbrain also begins to thin out, in a manner which suggests that the neural tube is 'opening out' in this region (Figure 12.4(b)). As described in Chapter 6, the brain and neural tube show a marked distinction between the ventral motor basal plates and the dorsal sensory alar plates. This means that the alar regions lie lateral rather than dorsal to the basal regions, with only a single cell layer forming the roof.

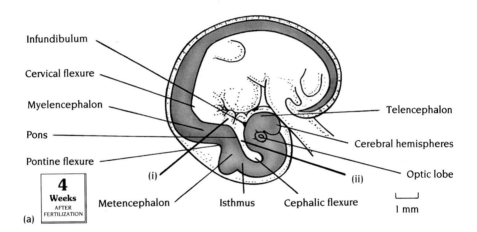

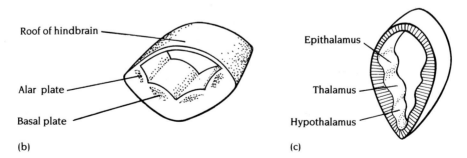

FIGURE 12.4 (a) As flexure of the embryo continues the brain continues to regionalize; (b) section through line marked (i); (c) section through line marked (ii).

Within each of these five regions (telencephalon, diencephalon, mesencephalon, metencephalon and myelencephalon) the cavity of the neural tube expands to form the primitive **ventricles** (Figure 12.5).

We will return to the regions of the brain later, to consider in more detail the structures to which each of the regions will contribute. Before this it is necessary to describe flexion of the brain, for the brain is not merely regionalizing, it is also changing its shape.

Flexures

During the fourth week a ventral-facing bend begins to develop in the mesencephalic region (Figure 12.3). This is known as the **cephalic flexure**. At about the same time the **cervical flexure** appears in the region between the rhombencephalon and the spinal cord.

During the fifth week, a dorsal-facing flexure appears between the metencephalon and the myelencephalon (Figure 12.4(a)). This is known as the **pontine flexure**. The mechanisms underlying development of these flexions remain to be elucidated, but may involve differential cell division and change of cell shape.

Further development of regionalization

The telencephalon

We have already seen how the optic vesicles arise from the telencephalon. As the vesicles approach the surface ectoderm of the head, they become concave, forming the **optic cups** (see Chapter 17). From about 5 weeks a substantial pair of lobes begins to grow out from the most cranial end of the telencephalon: these are the **cerebral hemispheres** (Figure 12.4(a)). From these beginnings they will grow dorsally and caudally to cover almost completely the original brain stem (see Figure 12.8). The rapid growth of the cerebral hemispheres causes folds and fissures to form on their surface. In addition to these most advanced of brain structures in terms of evolutionary status the telencephalon gives rise to the olfactory bulb and tract, which are among the most primitive.

The diencephalon

Inside the diencephalon, lying just cranial to the cephalic flexure, three paired structures begin to develop, growing in from the lateral walls (Figure 12.4(c)). These are (from dorsal to ventral as the flexed tube lies) the **epithalami**, the **thalami**, and the **hypothalami**. The thalami bulge out into the lumen of the diencephalon. The hypothalami meet and fuse to form the definitive **hypothalamus**: in many cases the thalami also meet in the midline and fuse, although the lumen of the brain is not completely occluded. A downward extension of the

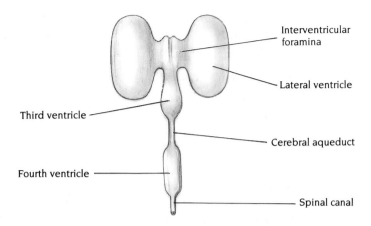

Interventricular
foramina

Lateral ventricle

Third ventricle

Cerebral aqueduct

Fourth ventricle

Spinal canal

FIGURE 12.5 Primitive ventricles, as seen in the brain of the embryo in Figure 12.4 after straightening out.

diencephalon, known as the **infundibulum**, represents what will become the stalk and the pars nervosa of the pituitary gland (Figure 12.4(a) and Chapter 15).

The mesencephalon

The mesencephalon stays comparatively unaltered in gross terms during development. However, an external median groove appears in the mesencephalic roof, which is subsequently crossed at right angles by a second groove. The four quadrants thus formed represent the superior and inferior **colliculi** (Figure 12.6). Each of the basal plates of the mesencephalon forms two motor nuclei, which innervate the eye musculature and the sphincter pupillary muscle.

Metencephalon and myelencephalon

The pontine flexure results in the roof of the metencephalon and myelencephalon adopting a rhomboidal shape rather in the way that a sharply flexed hose behaves. The edges of this rhomboid in the metencephalon will proliferate to form the **cerebellum** (Figure 12.6), which controls posture and movement. The basal plates of the metencephalon form three groups of motor neurons, containing the nuclei of the abducens, trigeminal and facial nerves and the nerves to the submandibular and sublingual salivary glands. The marginal layer of the basal plates forms the **pons** (Figure 12.4(b)), so named because it forms a bridge between the spinal cord and the cerebellar and cerebral cortices.

The myelencephalon will develop into the **medulla oblongata**. Motor nerve nuclei form in the basal plate and sensory nerve nuclei in the alar plate.

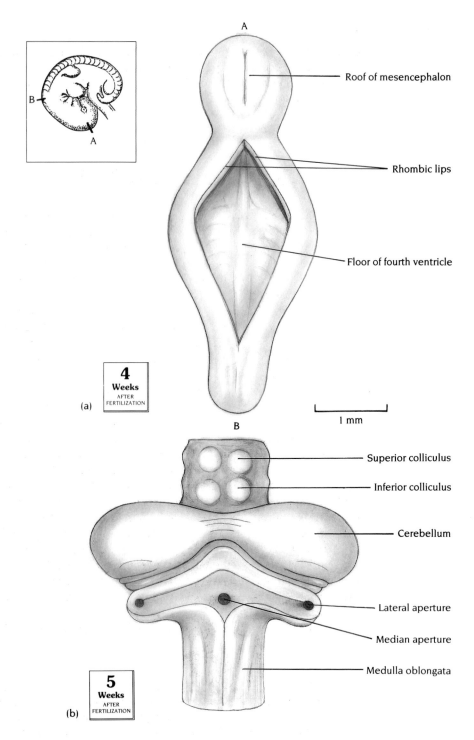

A

Roof of mesencephalon

Rhombic lips

Floor of fourth ventricle

4 Weeks
AFTER FERTILIZATION

(a)

1 mm

B

Superior colliculus

Inferior colliculus

Cerebellum

Lateral aperture

Median aperture

Medulla oblongata

5 Weeks
AFTER FERTILIZATION

(b)

Condensation of mesoderm

As described in Chapter 6, the brain and spinal cord are surrounded by mesoderm, which condenses around the brain and will eventually form three distinct layers: the pia mater next to the brain, the arachnoid mater, and the outer dura mater (see Figure 6.5).

Brain vesicles and cerebrospinal fluid

At the same time as these developments are taking place, the fluid-filled lumen of the neural tube is undergoing changes (Figure 12.5). As the cerebral hemispheres expand their central cavities also expand, and become the **lateral ventricles**. The cerebral hemispheres grow back and over the brain and the lateral ventricles change shape accordingly, to adopt an extended C-shaped form. The lateral ventricles communicate with the main neural cavity via narrow openings known as the **interventricular foramina (of Munro)**. The main cavity in the region surrounded by the diencephalon is described as the **third ventricle**. The cavity in the mesencephalic region narrows, and becomes the **cerebral aqueduct (of Sylvius)**. This in turn leads into the cavity of the rhombencephalon: the **fourth ventricle**.

Before fusion of the neural tube is complete the neural cavity is continuous with the amniotic cavity and amniotic fluid bathes the interior of the neural tube. When the tube has closed at both ends it is filled in the early stages with a simple filtrate of the fetal blood. Subsequently, the meningeal mesoderm above the dorsal aspect of the brain in several regions becomes richly vascularized, and from about 6 weeks special structures containing blood vessels become apparent, projecting down from the roof of the brain into the lumen of the neural tube (Figure 12.7). These are the **choroid plexuses** ('choroid' from their membranous appearance, which was thought to resemble the true chorion), and in the fetus and adult they are major producers of cerebrospinal fluid (CSF). There are four choroid plexuses altogether, projecting into the left and right lateral ventricles and the third and fourth ventricles. During the fetal period three openings appear in the thin roof of the metencephalon, one median and two lateral (Figure 12.6(b)). These allow CSF to pass from the lumen of the neural tube to the subarachnoid space.

Arachnoid villi protrude across the subdural space, through the dura and

FIGURE 12.6 (*opposite*)   (a) Rhomboidal roof of hindbrain, as seen in the dorsal view of the embryo in Figure 12.4. The cerebellum will develop from the rhombic lips. The median line between the alar plates, which gives rise to the formation of the collicular plate, is indicated, though it is unlikely yet to be visible externally. (b) Similar dorsal view of the cerebellum in the later human fetus.

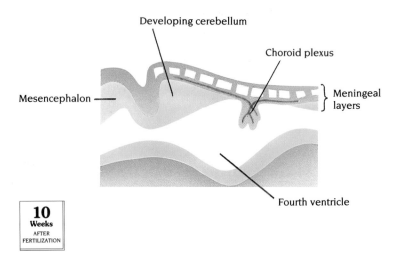

FIGURE 12.7   Sagittal section through hindbrain showing pons, developing cerebellum and choroid plexuses.

into the dural venous sinuses, through which CSF is reabsorbed into the venous blood, hence establishing a circulation.

Pressure of CSF aids the expansion of the brain vesicles: this drives the expansion of the bony plates of the skull. Abnormalities of CSF production or absorption will therefore lead to skull defects.

Clinical implications of brain development

The brain is a uniquely complex structure and it is therefore not surprising that many defects and variations can occur during its development. Formation of neural connections and maturation of neural and supporting tissues continues throughout the fetal period and into infancy and childhood, and can therefore be affected by environmental influences over a much wider timespan than most other structures. For example, the steroid hormones cause neural changes in sexual cell numbers and relationships during development, and may influence behaviour. It has even been suggested, though not proven, that homosexuality has an underlying basis in brain structure.

Many defects that are not apparent until long after birth may have a basis during the time of brain formation. Schizophrenia is perhaps one of the most mysterious of mental illnesses, and it has been speculated that underlying differences in brain structure between sufferers and control populations may relate to its aetiology.

The differentiation and survival of brain cells is believed to be controlled

Cerebral hemispheres

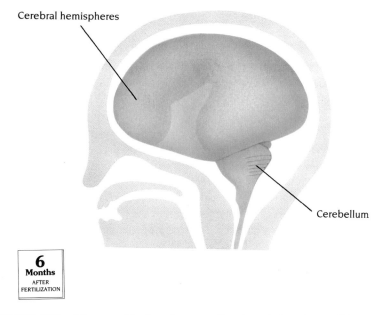

Cerebellum

6
Months
AFTER
FERTILIZATION

FIGURE 12.8.   Diagram of brain and surrounding tissue in later human fetus.

by growth factors, of which several are known to be involved in brain development. **Nerve growth factor** stimulates the survival of basal forebrain cholinergic neurones, while **brain-derived neurotrophic factor** stimulates the survival
of dopamine neurons. These are the cells that degenerate in Alzheimer's and
Parkinson's diseases respectively. Although it is not believed that these conditions are caused by failures of development, they could be treated using the
insights gained from development. The growth factors are difficult to administer
because they do not cross the blood–brain barrier but transplants of fetal brain
cells to affected patients have been reported, with some apparent success. Fetal
brain cells are difficult to obtain and their use controversial; a better strategy
would be to genetically engineer cells to manufacture nerve growth factors using
cells obtained from the patient in the first instance, so as to avoid immune rejection. It may be possible to obtain brain progenitor cells and to use immortalized
versions for therapeutic purposes.

  The brain and skull are intimately related during development (see Box
13.1 and Figure 12.8). As we will see in the next chapter, brain abnormalities
frequently lead to skull abnormalities. However, it is impossible to understand
these without first following the development of the skull.

Special Topic 6 Homoeobox genes

The fruit fly: a key to understanding human development

In recent years a major series of discoveries about developmental biology has been made using the fruit fly, *Drosophila melanogaster*, as a model system. These discoveries have unexpectedly shed light on the development of vertebrates, including mammals and humans. It is likely that these discoveries will revolutionize our views on human development in ways that we can only currently guess at.

It has been known for decades that dramatic spontaneous mutations (known as homoeotic mutations) can change one part of the fruit fly into another: an antenna can be converted into a leg, for instance. A number of such mutations were mapped to particular genes and these proved to be arranged in two major clusters in the *Drosophila* genome. Later studies indicate that these two clusters may have arisen from one ancestral cluster.

Even a single mutation in one of these genes can bring about large-scale changes in body pattern. Each of these genes must therefore act as a master gene, controlling many others.

When the sequences of the genes began to emerge, a further discovery was made. This was that one sequence was common to all of the genes within the cluster, no matter how widely they differed otherwise. This sequence was called the **homoeobox** (often spelt homeobox).

Probes for homoeotic genes

Knowledge of the homoeobox sequence enabled probes to be made that could identify homoeotic genes in other organisms without the time-consuming process of genetic analysis that had been necessary in *Drosophila*. Although the homoeotic genes were expected to be confined to clearly segmented animals such as insects, it emerged that clusters of homoeotic genes appear in the genome of all animals, including the unsegmented invertebrates and the vertebrates.

Gene clusters

Mutations in humans in which one part of the body converts into another do not seem to occur. One possible reason for this is that the original single ancestral cluster has reduplicated to give four versions of itself, all on separate chromosomes. For a given gene within a cluster, identifiable homologies can be observed with the corresponding gene in the other clusters so that, if a mutation does occur in one gene, another three genes can carry out something like its role. However, the same fact permits changes between clusters, so in evolutionary time they are slowly developing their own identities and roles.

Differential expression of genes in a cluster

The genes in a cluster are differentially expressed in space and time within the developing embryo in ways that seem to prefigure many interesting morphological events. These patterns of developmental expression have a truly startling feature: they often appear in sequence in the body, and the order in which they are expressed reflects their order on the genome. For example, genes at the 3' end (the 'right-hand end') of the cluster are expressed in cranial positions and genes to the left of this are expressed progressively more caudally down the embryo. Moreover, the pattern of spatial expression for corresponding genes is the same in all animals: if a particular gene is first switched on in the head of a fly embryo, the corresponding homologue gene will be switched on in the head of a chick, a mouse or a human embryo.

Neuromeres

The segmental pattern found in insect embryos is also reflected in mammalian embryos. In the developing brain segmental 'neuromeres' can be observed corresponding to the segmental pattern of the cranial nerves, but in an unexpected alternating manner (Figure 1). These segments are related to a segmental homoeobox gene expression pattern (Figure 1). It is possible that the branchial arches receive their segmental information from the expression of homoeobox-containing genes.

It is not yet known what establishes the pattern of expression of the neuromeres. However, retinoic acid (vitamin A) appears to be a likely candidate control molecule: as its concentration increases, the genes within a cluster are sequentially activated and if it is administered during development the pattern of gene expression and the morphology of the embryo alter.

Compartments

Another finding from fruit flies is that the body domains in which homoeobox genes are expressed need not correspond to any morphological landmarks on the body itself: the fruit fly is divided by invisible lines of gene expression into areas known as **compartments** which cells will not cross These compartments are like jigsaw pieces in some ways: the 'picture' runs across them, yet is built up by them. The same seems very likely in vertebrates, and if this is indeed the case we will have to rethink many of our ideas about development. Certainly cells seem unwilling to cross boundaries between adjacent neuromeres, preferring to migrate and divide within one neuromere, as if it was a 'compartment'.

Development of the limb bud

Another particularly interesting example of regionalized homoeobox gene expression can be seen in the development of the limb bud (Chapter 18) where a number of homoeobox genes are expressed during development. For instance, in the fourth gene cluster (*Hox*-4), five of the genes (4.4–4.8) are sequentially expressed in a 'skewed' pattern across the limb. At the caudal edge all of the genes are switched on (see Figure 18.12) but moving cranially the genes appear to be sequentially switched off in an order that corresponds to their order on the genome. As we will see in Chapter 18, the region of the limb in which all of the genes in the cluster are switched on has properties of considerable interest in development, even though it is morphologically indistinguishable from all the other tissues in the limb.

This pattern of gene expression appears to result from a gradient of retinoic acid (see Chapter 18). What then establishes the gradient of retinoic acid? Unfortunately there is no complete current answer to this question but the node (see Chapter 2) is a good source of similar retinoids, so perhaps this imparts signalling activity to the limb bud as the axis is formed.

A number of receptors for retinoic acid mediate its effect: cytoplasmic receptors may serve to 'mop up' excess retinoic acid; quite different nuclear receptors become activated by the presence of retinoic acid to switch on homoeobox genes, among others.

A gradient of homoeobox gene expression runs from the limb tip to its base, and this is thought to be involved in specifying proximodistal positions. This is considered again in Chapter 18.

Homoeodomains

The clue to the events following establishment of a gradient of homoeobox gene expression lies in the nature of the protein encoded by the homoeobox sequence. This **homoeodomain** binds to specific DNA sequences on the cellular genome. It can then activate or inhibit the expression of particular genes: in other words it acts as a transcription factor. This could in turn result in the initiation of a pattern of gene expression leading to differentiation and to changes in cellular properties such as cell division, growth, movement and death. These changes are presumably interpreted by the cells as instructions on how to form the elements of the limb.

Summary

To summarize, a local source of retinoic acid (or some similar activating material) must first be established in the limb and a gradient created by diffusion across the limb. At positions distant from the source only genes at the 3' end of the *Hox*-4 complex are activated. Closer to the source more and more genes in the cluster are activated until they are all switched on. Activation of different members of the *Hox* complex leads to activation

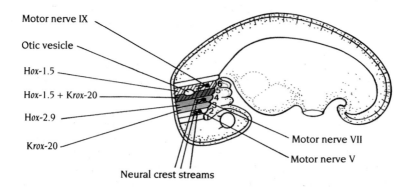

FIGURE 1 View of embryo indicating the neuromeres and their relationship with the branchial arches, neural crest streams, major motor nerves and homoeobox gene expression patterns.

of new sets of genes via the homoeodomain product, and these in turn lead to the acquisition of different craniocaudal positional values. These values are then somehow translated into morphological patterns. At the same time a separate gradient of homoeobox gene activation is established down the limb from tip to base and provides cells with a second axis of information. Much as latitude and longitude can specify positions on a map these two axes seem able to specify morphology in the limb.

This sketch still has large gaps and may need extensive revision, but it provides a plausible framework for thinking about morphogenesis: nor is it devoid of clinical implications (see Special Topic 7, pp. 259–60)

The discovery of these clusters of homoeobox-containing genes in *Drosophila*, where their roles can be elucidated with comparative ease, has been compared to the discovery of the Rosetta stone. The evolutionary implications of these findings are most profound. A set of gene components, intimately involved in establishing polarity of body pattern, have proved to be highly conserved across an astonishing range of animal species. This implies that these gene sequences were present in the ancestors common to all these animals and have come down to humans remarkably unchanged, reflecting our common kinship and their extraordinary importance. The presence of homoeobox-containing genes arranged in clusters has even been proposed as a definition of what constitutes an animal.

Homoeobox-containing genes could be used as a tool for retrospectively exploring evolution without waiting for rare fossil-finding events. For instance, the postulate that vertebrate limbs developed from fish fins seemed impossible to investigate in the conventional scientific sense, but it can now be shown that the pattern of expression of particular homoeobox genes in the region of the developing fin in fish matches exactly the expression of the corresponding gene in the developing limb bud in the amphibian *Xenopus laevis*.

Further reading

Gasser R.F. (1982). *Atlas of Human Embryos*. Hagerstown, Maryland: Harper & Row

Hamilton W.J., Boyd J.D. and Mossman H.W. (1962). *Human Embryology* 3rd edn. Cambridge: Heffer

Jiao S., Gurevich V. and Wolff J.A. (1993). Long term correction of rat model of Parkinson's disease by gene therapy. *Nature*, **362**, 450–3

Le Vey S. (1991). A difference in hypothalamic structure between heterosexual and homosexual men. *Science*, **253**, 1034–6

Muller F. and O'Rahilly R. (1980). The early development of the nervous system in staged insectivore and primate embryos. *J. Comp. Neurol.*, **193**, 741–51

Muller F. and O'Rahilly R. (1986). The development of the human brain and the closure of the rostral neuropore at stage 11. *Anat. Embryol.*, **175**, 205–22

Muller F. and O'Rahilly R. (1986). The development of the human brain from a closed neural tube at stage 13. *Anat. Embryol.*, **177**, 203–14

O'Rahilly R. and Muller F. (1987). *Developmental Stages in Human Embryos*. Carnegie Institution of Washington Publication 637

Toran-Allerand C.D. (1984). On the genesis of sexual differentiation of the central nervous system: morphogenetic consequences of steroidal exposure and possible role of alpha-fetoprotein. *Progr. in Brain Res.*, **61**, 63–75

Special Topic 6

De Robertis E.M., Oliver G. and Wright C.V.E. (1990). Homeobox genes and the vertebrate body plan. *Sci. Am.*, **253**, 26–32

Gehring W.J. (1985). The molecular basis of development. *Sci. Am.*, **253**, 152–62

Izpisua-Belmonte J.-C. *et al.* (1991). Expression of the homeobox HOX-4 genes and the specification of position in chick wing development. *Nature*, **350**, 585–9

Lumsden A. and Keynes R. (1989). Segmental patterns of neuronal development in the chick hindbrain. *Nature*, **337**, 424–8

Marshall H., Nonchev S., Sham M.H., Muchamore I., Lumsden A. and Krumlauf R. (1992). Retinoic acid alters hindbrain hox code, and induces transformation of rhombomeres 2/3 into a 4/5 identity. *Nature*, **360**, 737–9

Murphy P., Davidson D.R. and Hill R.E. (1989). Segment specific expression of a homoeobox-containing gene in the mouse hindlimb. *Nature*, **341**, 156–9

Slack J.M.W., Holland P.W.H. and Graham C.F. (1993). The zootype and the phylotypic stage. *Nature*, **361**, 490–2

Wilkinson D.G., Bhatt S., Chavrier P., Bravo R. and Charnay P. (1989). Segment-specific expression of a zinc-finger gene in the developing nervous system in the mouse. *Nature*, **337**, 461–4

13

The skull

Although the shape of the adult skull is complex, the development of the skull is less complicated than might be feared. The key to understanding skull morphology in evolution and development is the realization that it arises from the fusion of a number of simpler elements. These elements may be either **intramembranous** or **endochondral** in nature and may be derived from neural crest cells or the mesoderm (see Chapter 9). The elements can be classified into two major groups, the **neurocranium** and the **viscerocranium**, each of which may in turn be divided into subgroups. These groups represent differences in evolutionary as well as developmental origin.

Neurocranium

The neurocranium is composed of the **chondrocranium** and the **dermatocranium**.

- The elements of the chondrocranium represent the base of the skull.
- The elements of the dermatocranium cover and protect the dorsal aspect of the brain.

Chondrocranium

As the vertebrate brain evolved, the mesoderm surrounding the delicate sense organs of hearing, smell and sight that were being formed became cartilaginous (Figure 13.1) in order to protect and support them. This early cartilaginous condition prevails in primitive vertebrates such as hagfish and lampreys, and can be seen in the developing human embryo.

The supports form as endochondral bone, which is both mesodermal and neural crest in origin. The cartilage elements that were the most anterior neural arch vertebrae modify and are incorporated into the base of the skull. Figure 13.2 lists the component elements of the chondrocranium, deduced largely from evolutionary considerations: the rather rudimentary cartilage elements that form in the developing human skull (Figure 13.3) would be difficult to interpret without this insight. The trabeculae cranii and nasal capsules are associated with the olfactory lobes of the brain; the optic, otic and hypophyseal capsules are associated with the optic and otic vesicles and the pituitary or neurohypophysis, respectively. The parachordal cartilage and occipital sclerotomes represent cranial vertebrae. The parachordal cartilage perhaps represents the sclerotomes of the rhombomeres – the lost segments – of the hindbrain, even though it now shows no sign of segmentation.

These chondrocranial rudiments appear during week 6, well after the brain has started to differentiate: in fact, the brain tissue induces mesodermal condensations to form around it and the development of the skull should be considered in close association with that of the brain (see Box 13.1).

As shown in Figure 13.2, the chondrocranial rudiments begin to fuse while they are still cartilaginous. Once the cartilage has been replaced by bone they will form the combination bones known as the ethmoid and sphenoid and parts of the occipital and temporal bones. Figure 13.4 shows the chondrocranium at a more advanced stage.

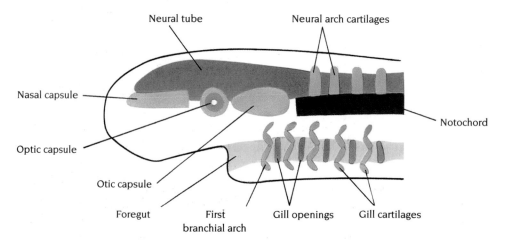

FIGURE 13.1   General disposition of cartilage in a hypothetical vertebrate ancestor.

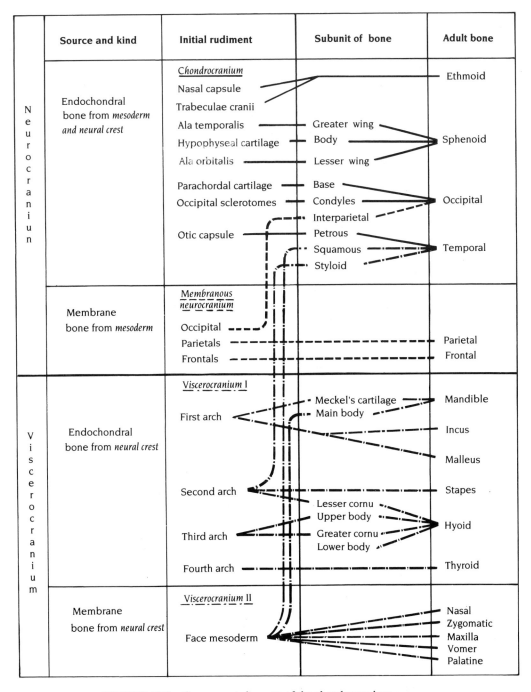

FIGURE 13.2   Component elements of the chondrocranium.

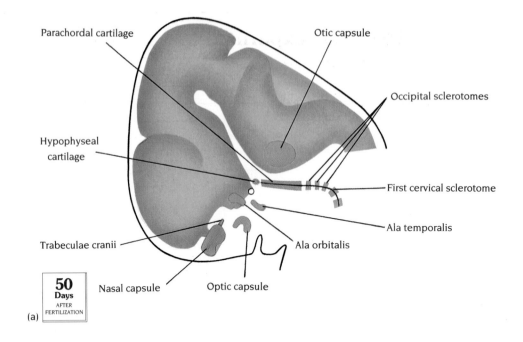

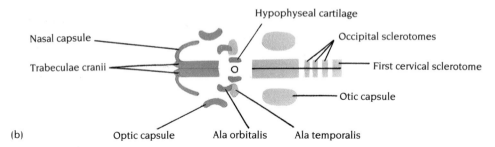

FIGURE 13.3 Early cartilaginous elements of chondrocranium seen (a) laterally and (b) from a dorsal view.

Dermatocranium

In evolutionary terms this component of the skull is believed to be derived from external dermal scales that served to protect the vulnerable top of the brain and that are thought to have come to lie under a superficial layer of skin. During human development mesoderm condenses around the brain (as described in Chapter 6) and membrane bone forms in the outermost, dural, layer of this condensation. This process begins during the fetal period, at about 12 weeks after fertilization, so the membranous neurocranium forms *after* the chondrocranium.

Five ossification centres form the vault of the skull: two frontal, two parietal and one occipital (Figure 13.4). The ossification plates extend towards each

Box 13.1 **Experimental analysis of skull formation**

It is important that a functional relationship be formed between the brain and the skull during development: the risks of specifying them by separate mechanisms would be too great. Certainly, study of the gradual appear-

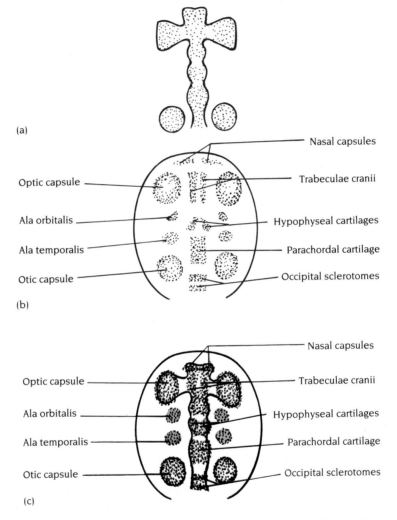

FIGURE 1 The underside of the brain and sensory organs produces collagen type II molecules, which are believed to initiate chondrogenesis. (a) Collagen type II molecules are shown on the underside of the brain. (b) A schematic view of the base of the skull after removal of the brain and top of the head. (c) Overlapping (a) and (b) shows the relationship between the two.

ance of the skull suggests that it is 'induced' by the brain in some way, but this does not directly indicate the underlying mechanisms.

Such information is now becoming available for the chondrocranium. It can be demonstrated that migratory neural crest cells must come into contact with the undersurface of the developing brain before they are able to differentiate into cartilage and form the chondrocranium. Further, a key component appears to be the extracellular matrix molecules secreted by the neural cells, rather than the cells themselves. Type II collagen, which may be capable of inhibiting movement of neural crest cells (Figure 1) plays a particularly important role.

It may be that the developing brain cells in particular regions secrete type II collagen. This then 'traps' the neural crest cells and induces them to differentiate into cartilage. In this way, the brain acts as a template around which the cartilage of the chondrocranium forms.

While the induction of the dermatocranium and viscerocranium has not yet been analysed in this detail, similar mechanisms may well operate.

other and where they meet a **suture** line is formed, at which the cells divide actively as long as the plates are under pressure from the expanding brain. Individual plates may be expanded outwards by osteoclasts removing bone from their inner aspect while osteoblasts produce new bone on the outer aspect. If the pressure exerted by the developing brain is abnormally high or low, the vault of the skull will be correspondingly larger or smaller.

Gradually the elements of the membranous neurocranium and the chondrocranium fuse to form a single large functional unit.

The occipital plate fuses to elements of the chondrocranium to become the definitive occipital bone (see Figure 13.2). The frontal plates will fuse after birth to form the frontal bone, and the parietal plates the parietal bones.

Viscerocranium

The viscerocranium is composed of an endochondral or **cartilaginous** part, and an intermembranous or **dermal** part.

- The elements of the cartilaginous viscerocranium represent primitive gill cartilages, and contribute to the jaws and middle ear bones among other structures.
- The elements of the dermal visceroranium represent the rudiments of the facial bones.

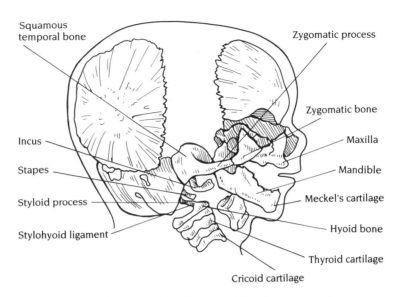

Squamous temporal bone

Zygomatic process

Incus

Stapes

Styloid process

Stylohyoid ligament

Zygomatic bone

Maxilla

Mandible

Meckel's cartilage

Hyoid bone

Thyroid cartilage

Cricoid cartilage

FIGURE 13.4   Later chondrocranial, viscerocranial and neurocranial condensations, from a model by Hertwig.

Cartilaginous viscerocranium

Primitive marine vertebrates were jawless but had cartilage supports for their gills (Figure 13.1). These cartilaginous rods in time evolved into jaws and a variety of other structures; several of them became re-inforced by intramembranous bone. The derivatives of these structures are of such importance that all of Chapter 14 is devoted to them.

Dermal viscerocranium

The facial bones will form from membranous bone (Figure 13.3), and they may be considered as forming a separate subgroup of the viscerocranium.

Postnatal events

Many important events in skull development occur after birth. The plates of the dermatocranium are not fused at birth, so they are able to overlap as the head is compressed. The head recovers its normal shape over the next 48 hours. The skull vault grows rapidly for the first 2 years, then more slowly until about 15 or 16 years. It is more difficult for an approximately spherical bony structure like the skull to grow quickly than it is for a long bone, which preserves localized growth zones.

Fusion of sutures

The sutures between the skull plates are unfused at birth and there is wide variation in the time at which they fuse. The frontal (metopic) suture begins fusing at
2–3 years and eventually disappears completely but others (and even the frontal
suture on occasion) may persist until adulthood, and may be mistaken for frac-
tures in radiographs.

Fontanelles

Where several membranous neurocranial plates meet, the interstices represent
membrane-covered openings in the forming bony skull at the time of birth.
These are known as **fontanelles**, and there are six in total (Figure 13.5):

- The paired posterior and sphenoid fontanelles are generally obliterated within
  2–3 months of birth.
- The mastoid fontanelle generally persists for about 1 year.
- The anterior (or superior) fontanelle may not close for several years.

Of these the anterior fontanelle is of the greatest significance. Its extent is
such that it provides a significant point of weakness in the infant skull. In addition, if the intracranial pressure is high (as may result from hydrocephalus (see
Chapter 13) or from the presence of a brain tumour or a haematoma), the skin
over the anterior fontanelle will bulge outward. Low intracranial pressure, found
in cases of dehydration, means that the region of the fontanelle may be
depressed. Finally, the orientation of the baby's head during birth can be
deduced by palpating the characteristic shape of the fontanelle.

Air spaces

The air spaces or **paranasal sinuses** of the skull are small or absent at birth and
they gradually enlarge during infancy and childhood. The solid appearance of
the skull may make this difficult to understand but, as described earlier, the bone
of the living skull is constantly being removed and replaced by osteoclasts and
osteoblasts as it grows. Small differences in the rates of these two processes lead
to marked reshaping, including the hollowing out of the sinuses.

Sinuses show considerable variation between individuals, and sinus shape
may be used for purposes of identification. The sinuses serve to lighten the skull;
they also alter the shape of the face and the sound of the voice, though this
seems unlikely to be their sole purpose.

The skull is penetrated by a number of openings and foramina that are related
to the presence of nerves and of neural tube derivatives such as the optic lobes.
Nerves are generally present before the cartilage elements begin to form, but the
precise mechanism by which foramina form – whether nerves repel cartilage, or
whether they induce it to become a sheath around themselves – remains unclear.

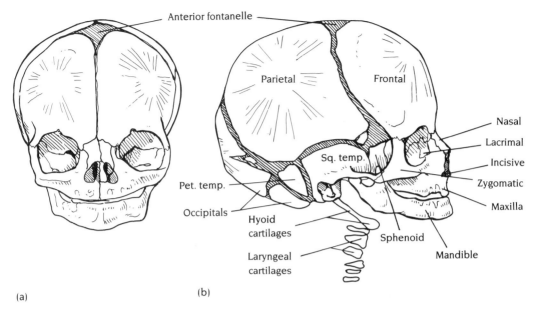

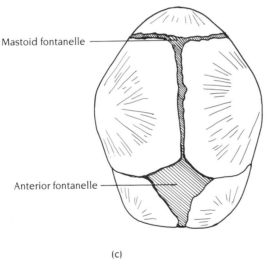

FIGURE 13.5 (a) Skull of a newborn infant. (b) Lateral view; (c) dorsal view, showing the fontanelles.

Defects of skull development

The shape of the skull, particularly the dermatocranium, is responsive to pressure – in fact, the ancient Persians bound the skulls of their infants to achieve a 'fashionable' head shape. Skull shape is dependent on the pressure exerted by the developing brain and, as a result defects of the brain and neural tube are often reflected in the shape of the skull.

Anencephaly has been considered in Chapter 6.

Hydrocephalus (hydrocephaly) This is not a dysraphic condition, although it is often associated with such defects. It is caused by increased pressure of CSF, perhaps due to a restriction in the neural tube lumen, to reduced drainage into the subarachnoid space or to reduced elasticity of the ventricles. The cerebral aqueduct may be involved, as this is the narrowest part of the continuous cavity within the brain. As pressure in the ventricles rises, the skull may expand faster than normal but the brain tissue may also be squeezed between the ventricles and the skull. The incidence of hydrocephalus is approximately 10 per 10 000 live births. An enlarged head can be detected in 30% of cases at birth, in 50% by 3 months and in 80% by the end of the first year. Other symptoms are a bulging, tense anterior fontanelle, dilated scalp veins and 'sunsetting' of the eyes. Remarkably, even major compression of the brain need not lead to mental retardation, although it often does. One individual with a rim of brain tissue inside the skull of only 1 cm gained a university degree in mathematics.

Hydrocephalus may be treated by using a shunt to reduce the pressure, usually a tube with a non-return valve leading from the affected ventricles to the abdomen or the right atrium. The prognosis is good in treatable cases; 80% of affected individuals survive to their fifth year, and 80% of these are of normal intelligence, or at least educable.

Encephalocoele This is rarer than spina bifida or anencephaly, with a European incidence of 1.7 per 10 000 pregnancies. A region of brain herniates through a congenital opening in the midline of the skull. It may be found occipitally or frontally, in which case it may appear as a mass at the medial wall of the orbit or projecting into the nasopharynx. An encephalocoele is generally covered with skin. If a substantial amount of brain tissue is included in the encephalocoele, mental retardation or neurological dysfunction may result.

Microcephaly Inadequate brain development leads to the formation of a small dermatocranium. This is a relatively rare condition, and figures for its incidence are unreliable.

Asymmetric defects

Hemifacial microsomia (This includes first and second arch syndrome and Goldenhar's syndrome). This group of conditions is present in about one in 3000 live births, affecting one side only in 70% of cases. In the others both sides are affected, but not in a symmetrical manner. The conditions affect the jaw outline, the ears and the eyelids. A possible explanation is that a haematoma forms at the developing ramus of the mandible as a result of damage to, or abnormality of, the stapedial artery and then destroys the mesodermal tissue to a degree depending on the size of the haematoma. The condition is difficult to correct surgically because so much of the mesodermal tissue has been destroyed that little is left for rearrangement.

Symmetric defects

Mandibulofacial dysostosis (Treacher Collins syndrome) This condition is much less common than hemifacial microsomia and affects both sides in a symmetrical manner. The palpebral fissures slant downward and the ears are often displaced, with associated deafness. The condition may be caused by failure of preotic neural crest cells to migrate to the otic and facial primordia. However, because the tissue has not been completely destroyed, it is easier to treat than hemifacial microsomia.

Craniosynostosis This is also a relatively rare condition. It is an abnormality of the shape and form of the skull rather than its size. It is often said to be caused by premature fusion of the skull plates, but it could be brought about by incomplete formation of the sutures. Surgery is successful for 75% of sufferers.

Holoprosencephaly Failure of the forebrain (prosencephalon) to form properly can lead to a spectrum of mental, skull and facial abnormalities, depending on the severity of the underlying condition. In milder forms the nose, palate, lip and/or jaw may be abnormal and in severe cases the midline structures of the face may fail to form altogether, giving cyclopia (Figure 13.6).

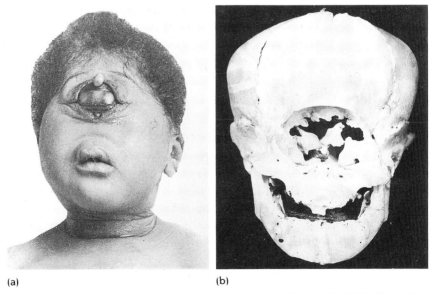

(a)   (b)

FIGURE 13.6   Case of cyclopia in a child who survived 5 hours after birth. (From the Anatomy Museum, University of St Andrews, by permission (a) Surface view just after death. (b) Skull.

Further reading

Bergsma D. (1979). *Birth Defects Compendium* 2nd edn. London: Macmillan

De Beer G. (1937). *Development of the Vertebrate Skull*. Oxford: Oxford University Press

Hamilton W.J., Boyd J.D. and Mossman H.W. (1962). *Human Embryology* 3rd edn. Cambridge: W. Heffer & Sons

Le Lievre C. (1978). Participation of neural crest derived cells in the genesis of the skull in birds. *J. Embryol. Exp. Morph.*, **47**, 17–37

Lewis W.J. (1920). The cartilaginous skull of a human embryo twenty-one millimetres in length. *Contrib. Embryol.*, **9**, 229–324

Noden D.M. (1978). The control of avian cephalic neural crest cytodifferentiation. I. Skeletal and connective tissues. *Dev. Biol.*, **67**, 296–312

McGrath P. and Sperber G.H. (1990). Floor of the median orbit in human cyclopia: an anatomical study in three dimensions. *J. Anat.*, **169**, 125–38.

Poswillo D. (1988). The aetiology and pathogenesis of craniofacial deformity. *Development*, **103** (suppl.), 207–12

Trenouth M.J. (1989). Craniofacial shape in the anencephalic human fetus. *J. Anat.*, **165**, 215–24

Box 13.1

Thorogood P.V. (1981). Neural crest cells and skeletogenesis in vertebrate embryos. *Histochem. J.*, **13**, 631–42

Thorogood P.V. (1987). Mechanisms of morphogenetic specification in skull development. In *Mesenchymal-Epithelial Interactions in Neural Development* (NATO ASI Series, Vol. H5) (Wolff J.R. *et al.*, eds), pp. 141–52. Berlin: Springer-Verlag

14

Branchial arches

EVOLUTION

The branchial arches in humans represent the evolutionary remnants of the gill arches of our fish ancestors. Fish gills possess a number of internal structures to enable them to carry out their respiratory functions: there are rods of cartilage to stiffen them so that water can flow through; muscles to move them slowly back and forth when the fish is stationary; nerves to supply these muscles; and, most importantly, a rich supply of blood vessels to facilitate gas exchange. Gill arch precursors form in all vertebrate embryos, but because in land animals they are no longer required for their original purpose they have been freed, in evolutionary terms, to be modified for other purposes.

Even before the vertebrates came on to land, the cartilage rods of the first arches had contributed to the evolution of jaws (Figure 14.1). The complex articulation of jaws in primitive terrestrial vertebrates later simplified, and this provided material for use in solving the problems of hearing in air rather than in water (Chapter 17).

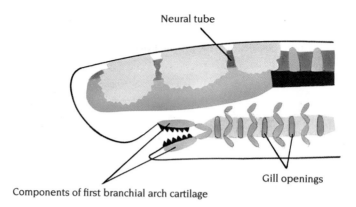

Neural tube

Gill openings

Components of first branchial arch cartilage

FIGURE 14.1 Formation of the jaw from the first branchial arch skeleton.

Growth and development of branchial arches in humans

The human branchial arches appear during a period of rapid growth of the face and head, so differential growth is a major factor behind the sequential changes described below (Figure 14.2). There are usually five, but sometimes six, identifiable pairs of arches, although only four at most are visible on the surface. They form in sequence during the early embryonic period, with the first pair appearing at about 24 days after fertilization and the remainder at approximately 2-day intervals thereafter. The five arches are conventionally numbered 1, 2, 3, 4 and 6; it is the fifth arch that is generally believed to be absent.

The first arch gives rise to the **maxillary prominence** (Figure 14.2). This may appear like a separate arch but is derived from the upper part of the cartilage core of the primitive first arch, which folds over during evolution (Figure 14.1).

In humans the openings between gills are never patent as they are in modern fish and our vertebrate ancestors (Figure 14.1). However, the ectoderm covering the head and the endoderm lining the mouth may approach each other very closely, with very little intervening mesoderm (Figure 14.3).

Cartilaginous fishes (sharks and rays) have exposed gills, while bony fish have evolved a gill cover – the operculum. Events crudely reminiscent of these are seen in humans; after the arches have formed, the second arch grows back to cover the others during the fifth week (Figure 14.4) and in normal circumstances will fuse completely over them.

Each arch possesses a core of cartilage, a blood vessel, a muscle component and its own innervation, which each possess a distinctive developmental history.

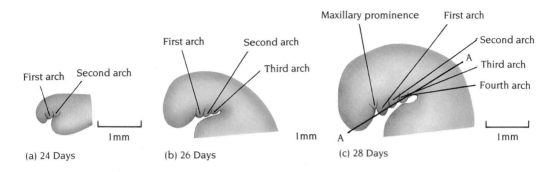

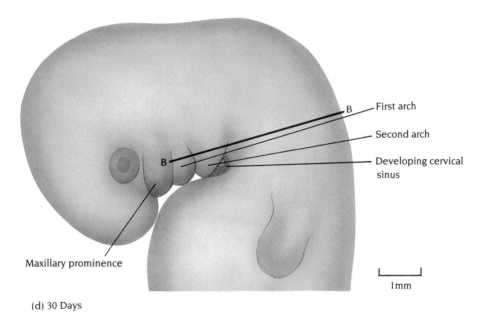

(d) 30 Days

FIGURE 14.2   Formation of the external branchial arches in the human. It is important to note the considerable amount of differential growth of the head during the embryonic period.

Derivatives of arch cartilage

The cartilage elements that form in the first three branchial arches are believed to arise from the neural crest cells of the midbrain and hindbrain. The remaining arch cartilages may derive from the arch mesoderm.

First arch

The cartilage core of the maxillary prominence once produced the upper jaw bone in evolutionary terms, but now it is believed to give rise only to a middle ear bone, the incus.

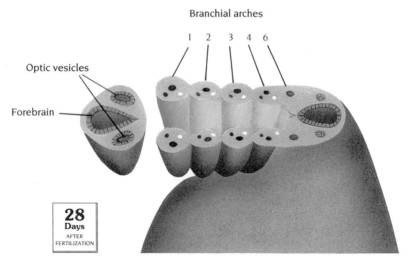

Branchial arches

1 2 3 4 6

Optic vesicles

Forebrain

28
Days
AFTER
FERTILIZATION

FIGURE 14.3 Section through line A–A on Figure 14.2.

The cartilaginous core of the ventral part of the first arch develops into a middle ear bone, the malleus, but also forms a long thin cartilage element (known as Meckel's cartilage) that will form the core of the mandible (Figure

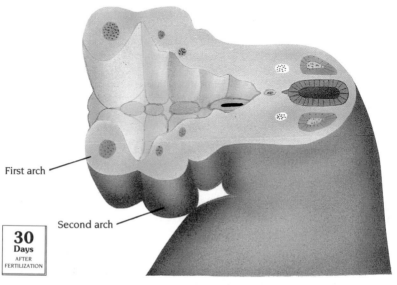

First arch

Second arch

30
Days
AFTER
FERTILIZATION

FIGURE 14.4 Section through line B–B on Figure 14.2.

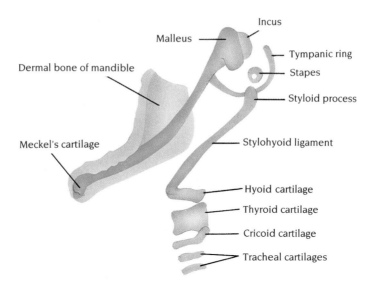

FIGURE 14.5 Cartilage derivatives of the branchial arches. Meckel's cartilage is being surrounded by dermal bone. The tympanic ring is also shown, although this is not derived from branchial arch cartilage.

14.5). The mandible will subsequently be enhanced by the condensation of dermal bone around Meckel's cartilage.

Second arch

The second arch cartilage gives rise to the stapes, the styloid process of the temporal bone, and part of the hyoid bone.

Third arch

The third arch cartilage produces the remainder of the hyoid.

Fourth and sixth arches

The fourth and sixth arches form the laryngeal cartilages, including the thyroid and cricoid cartilages.

Derivatives of arch muscle

Some head and neck muscles were once believed to derive from the mesoderm of the branchial arches but it now seems much more likely that all striated skeletal muscle comes from the paraxial mesoderm (see Chapter 8). Experiments using animal model systems have found that the somites of the head region do not reach their full differentiated state but are represented by somite-like bodies called somitomeres. These are the origin of the muscles in the head region, as shown by grafting experiments (Figure 14.6). There are good reasons to believe that this is also true in humans, although the facial muscles of the adult had previously been thought to arise from the branchial arches. It is possible that premyoblasts from the somitomeres make their way into the branchial arches before giving rise to the muscles indicated in Figure 14.6, and this may lend some degree of respectability to the conventional account.

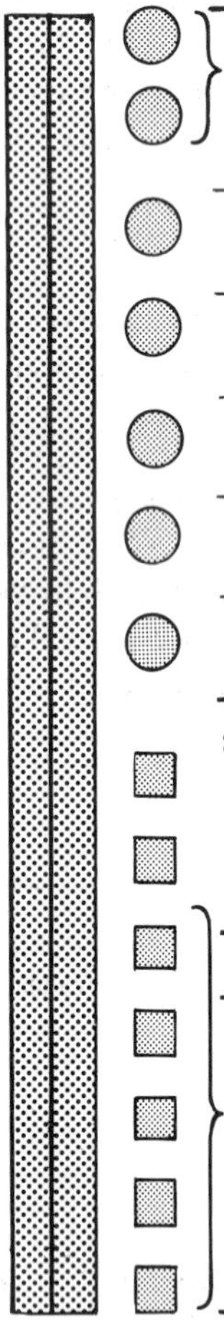

Somitomere	Gives rise to muscle(s)	Innervated by cranial nerve	Arch
1 2	Superior, inferior, and medial rectus	III (Oculomotor)	
3	Superior oblique	IV (Trochlear)	
4	Of mastication	V (Trigeminal)	1
5	Lateral rectus	VI (Abducent)	
6	Facial expression	VII (Facial)	2
7	Stylopharyngeus	IX (Glossopharyngeal)	3
Somite			4
1	Laryngeal muscles	X (Recurrent laryngeal branch of vagus)	
2	Palatoglossus	(Pharyngeal branch of vagus)	
		XI (Accessory)	
3–7	Tongue (except palatoglossus)	XII (Hypoglossus)	6

FIGURE 14.6 Muscle/somite/nerve relationships. This figure relates the head and neck muscles to the somites from which they originate. This clearly corresponds to the cranial nerves that supply them. The association between cranial nerves, muscles and branchial arches is a consequence of this relationship.

Nerves of the branchial arches

Altogether there are 12 cranial nerves, conventionally numbered I to XII (see Figure 14.6). Of these the special sensory nerves I, II and VIII (the olfactory, optic and otic nerves) are rather different from the others, and will be considered in Chapter 17.

The remaining nerves are conventionally divided into two series:

- nerves V, VII, IX, X and XI, which supply the branchial arches and
- nerves III, IV, VI and XII, which arise from the cells of the efferent column.

This division may reflect differences in later function, but probably does not reflect any differences at the time when the nerves originate. If the nerves in both series are listed with the muscles they supply (Figure 14.6), it is clear that they form one continuous segmented series, much like the nerves of the spine. This arrangement may reflect the primitive segmentation of the vertebrate head in evolutionary history: in other words, perhaps these are the nerves derived from the neuromeres of the brain.

The cranial nerves that supply the branchial arches are shown in Table 14.1 (see also Figure 14.7).

How do these cranial nerves become different from the other nerves in the original segmented cranial series? The answer is that streams of neural crest cells give rise to very substantial ganglia for these nerves (Chapter 11). For instance, cranial nerve V (the trigeminal nerve) is positioned near arch 1 (the maxillary prominence) and the eye. A large population of neural crest cells establishes this ganglion, making it much larger than the trochlear or abducent nerves on either side. However, this merely pushes the question back to an earlier stage: how do the neural crest cells know which ganglia to rally round in this way? The answer could lie in local expression of a particular set of genes in this region, as discussed in Special Topic 6 (pp. 174–7).

TABLE 14.1   Cranial nerves supplying the branchial arches.

Arch	1	2	3	4
Nerve	V	VII	IX	X and XI
Name	Trigeminal	Facial	Glossopharyngeal	Vagus

Blood vessels

Each arch attracts a blood vessel from the main system, as would be expected from the rules of interactive development (see Special Topic 5, pp. 153–7), but these blood vessels are not all present at the same time (Figure 14.7). They appear in sequence with the arches, but by the time the last arches appear the first blood vessels are already highly modified.

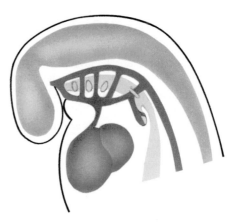

FIGURE 14.7 Indication of the aortic arch blood vessels. The pharyngeal pouches lie between the blood vessels.

Each pair of arches takes its supply from the outlet of the heart, the **aortic sac**. Blood runs cranially and dorsally through the arch blood vessels to the paired dorsal aortae and then caudally down the length of the body.

For the sake of simplicity all the blood vessels are shown as present at one time in Figure 14.8. Also shown are the seventh pair of somitic arteries, although a similar pair grows out between each pair of somites.

The lungs are growing ventrally and caudally from the foregut at this time (Chapter 20) and attract sprigs of blood vessels (which will in time be the pulmonary arteries) from the sixth arch arteries.

The blood vessels running through the first and second arches do not persist: their remnants become the stapedial and maxillary arteries. The arteries running through the third and fourth arches do persist, however (Figure 14.8), but the connection between the third and fourth at the level of the dorsal aorta vanishes. The blood now runs cranially to the head and neck from the third arch. On the right side, the connection between the pulmonary artery and the dorsal aorta also vanishes but it persists on the left. (This asymmetry between right and left is part of a very puzzling problem, discussed further in Special Topic 8, pp. 295–6.)

The stretch of the right dorsal aorta between the right seventh intersegmental artery and the meeting of the dorsal aortae also disappears.

At this time, septae begin to divide the cranial part of the primitive heart: these then twist as they proceed cranially (see Chapter 21). This is part of the process of septation of the heart, which alters the blood outflow so that the right ventricle supplies the pulmonary circulation. This circulation is largely short-circuited by the **ductus arteriosus**, as the remnant of the left sixth arch is called (see Chapter 7). At birth the ductus arteriosus becomes the **ligamentum arteriosum**. The seventh segmental arteries will become the left and right **subclavian arteries**. The left and right recurrent laryngeal nerves will adopt different routes on each

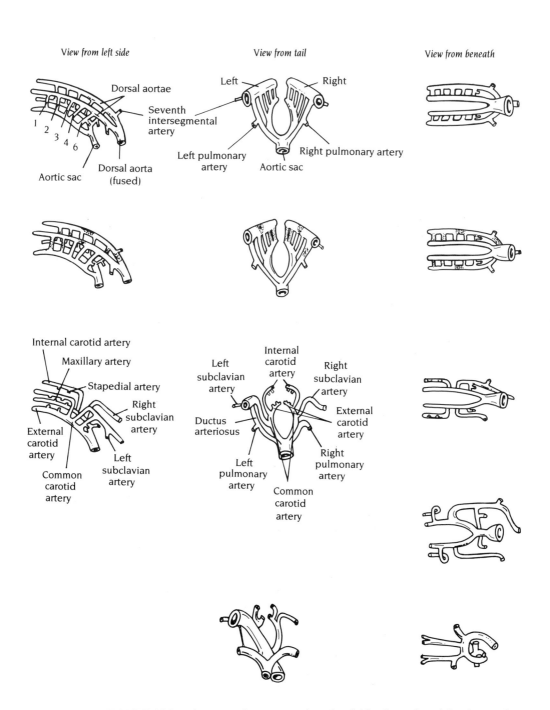

View from left side

View from tail

View from beneath

Dorsal aortae

Left

Right

Seventh
intersegmental
artery

1
2
3
4 6

Aortic sac

Dorsal aorta
(fused)

Left pulmonary
artery

Right pulmonary artery

Aortic sac

Internal carotid artery

Maxillary artery

Stapedial artery

Right
subclavian
artery

External
carotid
artery

Left
subclavian
artery

Common
carotid
artery

Left
subclavian
artery

Internal
carotid
artery

Right
subclavian
artery

Ductus
arteriosus

External
carotid
artery

Right
pulmonary
artery

Left
pulmonary
artery

Common
carotid
artery

FIGURE 14.8 Diagrammatic representation of arch blood vessels and the changes they
undergo.

side of the body because they initially loop round the sixth arch artery. However, because the sixth arch will disappear on the right hand side only, the course of the recurrent laryngeal nerves differs between left and right (Figure 14.8).

Defects of branchial arch development

A number of defects may arise. Those affecting the blood vessels are considered in Chapter 21. Those affecting other structures derived from the arches are best considered after the events involving the intervening pharyngeal pouches have been described in Chapter 15.

Further reading

De Beer G. (1937). *Development of the Vertebrate Skull.* Oxford: Oxford University Press

Friant M. (1958). Sur les premiers stades d'ossification du cartilage de Meckel. *Acta Anat.*, **32**, 100–14

Hamilton W.J., Boyd J.D. and Mossman H.W. (1962). *Human Embryology* 3rd edn. Cambridge: Heffer

Hildebrand M. (1982). *Analysis of Vertebrate Structure* 2nd edn. New York: John Wiley & Sons

Hughes G.M., ed. (1976). *Respiration of Amphibious Vertebrates.* New York: Academic Press

Noden D.M. (1984). Craniofacial development: new views on old problems. *Anat. Rec.*, **208**, 1–13

Noden D.M. (1986). Origins and patterning of craniofacial mesenchymal tissues. *J. Craniofac. Genet. Dev. Biol.*, **2**, 15–31

Noden D.M. (1988). Interactions and fates of avian craniofacial mesoderm. *Development*, **103** (suppl), 121–40

Piiper J. (1982). Respiratory gas exchange at lungs, gills and tissues: mechanisms and adjustments. *J. Exp. Biol.*, **100**, 5–22

15

Branchial grooves and pharyngeal pouches

As described earlier, the openings between the gill arches in fish are never normally patent in humans. They are represented by internal and external grooves. Seen from the outside these grooves are the **branchial grooves**: from the inside they are known as the **pharyngeal pouches** (Figure 15.1). They are numbered in accordance with the arch cranial to them. The ectoderm of the head and the endoderm from the foregut approach very closely between the arches, with almost no mesoderm in between.

A number of structures develop in the mouth and foregut region during the early embryonic period. Initially, the mouth opening is covered by the **oropharyngeal membrane**, which will rupture at about 24 days after fertilization. A viewpoint from just inside the mouth following this rupture, looking in a caudal direction, would reveal four pairs of alcoves in the sides of the foregut (Figure 15.2): these are the pharyngeal pouches. A number of protuberances in the floor of the mouth region will contribute to the formation of the tongue, as described in Chapter 16. A thickened plaque in the floor represents the first stage in thyroid development (see p. 205). Further along the foregut, a shallow trench runs craniocaudally in the midline of the floor: this is the beginning of lung development (see Chapter 20). In the roof, where the gut begins to curve, is a thickening of ectoderm. This will contribute to the formation of the pituitary gland, as described later in this chapter.

It is convenient to deal with the first branchial groove and first pharyngeal pouch together and then to consider the fate of the remaining branchial grooves before returning to the inside of the mouth to deal with the other pharyngeal pouches.

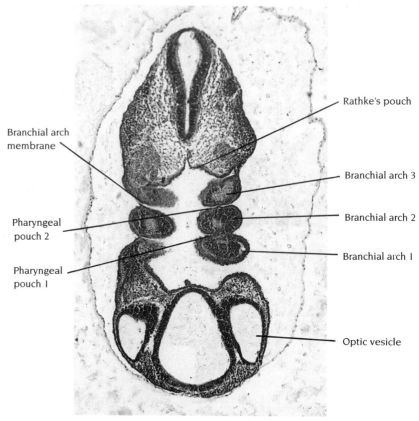

FIGURE 15.1 Section through branchial region of 27-day human embryo. Compare with Figure 15.2 for orientation.

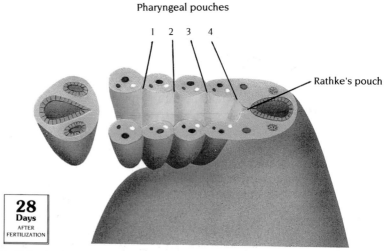

FIGURE 15.2 Section through branchial region of 28-day embryo. See also Figure 14.2.

Branchial groove 1 and pharyngeal pouch 1

As the head undergoes the rapid growth characteristic of this period the first pharyngeal pouch elongates into a large opening directed laterally (Figure 15.3). At its far end it will expand to form the **tubotympanic recess** and the connection with the foregut will then become the developing **auditory tube** (Figure 15.5(b)). The corresponding branchial groove also deepens and elongates. This will become the **external auditory meatus** (Figure 15.3), and by the fifth week after fertilization all of these structures are sufficiently well marked to be known by their definitive names. At this time the cartilaginous precursors of the middle ear bones are growing from neural crest cells in the mesoderm of arches 1 and 2 (as described in Chapter 14). The tubotympanic cavity will penetrate into these arches so that during the fetal period the cartilage rudiments become suspended in the recess. They are wrapped around by the endoderm that once lined the tubotympanic recess and have yet to ossify. The erosion of the mesoderm will continue dorsally, producing the rather variable spaces known as the **mastoid air cells** (see Chapter 17).

Branchial grooves 2–4

These grooves are covered over by the caudal growth of the second arch (Figure 15.3), in a manner reminiscent of the development of the gill cover in modern fish. Initially, this creates a space called the cervical sinus, which is usually obliterated by the beginning of week 7. This series of events may occur in an abnormal manner, causing cysts or sinuses (see below).

Inside the mouth

Pharyngeal pouch 2

The second pharyngeal pouch does not expand in the way that the first pouch does. The internal endoderm lining the alcove begins to divide, largely obliterating the lumen of the pouch. The endoderm also forms buds, which push into the underlying mesoderm (Figures 15.4 and 15.5(c)) and in turn hollow out to form crypts. During the early fetal period, the surrounding mesoderm becomes lymphoid: the structure thus formed is the **palatine tonsil**. Other tonsillar plaques form in a similar manner in the first pouch, on the tongue and on the dorsal wall of the foregut: these last structures are known as the **adenoids**.

Developing tubotympanic recess

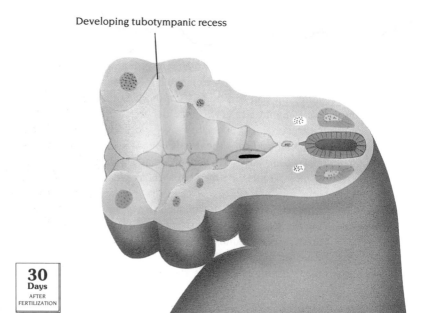

30 Days AFTER FERTILIZATION

FIGURE 15.3   Section through branchial arch region of 30-day embryo. Compare with Figure 14.4. See also Figure 15.5(b) for development of the first pharyngeal pouch.

Pharyngeal pouch 3

The dorsal and ventral parts of the third pair of pouches have different fates but at first each pouch gradually pinches off until it loses its connection with the gut (Figure 15.5(d)). Cell division in the endodermal wall then leads to the internal space being obliterated by week 6. The dorsal and ventral parts then separate. Both components will gradually change their position relative to the gut, probably because of differences in relative growth rate, rather than active burrowing through the surrounding tissues. In any case, both portions shift to more ventral and medial positions underneath the gut and become more caudal (Figures 15.5(d) and 15.6). The dorsal components develop into the **inferior parathyroid glands** in their new position. The ventral parts shift so far ventrally that, towards the end of the embryonic period, they meet in the midline: they will subsequently fuse to form the **thymus gland**. This is a large and important organ in the fetus, with a key role in the development of the immune system. Even after birth, the thymus may continue to grow; but it regresses at puberty.

Pharyngeal pouch 4

An initially similar series of events occurs with the fourth pouches (Figure 15.5(d)). After separation, the dorsal parts become the **superior parathyroids** (note that the third arch parathyroids have moved past those of the fourth arch to

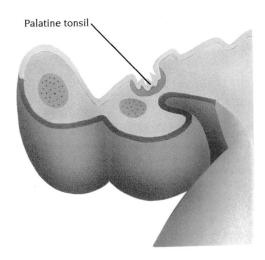

Palatine tonsil

FIGURE 15.4 The palatine tonsil is derived from the second pharyngeal pouch. See also Figure 15.5(c).

lie inferiorly in the adult) (Figure 15.6) and the ventral parts become the **ultimo-branchial bodies**. These fuse with the thyroid and provide the calcitonin-secreting cells (C cells). The C cells are believed to originate in the neural crest.

Thyroid

In evolutionary terms the thyroid is very ancient, at least as old as the gills. It controls growth by its secretions and is active from an early time in the embryo. The thyroid originates in the floor of the pharynx at about 24 days as a thickening of the endoderm in the midline between the left and right second arch. This gradually becomes a depression, which continues to deepen due to differential growth rates with neighbouring tissues. Eventually the depression will form the **thyroglossal duct** (Figure 15.6). The hyoid bone lies between the thyroglossal duct and the larynx.

By about 7 weeks the thyroid reaches its adult position inferior to the cricoid cartilage although, as the head lifts up in later development, it will come to lie even further from its origin. Two lobes generally form, but frequently a tail or 'pyramidal lobe' is also present. Small islands of accessory thyroid tissue may continue to develop along the path of the thyroglossal duct, or short regions of duct may remain patent. The origin of the thyroid in the tongue remains detectable as the **foramen caecum** or 'blind opening'.

Pituitary

This is first evident at 24 days as a thickening in the roof of the mouth opening, just external to the oropharyngeal membrane (Figure 15.6). This thickening will

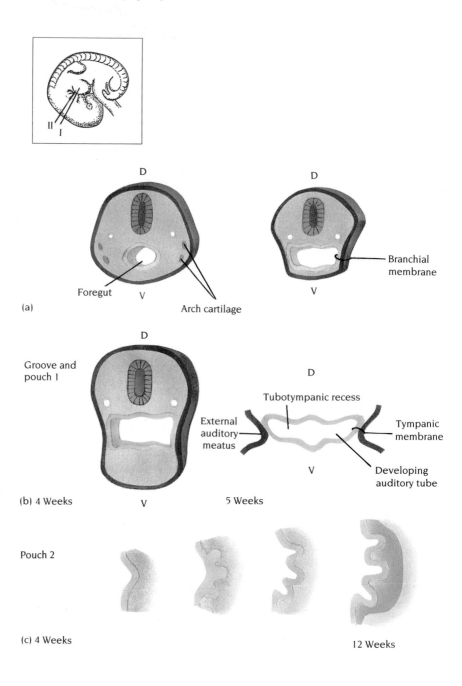

FIGURE 15.5 (a) Section through branchial arch (line marked I) and a similar section through first pharyngeal pouch II. (b) Expansion of first pouch to form tubotympanic recess. (c) Development of second pharyngeal pouch to give palatine tonsil. Rearrangement of the components of the third and fourth pharyngeal pouches.

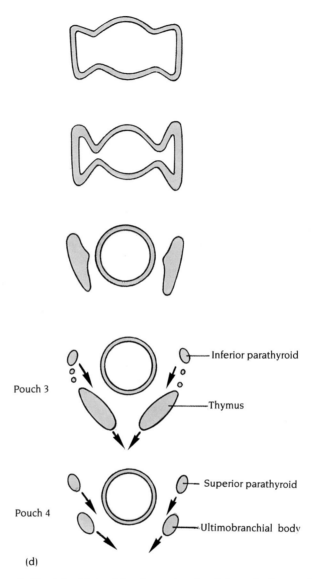

(d)

FIGURE 15.5 (*cont*) (d)   The third and fourth pouches detach from the foregut, filling in as they do so. The solid pouches now split into a dorsal and ventral component. In the third pouch, these form the inferior parathyroid and thymus rudiment respectively. Pouch four gives rise to the superior parathyroids and ultimobranchial bodies. These will move medially, ventrally and caudally (see Figure 15.6).

go on to form a pit (known as **Rathke's pouch**). After the membrane has ruptured, this pit marks the junction between the head ectoderm and the gut endoderm: as the oral cavity deepens it comes to lie further inside the mouth. The pit continues to extend in the direction of the diencephalon and will eventually lose

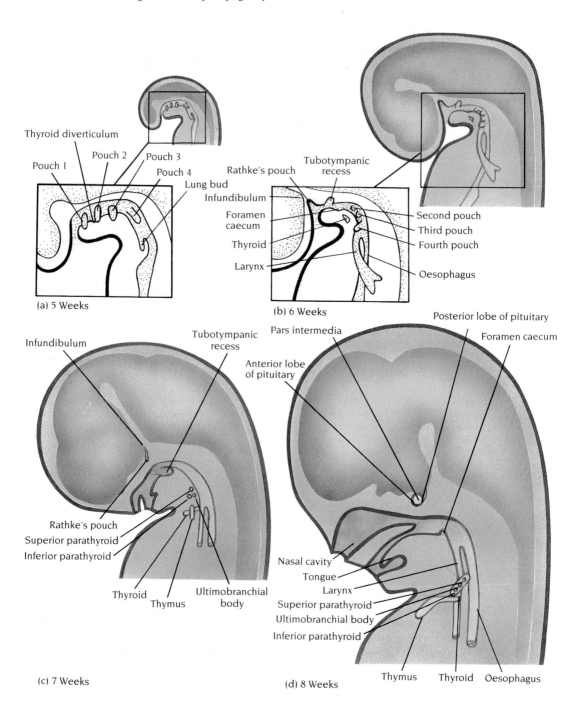

FIGURE 15.6 (a–d) Alterations in the position of the pharyngeal pouch and foregut derivatives. These shifts take place against a background of considerable relative growth.

its connection with the foregut. A downgrowth of the diencephalon, the **infundibulum**, descends towards the pouch and the two fuse at about 5 weeks. The pouch-derived part forms the anterior lobe of the hypophysis (or **adenohypophysis**), which gives rise to the **pars intermedia** and **pars tuberalis** of the adult pituitary; the brain-derived part becomes the **stalk** and **pars nervosa**. The sphenoid bone subsequently forms from chondrocranium underneath the pituitary and pituitary remnants are sometimes found ventral to this, in the pharyngeal tissue or occasionally even in the sphenoid bone.

Larynx

At about 28 days the laryngotracheal groove is present as an elongated depression or 'trench' running craniocaudally in the floor of the foregut, commencing at the level of the fourth branchial arches. However, in the foregut the **arytenoid swellings** will develop on either side of the cranial end of the laryngotracheal tube at about day 35 (see Figure 17.8) and will become the **arytenoid cartilages**. The epiglottal cartilages form much later, not until well into the fetal period. Although they appear in the general area of the fourth arch, they probably originate from lateral somatic mesoderm rather than from original arch cartilages. Two pairs of folds will develop inside the larynx: the **vestibular** or **vocal folds**.

At 10 weeks, the larynx is occluded by endodermal cells. It will recanalize later: if not, the rare condition known as persistent laryngeal web will occur.

Defects of the branchial grooves and pharyngeal pouches

Branchial sinus If the cervical sinus formed by the backward growth of the second arch is not completely obliterated, an external branchial sinus may be formed. This causes a discharge in the neck along the anterior border of the sternocleidomastoid muscle.

Branchial cyst If a branchial sinus has no external opening a branchial cyst will form. This appears as a painless, mobile, slowly enlarging mass in the neck in the same areas that external sinuses are found. In young children it may inhibit breathing. A cyst of this type may drain to the inside of the neck, often exiting at the palatine tonsil causing a persistent bad taste in the mouth.

Branchial fistula Alternatively the cyst may drain both to the outside and to the inside, forming a branchial fistula. This may result from infection or incomplete surgical removal of a cyst.

Accessory cartilage Accessory cartilage structures may develop from branchial arches. These are generally symptomless.

The incidence of these conditions is uncertain, because they are treated as minor procedures and are not centrally recorded.

Accessory glands It is clear from consideration of their development that accessory, often functional, remnants of pituitary, thymus and thyroid tissue may be found in characteristic ectopic sites. These may secrete material and could confuse surgery of the region.

Craniopharyngioma Of these remnants craniopharyngioma, arising from ectopic islands of pituitary tissue, is perhaps the most serious. A piece of pituitary tissue may be trapped underneath or within the chondocranium as it forms and may prove extremely difficult to remove completely.

Thymic agenesis (DiGeorge syndrome) The incidence of this is uncertain. It is believed to result from defective formation of the third and fourth branchial arches. A spectrum of defects results with very variable degrees of expression. The eyes may be further apart than normal, and the ears low set and abnormal; the thymus may be reduced or absent, as may the parathyroid glands; there may be abnormalities of the great vessels of the heart and of the heart itself. The reduction of the thymus leads to inadequate immune function and the child is prone to infections. The condition may be alleviated by transplantation of fetal thymus tissue. The absence of the parathyroids is compensated for by injections of hormones, calcium and vitamin D.

Further reading

Albers G.D. (1963). Branchial anomalies. *JAMA*, **183**, 399–409

Conley M.E., Beckwith J.B., Mancer J.F.K. *et al.* (1979). The spectrum of the Di George syndrome. *J. Pediatr.*, **94**, 883–90

Goodman R.M. and Gorlin R.J. (1977). *Atlas of the Face in Genetic Disorders* 2nd edn. New York: McGraw-Hill

Lobach D.F. and Haynes B.F. (1987). Ontogeny of the human thymus during development. *J. Clin. Immunol.*, **7**, 81–97

Moseley J.M., Matthews E.W., Breed R.H., Galante L., Tse A. and McIntyre I. (1968). The ultimobranchial origin of calcitonin. *Lancet*, **i**, 108–10

O'Rahilly R. (1978). The timing and sequence of events in the development of the human digestive system during the embryonic period proper. *Anat. Embryol.*, **153**, 123–35

O'Rahilly R. (1983). The timing and sequence of events in the development of the human endocrine system during the embryonic period proper. *Anat. Embryol.*, **166**, 439–51

Robinson H.B. (1975). DiGeorge's or the III–IV pharyngeal pouch syndrome: pathology and a theory of pathogenesis. In *Perspectives in Pediatric Pathology*, Vol. II (Rosenberg H.S. and Bolande R.P., eds), pp. 173–206. Chicago: Year Book Medical Publishers

Skandalkis J.E., Gray S.W. and Rowe J.S. (1983). *Anatomical Complications in General Surgery*. New York: McGraw-Hill

Weller G.L. (1933). Development of the thyroid, parathyroid and thymus glands in man. *Contrib. Embryol.*, **24**, 93–139

Zaw-Tun H.A. (1985). Re-examination of the origin and early development of the human larynx. *Acta Anat.*, **122**, 163–84

16

The face and palate

The development of the face and palate is complicated, and complex developmental events are more likely to go wrong than simple ones. As a result, approximately one in 600 children has a marked facial deformity. Although these are generally not life threatening, they have an effect out of all proportion to the clinical risk they represent, because we respond emotionally to faces and facial expression. Even minor variations such as the height of the brow or the distance between the eyes are taken to be associated with moral qualities such as intelligence, shiftiness, or frankness: the same is not asserted of, for instance, the kidneys. However, even in quite severe abnormalities the prognosis may be very good after repair: the face has a great capacity for regeneration. Operations to correct facial abnormalities have even been carried out before birth, when healing powers are at their maximum.

The facial prominences and their fusions

The face arises from five facial prominences in the embryo. At the beginning of the fourth week these prominences are marked out by grooves on the surface (Figure 16.1) but the grooves do not penetrate all the way through to the oral cavity. The prominence lying just in front of the forebrain is the **frontonasal**

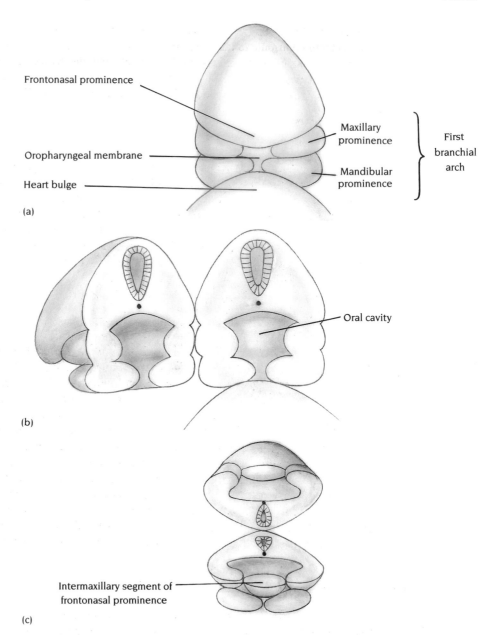

Frontonasal prominence

Maxillary prominence

First branchial arch

Oropharyngeal membrane

Mandibular prominence

Heart bulge

(a)

Oral cavity

(b)

Intermaxillary segment of frontonasal prominence

(c)

FIGURE 16.1 (a) The facial prominences early in the fourth week. In this view, the remaining branchial arches are hidden behind the heart bulge; (b) a section through (a) in the plane of the page has been hinged open to show the oral cavity from the inside; (c) a section through the maxillary prominence and frontonasal prominence, hinged upwards.

prominence. Neural crest cells migrate between the brain and the surface ectoderm and will contribute to the structures formed by the frontonasal prominence. The paired **maxillary prominences** lie cranial, and the paired **mandibular prominences** just caudal to, the mouth opening (Figure 16.1). Both sets of prominences are derived from the first branchial arch, as shown in Chapter 14.

Mouth

The opening of the mouth, the **stomodeum**, is initially covered by the **oropharyngeal** (or oral) **membrane**, consisting of ectoderm in contact with endoderm without intervening mesoderm (see p. 201). The hind end of the gut is similarly sealed off by the **cloacal membrane** (see p. 315). The gut and yolk sac are therefore at first sealed off from the amniotic cavity but the oral membrane ruptures towards the end of the fourth week, and the cloacal membrane a little later. The embryo is then able to swallow amniotic fluid. (Very rarely the oropharyngeal membrane may persist in whole or in part as an abnormality.)

Nose

At the end of the fourth week two thickenings develop in the ectoderm of the frontonasal prominence: the **nasal placodes** (Figure 16.2(a)). Subsequently, depressions (the **nasal pits**) begin to form as the placodes sink beneath the surface, possibly as a result of differential relative growth rather than active invasiveness. The walls of these pits are not quite complete in that there is an opening towards the mouth (Figure 16.2(b)). In a transverse section (Figure 16.2(c)), the walls appear as separate median and lateral 'prominences' or swellings, but they are in fact continuous from medial to lateral: their appearance as separate structures is therefore an artefact of the plane of section. Perhaps it is better to describe these swellings as the median and lateral parts of the **nasal rim**.

The nasal pits continue to deepen until they break through the frontonasal process into the oral cavity (Figure 16.2(d)). The walls will fuse in the midline to form the fleshy nasal septum; their lateral regions will form the alae of the nostrils.

Fusion of the prominences

The five prominences and their derivatives undergo a critical series of 'fusions' (Table 16.1). If these fail to occur, a corresponding defect will arise (see below). Because the elements are not truly separate from each other, but merely marked out by surface grooves for the most part, no ectodermal coverings are broken down. However, the defects that result from failure of even this degree of fusion may form complete patent clefts. A secondary breakdown of tissue must therefore occur in some manner.

The first fusion (during week 4) is that of the mandibular prominences in the midline (Figure 16.3). The developing mandibular elements lying inside each of

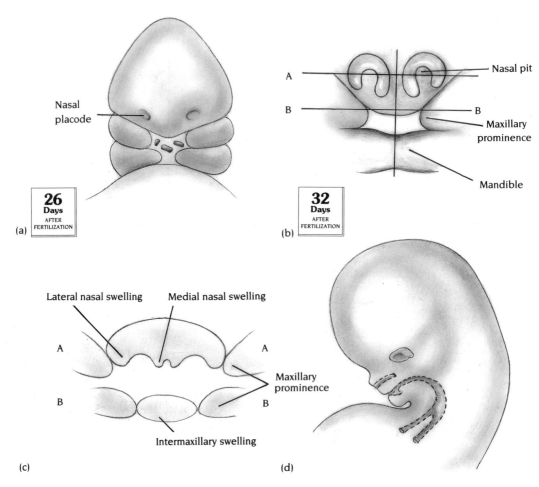

FIGURE 16.2 (a) The nasal placodes form on the frontonasal prominence and begin to sink in, forming an incompletely walled pit (b). Sections through the lines A–A and B–B show the appearance described as the medial and lateral nasal prominences (c). The pits continue to sink under the surface until they break through to the oral cavity (d).

TABLE 16.1 Fusions of the facial prominences.

Time after fertilization (weeks)	Fusion	Defect
4	Mandibular prominences	Median cleft of mandible or lower lip
5	Mandibular to maxillary prominences	Macrostomia/microstomia
5+	Maxillary to frontonasal prominences	Oblique facial cleft
5+	Medial nasal swellings	Median cleft of the upper lip
5+	Medial nasal swelling to lateral nasal swelling	Cleft lip
7+	Lateral palatine shelf	Secondary cleft palate
7+	Lateral palatine shelf to primary palate	Primary cleft palate
7+	Lateral palatine shelf to nasal septum	Secondary cleft palate

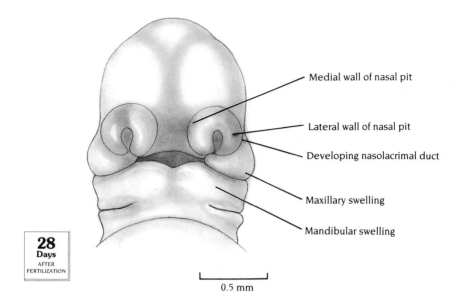

FIGURE 16.3   Development of the face during the later part of the fourth week.

the prominences also fuse to form a single mandible. Early in week 5 the mandibular prominences fuse to the maxillary prominences where they are in contact (Figure 16.4). Later in the fifth week the cranial edge of the maxillary prominence fuses to the lateral rim of the wall of the nasal pit, and to the remainder of the frontonasal prominence with which it is in contact. Along this line of contact a

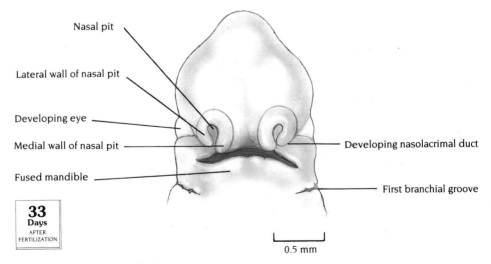

FIGURE 16.4   Development of the face during the fifth week.

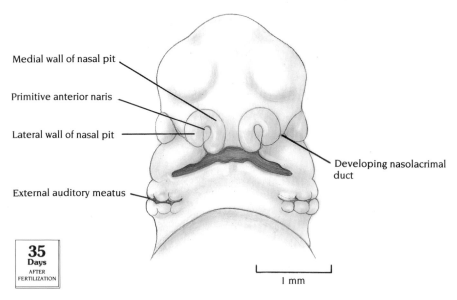

Medial wall of nasal pit

Primitive anterior naris

Lateral wall of nasal pit

Developing nasolacrimal duct

External auditory meatus

35 Days AFTER FERTILIZATION

I mm

FIGURE 16.5 Development of the face during the sixth week: the frontonasal prominence and maxillary prominences come in close contact before fusing.

cord of ectoderm forms and starts to sink beneath the surface. Eventually, it will detach from the surface ectoderm and forms a hollow tube underneath the surface,

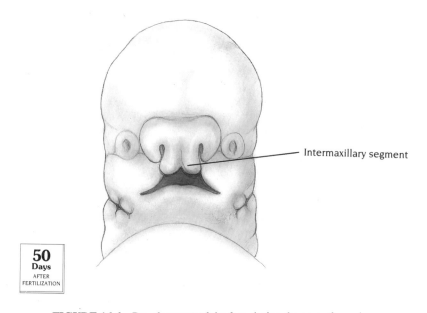

Intermaxillary segment

50 Days AFTER FERTILIZATION

FIGURE 16.6 Development of the face during the seventh week.

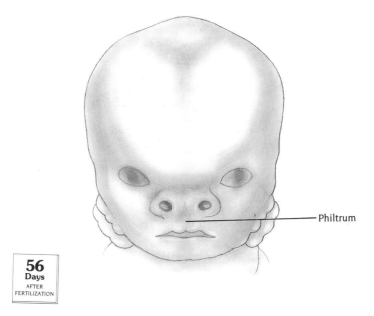

Philtrum

56
Days
AFTER
FERTILIZATION

FIGURE 16.7   The intermaxillary segment and the philtrum. See also Figures 16.1(c) and 16.2(c).

which will develop into the **nasolacrimal duct**. The end of the duct nearest the eye widens out to form the **lacrimal sac**. The lacrimal duct will drain internally into the nasal cavity. A little later as the nasolacrimal duct develops the medial parts of the walls of the nasal pits begin to fuse in the midline (Figures 16.5 and 16.6) and the wall of the nasal pit at the lateral aspects of the frontonasal prominence also fuses with the maxillary prominence (Figures 16.4 and 16.5).

Formation of the palate

Primary palate

That part of the frontonasal prominence which lies between the maxillary prominences is known as the **intermaxillary segment** (Figure 16.1). On the surface of the face this will form the **philtrum** of the lip (Figure 16.7); deep to this it forms the premaxillary part of the maxilla, which carries the incisor teeth, and the **primary palate**. The incisors therefore have separate evolutionary and developmental origins from the other teeth, and may undergo changes that the other teeth do not.

Secondary palate

The rest of the palate is derived from the maxillary prominences. **Lateral palatine shelves** develop on the inside (or oral cavity) aspect, pointing down ventrally to the floor of the mouth (Figure 16.8). At this time the tongue is forming

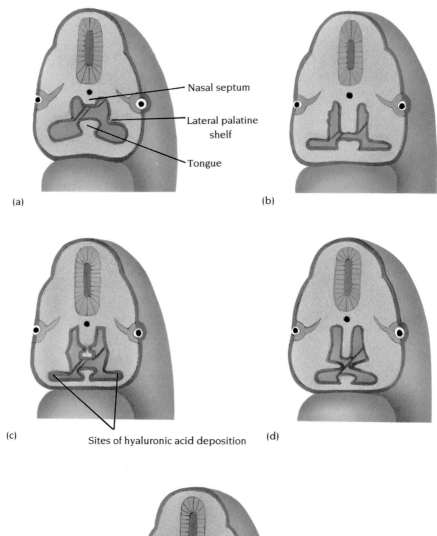

Nasal septum

Lateral palatine shelf

Tongue

(a)

(b)

(c)

Sites of hyaluronic acid deposition

(d)

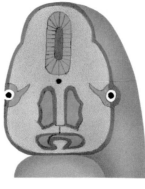

(e)

FIGURE 16.8 (a–e) Successive stages in the meeting and fusion of the palatal shelves.

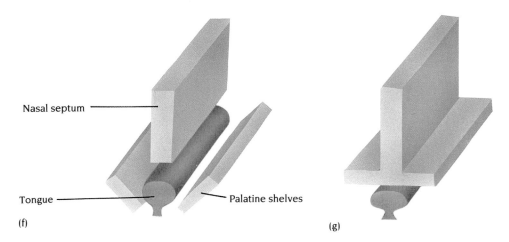

Nasal septum

Tongue

Palatine shelves

(f)

(g)

FIGURE 16.8 (*cont.*) The 'trapdoor'-like closure of the shelves is indicated in (f) and (g).

from protuberances in the floor of the pharynx and the **nasal septum** is growing down from the oral aspect of the frontonasal prominence. In the seventh week the palatine shelves swing up rapidly to meet in the midline (Figure 16.8). This process takes place very quickly even in developmental terms, and therefore cannot be due to cell division or cell movement alone. It could be caused by hyaluronic acid (produced by cells in the acute angle between the palatine shelves and the maxillary prominences) becoming hydrated and expanding rapidly, raising the shelves to their new position by physical pressure.

The palatine shelves fuse in the midline and with the intermaxillary segment at about 7 weeks in males and 8 weeks in females. The fusion is mediated by the underlying mesoderm (see Box 16.1). Any delay in the meeting of the shelves means that the critical period for fusion has passed and that the shelves will remain separate. This process is sensitive even to small errors in the timing of these interrelated events. The posterior part of the palatine shelves forms the uvula. The bony **hard palate** forms in the ventral part of the secondary palate by endochondral ossification. The **soft palate** develops in the dorsal part.

The nasal septum grows down from the frontonasal process and fuses with the secondary palate (Figure 16.8).

Box 16.1 Experimental analysis of palate development

It should by now be no surprise that light should be shed on human palate development by the study of animal model systems and, in the case of palate development, the improbable pairing of the mouse and the crocodile provides the required clues. The mouse undergoes a process of palatal fusion not unlike that in the human: the crocodile, by contrast, shows an anterior to posterior fusion pattern of the palatal shelves, with the ectoderm cells migrating away from the edge rather than dying in place. Histological study of the mouse palatal shelves reveals that the ectoderm covering them dies just before fusion, so that the fusion actually occurs between the mesoderm of the shelves. Crocodiles show no such ectodermal death over their palatal shelves.

Does the ectoderm die naturally in the mouse, or is it killed by the neighbouring tissue? Mouse palatal ectoderm can be combined in culture with crocodile palatal shelf mesoderm, and vice versa. In the combination of mouse mesoderm and crocodile ectoderm the ectoderm dies at the time appropriate for mouse development but in the combination of mouse ectoderm and crocodile mesoderm the mouse ectoderm, which would normally die, now survives. This indicates that the mesoderm somehow induces the death of the overlying ectoderm, and even hints that if the ectoderm does not die incomplete palatal fusion will ensue.

Defects of the face and palate

This series of fusion events represents a family of potential defects. If surface fusion fails to occur the groove may become patent all the way through to the oral cavity, resulting in a major clefting abnormality. Failure of fusion may be related to abnormal development of the rudiments.

Fusion defects may be triggered by an environmental factor but some individuals seem to have a hereditary predisposition. For example, some strains of rats have similar spontaneous rates of facial clefting but react very differently to the same teratogenic insult.

Anything that disturbs any part of the fusion process will throw the rest out of synchrony. For this reason, the same outcome may be generated by a number of different teratogens and, equally, a particular teratogen could generate a spectrum of defects (see Special Topic 9, pp. 369–74).

Because of genetic predisposition the frequency of defects varies considerably. If all the minor variants (such as cleft uvula) were identified, they might occur in approximately 100 per 10 000 live births, but these would not all be defects in the usual sense of the word. Overall, the incidence of serious facial clefts probably approaches 15 per 10 000 live births. An indication of the range of frequencies observed for particular conditions is given below.

Facial abnormalities are often present in association with other conditions, because a generalized insult or deficiency will affect many events simultaneously.

Cleft lip/cleft lip with cleft palate (Figure 16.9) Incidence of this condition is variable, as might be expected from the foregoing discussion: in Japan the incidence is 20 cases per 10 000 live births; among African Americans and Europeans it is five per 10 000. Sex differences may occur within a population, but there is no *overall* sex difference in incidence. The condition results from failure of the maxillary prominence and the frontonasal prominence (and its derivatives) to fuse completely. If the lateral wall of the nasal pit fails to fuse to the maxillary prominence there will be a cleft in the lip extending into the nostril. As the severity of the cleft increases, it may extend between the primary palate and the secondary palate (see anterior cleft palate, below). When this occurs the teeth on the intermaxillary segment may be very abnormal in their development, which results in marked difficulties with speech.

Cleft palate The incidence of cleft palate varies, but the median incidence is probably about 5–10 per 10 000 live births. It includes clefts of the

- **Anterior or hard palate** This condition arises if the primary palate fails to fuse with the lateral palatine shelves. It is often present in association with cleft lip, but can occur on its own. It may be unilateral or bilateral.
- **Posterior or soft palate** If the lateral palatine shelves fail to fuse to each other a midline cleft will develop in the soft palate. The defect frequently continues anteriorly. Mild forms of clefting may be present as cleft uvula.
- **Median cleft of the lower lip (or mandible)** This rare condition results from incomplete fusion of the mandibular processes.
- **Macrostomia (or lateral facial cleft)** This uncommon condition is apparent as a widening of the mouth, perhaps as a result of failure of surface fusion of the maxillary and mandibular prominences. It may be unilateral or bilateral. Its incidence is uncertain, but it may be as rare as one per 100 000 live births.
- **Oblique facial cleft** This is also a rare condition. It may result from a failure of the maxillary prominence to fuse to the frontonasal prominence. In this case the cleft will skirt the alae of the nose and run up towards the eye, perhaps leaving nasolacrimal tissue exposed on the surface. 'Oblique facial clefts' can also occur in other locations, and probably do not represent a fusion defect.
- **Median cleft of the upper lip** Again, this is a rare condition. Failure of complete fusion of the medial walls of the nasal pits may result in a cleft which may extend into the lip or the nose.

These last four conditions may be uncommon because the relevant facial prominences lie next to each other. Where there is a greater distance between prominences, the likelihood of defects is greatly increased.

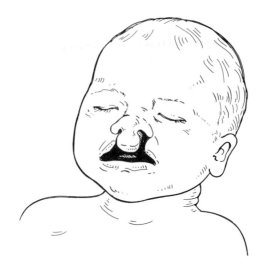

FIGURE 16.9   Bilateral cleft lip.

Median cleft of the face This condition is believed to arise from inadequate migration of neural crest to form the ectomesenchyme of the frontonasal process. The eyes are further apart than normal and a midline defect affects the bridge of the nose, sometimes extending as far as the frontal bones. These may not fuse properly, leading to the formation of a frontal encephalocoele. Whatever the initial cause of the defect, it is likely to be exacerbated by abnormal stress patterns generated on the remaining cartilage elements: a defective muscle, for instance, may exert a reduced pull on a cartilage element or bone, thereby altering its shape.

Further reading

Ferguson M.W.J. (1988). Palate development. *Development*, **103** (suppl), 41–60

Gorlin R.J., Pinborg J.J. and Cohen M.M. Jr. (1976). *Syndromes of the Head and Neck* 2nd edn. New York: McGraw-Hill

Hall B.K. (1982). Mandibular morphogenesis and craniofacial malformations. *J. Craniofacial Genet. Dev. Biol.*, **2**, 309–30

May H. (1962). Transverse facial clefts and their repair. *Plast. Reconstr. Surg.*, **29**, 240–9

Noden D.M. (1984). Craniofacial development:new views on old problems. *Anat. Rec.*, **208**, 1–13

Poswillo D. (1988). The aetiology and pathogenesis of craniofacial deformity. *Development*, **103**, 207–12

Pratt R.M. and Christiansen R.L., eds (1980). *Current Research Trends in Prenatal Craniofacial Development*. New York: Elsevier, North-Holland

Wedden S.E., Ralphs J.R. and Tickle C. (1988). Pattern formation in the facial primordia. *Development*, **103**, 31–40

Box 16.1

Ferguson M.J.W. and Honig L.S. (1984). Epithelial–mesenchymal interaction during vertebrate palatogenesis. In *Current Topics in Developmental Biology 19: Palate Development: Normal and Abnormal, Cellular and Molecular Events.* (Zimmerman E.F., ed.), pp 137–64. New York: Academic Press

17

The sense organs

The sense organs have an essential similarity of function in that they are all based around systems that detect external influences (albeit of many different kinds) and transduce these influences into nerve impulses. The nerve impulses are transmitted into the brain, which uses them to construct a model of the outside world. However, the sense organs carry out these functions via a wide variety of forms. Generally, the delicate primary detection systems are assisted and protected by a variety of secondary structures.

Humans are sensitive only to some of the possible stimuli available. Some animals can see in the infra-red or ultra-violet parts of the spectrum, others have remarkable capabilities for odour detection, or can respond directly to electromagnetic fields.

Sight

EVOLUTION

When light detection systems evolved in the central nervous system of vertebrates they did so on the inner aspect of the neural tube rather than the outer. This may imply that the vertebrates were rather small and transparent at that time. As vertebrate size increased special outpushings of the brain were required to keep the light-sensitive cells near the surface and the skin over these outpushings had to be transparent. Quite simple thickenings in the ectoderm would act as a lens, and the outpushings became concave so that the image thus formed would be in focus. Undoubtedly increasing complexity went hand in hand with increasing development of the brain to process the information gathered. When dinosaurs ruled the earth, our mammalian ancestors were forced to become nocturnal. Rapid response to light was therefore not necessary, and iris closure was achieved by smooth muscle rather than by the faster-acting striated muscle used by dinosaurs. However, birds, like the dinosaurs from which they are descended, still have striated irideal muscles.

Development

Even before the neural tube has closed cranially at about day 24 the forebrain has developed paired outpushings – the optic sulci (see Figure 12.2). As the forebrain closes these produce projections from the brain: the **optic vesicles** (Figure 17.1(a)). Gradually each vesicle indents to form an **optic cup** and the connection with the brain becomes relatively narrower to become the **optic stalk** (Figure 17.1(b,c)). The optic cup lies close to the surface ectoderm and at about 30 days after fertilization this ectoderm begins to thicken and develop the **lens placode** (Figure 17.1(b)). Subsequently, the placode will sink in and pinch off to form the hollow **lens vesicle** (Figure 17.1(c)) and finally the **lens** (Figure 17.2). The optic vesicle is involved in inducing lens formation (see Box 17.1). The ectoderm overlying the lens gives rise to the transparent **cornea**.

The lens

The cells of the lens vesicle nearest the optic cup elongate to form the primary lens fibres, which gradually obliterate the cavity of the lens vesicle. The 'anterior' epithelial cells on the corneal face of the lens will produce secondary lens fibres that wrap around the primary fibres. The fibre cells produce lens crystallins and cease to divide as they differentiate. In consequence, the core of the adult lens contains material laid down before birth.

Blood supply

The growing lens is supplied by the **hyaloid artery**, a branch of the **ophthalmic artery** (Figure 17.3(a)). This and its companion vein lie ventral to the optic stalk. As the stalk expands it encloses the artery and vein, which are then said to lie in the **optic fissure** (Figure 17.3(b)). This will largely close up, trapping the artery and vein in the optic stalk.

The stalk of the optic cup will become the **optic nerve**, as axons grow back down it from the inner layer of the optic cup. As a result the hyaloid artery and vein (now known as the central artery and vein) run in the middle of the optic nerve. The central artery also supplies the inner layer of the optic cup. As the

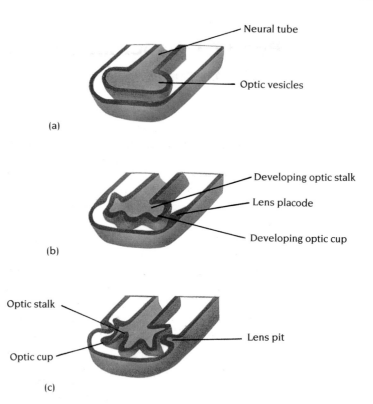

FIGURE 17.1 (a–c) The development of the optic vesicle and the lens.

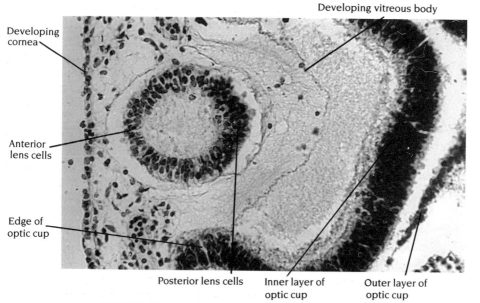

FIGURE 17.2 Human lens after budding from the surface.

Box 17.1 Experimental analysis of lens development

It is obviously essential that the lens and the retina should form in the correct relationship, and it is therefore to be expected that the lens and the optic cup will interact during their development. In amphibian embryos, where the appropriate developmental stages are easily studied, early removal of the optic cup prevents a lens being formed, and combination of the optic cup with early ectoderm from other sites results in formation of a lens from that ectoderm. From these results it was concluded that the optic cup 'instructs' the ectoderm specifically to form a lens. This was viewed as an *induction* event. As it could be shown that the ectoderm responds to the optic cup even if a filter is placed between them, a specific diffusible molecule was thought to carry the instructive information.

However, the situation proved to be more complex. The ability to induce and be induced decreases with developmental age. In amphibian embryos maintained at low temperatures, lenses could form even in the absence of optic cups. In experimental situations lenses could also be induced from ectoderm by tissues from nearby regions, and even by non-embryonic tissues such as boiled liver and heart. Similar results were obtained using avian and mammalian embryos.

It is possible to interpret all these results consistently. Early ectodermal cells have the option of differentiating into a number of cell types, including lens cells. A variety of influences, which need not be highly specific in themselves, can act to select one of these outcomes. In the natural situation the near and continued presence of one source of such influences, the optic cup, results in the development of a lens in the appropriate place.

This ability of ectoderm to respond to influences may decrease with time, perhaps because the cells come under the influence of other signals and make other choices. However, it need not be lost entirely: in many species of newt a lens will regenerate if the normal lens is removed. Surprisingly, the new lens is formed not from the head ectoderm but from the pigmented retinal epithelium. Although birds and mammals will not regenerate a lens spontaneously, the corresponding pigmented retinal cells can, in culture, become lens cells. Of course, retinal cells originate from the ectoderm via the neural tube and forebrain and seem to retain developmental plasticity in this regard.

Once the lens develops, it induces the overlying ectoderm to become the transparent cornea. It also reciprocally affects the retina; without a lens the retina becomes abnormal. These interactions mean that failure of any one step could lead to sequential failure in others, resulting in conditions such as **microphthalmia**, where the eye is smaller than normal.

The underlying molecular mechanisms for these events have remained obscure for many decades. However, evidence is accumulating that they are moderated by the action of growth factors (see Special Topic 10, pp. 384–5): for instance, fibroblast growth factor modulates lens fibre differentiation, while lens growth and transparency are controlled by platelet-derived growth factor.

Although the basis for induction of the inner ear is not well understood, it could operate in the same way as eye development.

lens cells gradually cease to divide the lens loses its blood supply, although a remnant may be observed in some adults.

Retina

The optic cup forms the **retina** (Figure 17.4). The outer layer becomes pigmented and the light receptors lie in the inner layer, but rather perversely light must pass through the cell bodies to reach them. The pigmented layer absorbs stray light: on the same principle cameras generally have black internal surfaces. An intraretinal space lies between the neural and pigmented layers until the end of the fifth week after which the layers become very closely apposed, but could easily come apart again – after a blow to the head, for instance. This is described as a detached retina.

Epithelium

The edge of the optic cup forms the **iris epithelium** and the **ciliary epithelium** (hence the dilator and sphincter muscles are derived, remarkably, from neurecto-

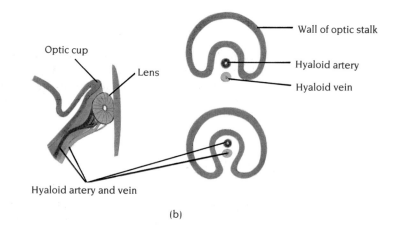

(a)   (b)

FIGURE 17.3 (a,b) The lens vascularization runs in the optic fissure and becomes the hyaloid artery and vein.

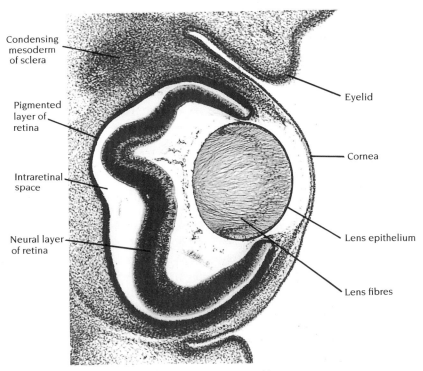

FIGURE 17.4   Later view of retina and lens.

derm). Mesoderm begins to condense around the stalk and pigment layer, forming an inner vascular layer and an outer fibrous layer. These are the continuations of the pia-arachnoid mater and the dura mater of the brain, respectively (see Chapter 6).

Eyelids

The eyelids appear as ectodermal folds containing mesoderm at 6 weeks after fertilization. These folds fuse at about 10 weeks, completely covering the eye, and separate at about 26 weeks. Eyelashes develop in the lid margins.

Hearing and balance

Hearing requires the transduction of compression waves in air into nerve impulses, and this is achieved by means of cells with delicate hairs on their surface. When these hairs are deflected the cell membrane depolarizes to initiate a nerve impulse. The hairs project into a fluid-filled space which in mammals is some way from the surface of the head; complex structures have therefore evolved to transmit sound from the outside to the hearing apparatus.

The same system is used to provide information on spatial orientation of the head, giving rise to the sense of balance.

EVOLUTION

In modern fish, like our marine ancestors, movement relative to the surrounding water is detected via the lateral line – a trough or channel running along the length of the animal. This channel contains hair cells, which fire nerve impulses when deflected. If part of the channel is closed off the animal is able to distinguish its movement relative to its environment from movement of the environment relative to itself (for example pressure waves in the water).

*This system works well in water, where vibrations have low amplitude and high energy, but in air vibrations have large amplitude and low energy, so they cannot readily pass through intervening tissue (also the lateral line system cannot operate effectively in air: the delicate hair cells operate best in a fluid environment). So in terrestrial animals hearing and detection of movement are both carried out in a sealed fluid-filled pouch (the **inner ear**) deep to the surface.*

The branchial grooves and pharyngeal pouches were also available for modification in air-breathing animals, so the first groove and pouch were adapted to help conduct sound to this deep pouch. The closely apposed ectoderm and mesoderm of the groove formed a membrane which vibrates as air moves, transmitting impulses via bones to the inner ear. In amphibians this is achieved by a single bone: mammals have a more sophisticated system in which a series of small bones act as levers in reverse to convert the low-energy, high-amplitude pressure waves found in air to high-energy, low-amplitude waves reminiscent of those in water. These bones are modified jaw articulation elements (see Chapter 14 and Figure 13.1).

Development of the hearing apparatus

Early in week 4 a thickening – the **otic placode** – forms on each side of the head (Figure 17.5(a–c)), possibly in response to signals from the underlying brain. Later during this week the **otic pits** develop from the placodes, which in turn become the **otic vesicles**.

Middle and inner ear

As indicated in Chapter 15, the first pharyngeal pouch forms the tubotympanic recess, which expands to form the middle ear cavity and the auditory tube. The apposed endoderm and ectoderm between the pouch and the groove will contribute to the **tympanic membrane**.

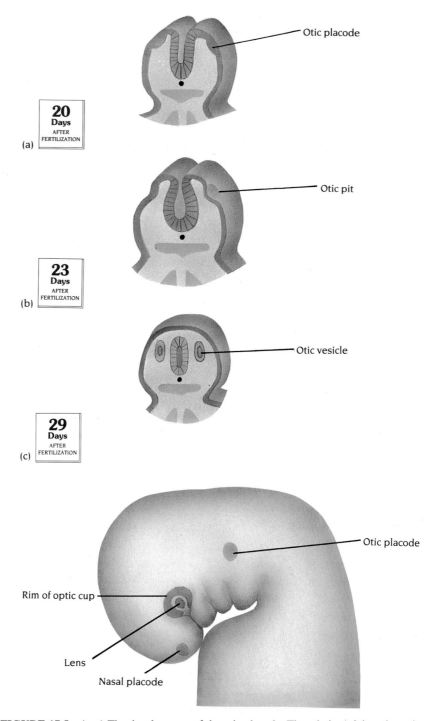

FIGURE 17.5   (a–c) The development of the otic placode. The relation of the otic vesicle to the other sensory structures is shown in (d).

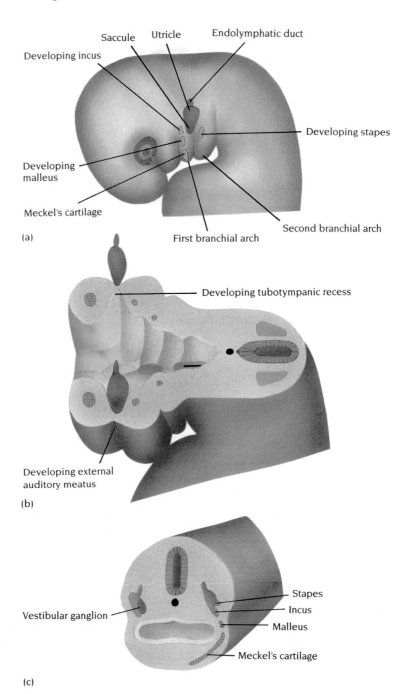

Saccule   Utricle   Endolymphatic duct

Developing incus

Developing stapes

Developing
malleus

Meckel's cartilage

(a)   First branchial arch

Second branchial arch

Developing tubotympanic recess

Developing external
auditory meatus

(b)

Stapes
Incus
Vestibular ganglion
Malleus

Meckel's cartilage

(c)

FIGURE 17.6   Later development of otic placode. (a)–(c) The developing placode in relation to the branchial arches and their cartilages.

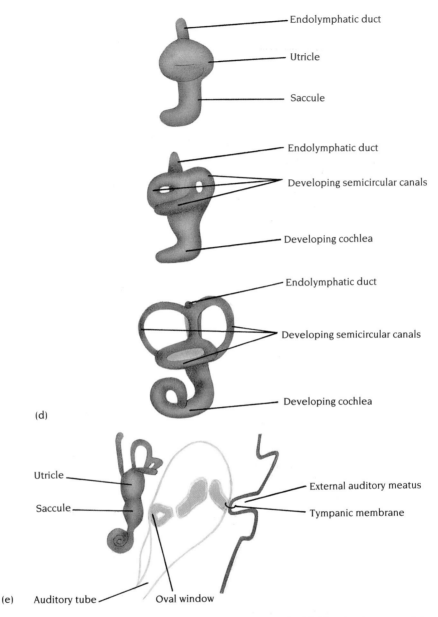

FIGURE 17.6 *(cont.)* Later development of otic placode. (d) The development of the inner ear. (e) The later development of the inner ear in relation to the middle air cavity and external auditory meatus.

Over the next few weeks (up to week 8) the cartilaginous precursors of the middle ear bones form from neural crest cells in the first and second branchial arches, and the morphology of the otic vesicle develops in a complex manner

(Figure 17.6). Two distinct regions become recognizable: the more dorsal is known as the **utricle**, and the more ventral as the **saccule** (Figure 17.6(d)). A long process, the **endolymphatic duct**, extends from the utricle. Three flat, mutually orthogonal projections grow out from the utricle: these will hollow out to become the **semicircular canals**. A long coiled tube from the saccule becomes the **cochlea** (Figure 17.6(d)). Meanwhile, in the same way as mesoderm condensed round the brain to give the dura mater or round the optic cup to give sclera, so it condenses round the inner ear and begins to ossify. In the cochlear region two windows (the oval and round windows) persist to provide access to the inner ear.

The tubotympanic recess expands into the branchial arches to include the middle ear ossicles; as a result these are covered in endoderm. The **temporal ring** surrounds the external auditory meatus, but is initially incomplete and small. The **mastoid antrum** will also expand, and air cells will form in late fetal and postnatal life: these are lined with endoderm. Gradually the bony covering of the inner ear will become locked into the temporal bone.

The external auditory meatus becomes occluded following division of the lining cells, but reopens during fetal life: failure to do so results in congenital deafness.

External ear

The external ear develops from the **auricular hillocks**. Six of these form round the first branchial groove and are derived from the first and second arches (Figure 17.7).

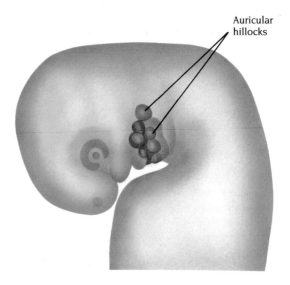

Auricular
hillocks

FIGURE 17.7 Development of the external ear.

Smell

Smell is the detection of airborne chemicals. A 'shaped' receptor on the cell surface is thought to initiate a nerve impulse when it is occupied by a molecule of appropriate shape, which runs to the olfactory bulb of the brain.

EVOLUTION

These tissues are very ancient, as might be expected. Patches of specialized and thickened ectoderm bearing the receptors formed in the head region, and frequently sank in to form nasal pits. Molecules would circulate inside these pits so that they had more time to bind to the receptor. This arrangement is still found in many vertebrate species; however, in higher vertebrates the pits break through into the primary oral cavity, as described in Chapter 16.

Development

The nasal placode forms a pit, which in turn becomes a channel to the oral cavity (see Figure 16.2(d)). The nasal septum grows down into the oral cavity and meets the palatine shelves, thus dividing the primary oral cavity into communicating oral and nasal cavities. The cells bearing receptors for smell develop in patches of specialized epithelium inside the nasal cavities. Olfactory nerve fibres are unique in that they grow *from* this nasal epithelium *to* the brain, and are therefore derived from oral ectoderm rather than from the nervous system. The cribriform plate subsequently develops *around* these fibres, giving it the characteristic sieve-like structure for which it is named.

Vomeronasal organs on the nasal septum develop – these are associated with sex scents in most mammals: in humans they generally degenerate, but may persist in some individuals.

Choanae or ledges appear on the lateral walls of the nasal cavity to create turbulence, and retain air for longer. The cavity walls secrete mucus, in which trace molecules will dissolve and remain longer in the vicinity of the cell receptors.

Taste

The sense of taste is believed to operate in essentially the same way as the sense of smell, although it is more limited in its capabilities.

EVOLUTION

Taste and smell are related in evolutionary terms. Patches of specialized epithe-lium are often found outside the mouth in lower vertebrates: however, in humans they are confined to the dorsal surface of the tongue.

Development

Towards the end of the fourth week after fertilization, three protrusions begin to form in the midline of the floor of the mouth.

- The more cranial of these, lying between the caudal ends of the first branchial arch, is known as the **tuberculum impar**.
- The **copula** lies between the second branchial arches.
- The third bud, lying between the ends of the third and fourth arches, is the **hypobranchial eminence** (Figure 17.8), which soon overgrows the copula.

The medial parts of the first branchial arches, known as the medial or distal **tongue buds**, overgrow the tuberculum impar. Hence the anterior two-thirds of the tongue in the adult arise from the median parts of the first arch. The tuberculum impar makes only a small contribution to this part of the tongue. The foramen caecum, marking out the origin of the thyroid gland, lies just behind the tuberculum. The posterior third of the tongue derives from the hypobranchial eminence.

Innervation

Since the anterior part of the tongue largely develops from the first branchial arch it is supplied by the trigeminal nerve (mandibular division). The posterior part of the tongue is supplied by the nerve of the third arch, the glossopharyngeal nerve, because the third arch has overgrown the second.

The tongue also contains striated skeletal muscle that has migrated forward from the occipital somites, which is supplied by the hypoglossal nerve: the palatoglossus, however, is supplied by the pharyngeal branch of the vagus nerve.

Separation from floor of mouth

The tongue gradually separates from the floor of the mouth as the grooves on either side begin to deepen. In the midline a line of tissue, the **frenulum**, remains to connect the tongue to the floor. If this persists in an extensive form (tongue-tie), the child has difficulty in speaking.

Taste receptors

Taste receptors are found in crypts in the tongue known as **taste buds**. Taste buds are directly induced from tongue epithelium by nerve fibres. Because the epithelium is derived from the branchial arches the innervation of the taste buds

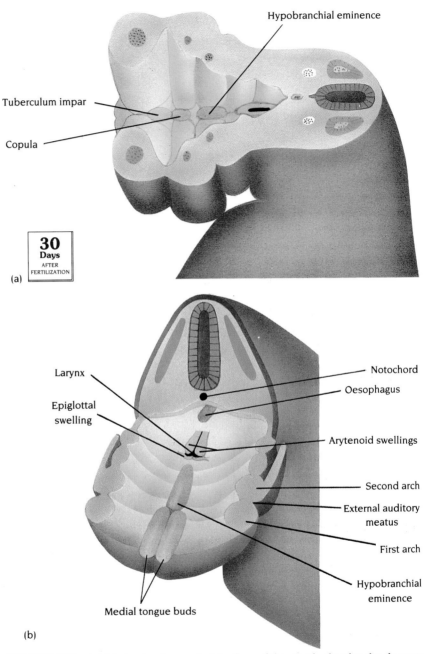

FIGURE 17.8 (a,b) Later development of the floor of the mouth, showing the elements that will contribute to the tongue.

on the anterior two-thirds of the tongue is supplied by the lingual branch of the mandibular division of the trigeminal nerve. The posterior third is supplied by the chorda tympani (a branch of the facial nerve).

If the nerve supplying a taste bud is cut the taste buds will degenerate but if the nerve regrows to another part of the tongue the epithelial cells will redifferentiate into a taste bud.

Defects of the eye and ear

The European baseline incidence of eye abnormalities is about six per 10 000 live births, although again, this may vary – Glasgow has an incidence of twice this figure.

Irideal coloboma If the optic fissure fails to close a gap persists. This is described as a coloboma.

Microphthalmia In this condition one or both eyes may be reduced in size.

External ear defects Defects arising from incorrect fusion of the auricular hillocks are not uncommon, but may not cause hearing loss. The European incidence is in the region of 6–7 cases per 10 000 live births. Hearing defects are reported as only one or two per 100 000 live births, but are rarely diagnosed until infancy and therefore are not recorded as congenital abnormalities. Their incidence is almost certainly much higher than this.

Further reading

Davis J.A. and Dobbing J., eds (1974). *The Scientific Basis of Paediatrics*. Philadelphia: W.B. Saunders

Gasser R.F. (1982). *Atlas of Human Embryos*. Hagerstown, MD: Harper & Row

Hamilton W.J., Boyd J.D. and Mossman H.W., (1962). *Human Embryology* 3rd edn. Cambridge: Heffer

Hildebrand M. (1982). *Analysis of Vertebrate Structure* 2nd edn. New York: John Wiley & Sons

Kanagasuntheram R. (1967). A note on the development of the tubotympanic recess in the human embryo. *J. Anat.*, **101**, 731–41

O'Rahilly R. (1963). The early development of the otic vesicle in staged human embryos. *J. Embryol. Exp. Morph.*, **11**, 741–55.

O'Rahilly R. and Muller F. (1987). *Developmental Stages in Human Embryos*. Carnegie Institution of Washington Publication, **637**

Proctor B. (1964). The development of the middle ear spaces and their surgical significance. *J. Laryngol. Otol.*, **78**, 631–42

Box 17.1

Brewitt B. and Clark J.I. (1988). Growth and transparency in the lens, an epithelial tissue, stimulated by pulses of PDGF. *Science*, **242**, 777–9

Chamberlain C.G. and McAvoy J.W. (1989). Induction of lens fibre differentiation by acidic and basic fibroblast growth factor. *Growth Factors*, **1**, 125–34

Clayton R.M. (1970). Problems of differentiation in the vertebrate eye. *Curr. Top. Dev. Biol.*, **5**, 115–80

Clayton R.M., Thompson I. and De Pomerai D.I. (1979). Relationship between crystallin mRNA expression in retina cells and their capacity to re-differentiate into lens cells. *Nature*, **282**, 628–9

Cuny R. and Malaconski G.M. (1986). Axolotl retina and lens development: mutual tissue stimulation and autonomous failure in the eyeless mutant retina. *J. Embryol. Exp. Morph.*, **96**, 151–70

Hay E. and Meier S. (1976). Stimulation of corneal differentiation by interaction between cell surface and extracellular matrix. II. Further studies of the nature and site of transfilter 'induction'. *Dev. Biol.*, **57**, 141–57

Jacobson A.G. (1966). Inductive processes in embryonic development. *Science*, **152**, 25–34

Karkinen-Jaaskelainen M. (1978). Permissive and directive interactions in lens induction. *J. Embryol. Exp. Morph.*, **44**, 167–79

Reyer R.W. (1977). The amphibian eye: development and regeneration. In *Handbook of Sensory Physiology, Vol. VII/5. The Visual System in Vertebrates* (Cressetali, F., ed.), pp. 309–90. Berlin: Springer-Verlag

LIMBS

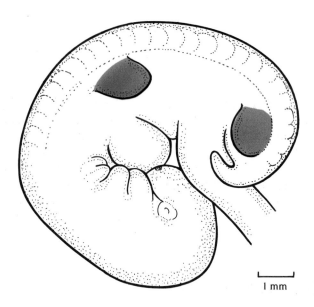

1 mm

18

The limbs

Defects of limb development are the most common single category of birth abnormality observed in Europe: nearly a quarter of all defects fall under this heading. Development of the limbs is therefore of major clinical importance. In addition, limb development is of great general interest because the limb displays all the main features of development – growth, differentiation and the formation of spatial patterns in a structure that is not essential to survival, and which can be experimented upon with comparative ease. Limb development has therefore been used as a study system for general developmental mechanisms.

Human limb development

Essentially, all the key events in limb development occur during the embryonic period, by the end of which a miniature version of the limb has formed, although it has to grow and mature and the cartilage elements have to be replaced by bone.

External appearance

The limbs appear as buds growing out from flanks at the beginning of the embryonic period. In humans the arm buds appear first and continue to develop

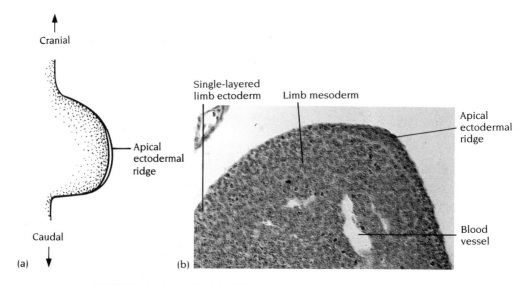

FIGURE 18.1 (a) Profile of human limb bud; (b) section through equivalent chick embryo limb bud showing the apical ectodermal ridge.

a little before the legs. This is sometimes ascribed to the proximity of the upper limbs to the heart, but in some vertebrates the legs grow faster than the arm.

The limb buds are composed of a layer of ectoderm containing somato-pleural mesoderm, which is at first quite undifferentiated. The ectoderm is mainly in the form of a layer one cell thick covering the mesoderm. However, it is raised at the tip into a ridge several cells thick: this is known as the **apical ectodermal ridge** (AER) (Figure 18.1).

The limb gradually elongates and the distal end becomes paddle-shaped (Figure 18.2). At about 38 days after fertilization in the arm and at 44 days in the leg grooves appear between the sites of digit formation, and will eventually sep-arate. By the end of the embryonic period the limb appears externally like a miniature of the adult form, although it is only 1 cm in length. The timings of the main events are summarized in Table 18.1. Nails and fingerprints are dealt with in Chapter 10.

Tissue differentiation

Cartilage

Cartilage elements begin to emerge from the mesoderm about half-way through the embryonic period. They are indistinct at first, with fuzzy edges like an out-of-focus picture, but they slowly become more sharply defined (Figure 18.3). The cartilage elements differentiate directly from the limb somatopleural meso-derm. Initially, the proportions of these elements are such that they appear wide

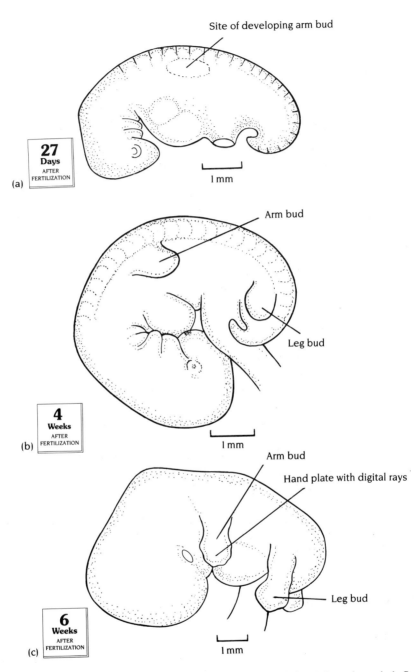

FIGURE 18.2 (a–c) Changing limb morphologies during the embryonic period. See also Figure 18.6.

TABLE 18.1 Summary of the main events in limb formation (chronology largely based on Lewis (1902)).

Time after fertilization (days)	Event
24	Muscle cells enter prospective limb mesoderm from somites
26	First appearance of limb buds. Blood vessel network starts to form
33	Cartilage begins to condense in the mesoderm
35	Nerves start to enter limb
40	Muscles begin to condense visibly
40	Fingers begin to be detectable from the outside
44	Toes can be identified (front limbs develop faster in humans – important for teratology)
45	Rotation of limbs
49 on	Ossification begins in the middle of cartilage elements

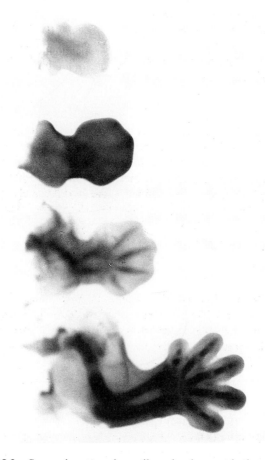

FIGURE 18.3 Successive stages in cartilage development in the mouse limb bud. (Courtesy of Dr G.B. Shellswell.)

for their length, but by the end of the embryonic period they have acquired the form of the adult bones. The cartilage is replaced by bone during the fetal period and after (see Chapter 9).

Muscle

Muscle cells invade from the somites (see Chapter 8). They form indistinct blocks of muscle lying dorsally and ventrally, which split up to form the individual adult muscles of the extensor and flexor compartments respectively (see Figure 8.2).

Nerves

Nerve cells, like the muscle cells, are invasive. Nerve 'roots' grow out between each somite pair all the way down the neural tube (see Chapter 6). Opposite the limbs, these grow into a plexus (Figure 18.4). About half-way through the embryonic period, when the limb is already well formed, nerve trunks leave the plexus and invade the limb down paths corresponding to those taken in the adult. From the first, these nerve trunks contain fibres from a number of roots. The limb is *never* innervated in a simple segmental pattern.

The limbs begin to move from week 7 onwards. These movements arise from firings of motor nerves, and are essential to the normal development of the joints.

Blood vessels

Blood vessels also connect to an external source – the dorsal aortae (see Chapter 7). Initially a random net of small blood vessels is present throughout the limb; later a central artery develops in the core of the limb with a peripheral vein running round the margin. Finally, as the other tissues of the limb take on their mature forms, they influence the blood vessels to grow to supply them (see Special Topic 5, pp. 153–7). The expression of these influences varies slightly between individuals and blood vessel pattern is thus more variable than that of the other tissues.

Tendons

Tendons, like cartilage, appear to differentiate directly from the somatopleural mesoderm. They condense as elongated cellular aggregates, which will interdigitate with muscles at one end but gradually become continuous with cartilage elements at the other, suggesting that they are related to cartilage in terms of their differentiation class.

Limb rotation

Initially the limbs of all vertebrate embryos project out from the body with the first digit (the thumb and big toe) on the cranial margin. In evolutionary terms

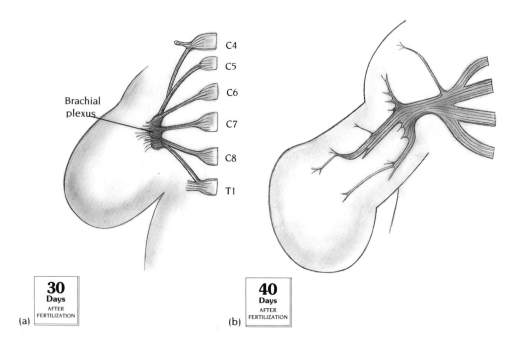

C4
C5
C6
C7
C8
TI

Brachial
plexus

30
Days
AFTER
FERTILIZATION

(a)

40
Days
AFTER
FERTILIZATION

(b)

FIGURE 18.4 Nerves growing into the limb from the spinal nerve roots. (a) 30-day embryo (b) 40-day embryo. Based on Bardeen (1906), Gasser (1975) and Bennet *et al.* (1980).

land tetrapod limbs are believed to have first flexed ventromedially at the elbow and dorsolaterally at the wrist, so that they could support the weight of the body (Figure 18.5(a)) and then twisted cranially at the wrist and ankle to aid locomotion (Figure 18.5(b)). (This means that the radius and ulna in the forelimb, and the tibia and fibula in the hindlimb, cross during development.) Next the elbows swing medially under the body in a caudal direction while the knees move in under the body in a cranial direction (Figure 18.5(c)), uncrossing the tibia and fibula but not the radius and ulna. Finally our ancestors stood erect, with the arms falling by the sides.

In the human embryo the limbs begin to swing medially from their initial position during week 5, to lie along the flanks of the embryo. The limbs also develop a slight caudal orientation. During weeks 6–7, the wrists rotate so that thumbs point medially and the radius and ulna cross. A caudal flexion at the elbow becomes evident (Figure 18.6). Within a few days the knees develop a cranial flexure.

Although the underlying causes of limb rotation are unclear, it has been proposed that the initial changes in limb position are caused by increased local cell division. Defects of rotation may contribute to a number of limb defects.

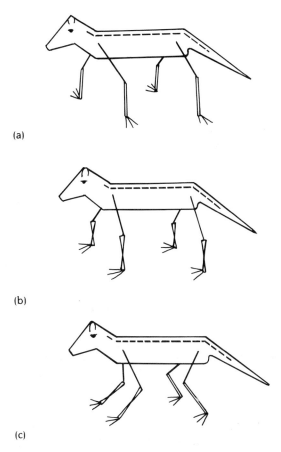

(a)

(b)

(c)

FIGURE 18.5   (a–c) Evolutionary stages of limb rotation. See text for details.

Controls of limb development

Development of the limb is understood at a more detailed level than perhaps any other structure in the body. In this chapter, therefore, it is possible to integrate the description of what happens during limb development with an account of the mechanisms that make it happen. This is most conveniently shown separately for the proximodistal and craniocaudal axes.

Distalization

At the distal tip of the limb bud is the AER. This appears just as the limb bud starts to form; it flattens and disappears when the limb is complete. This raises the possibility that it is involved in development, and this can be tested by experiment.

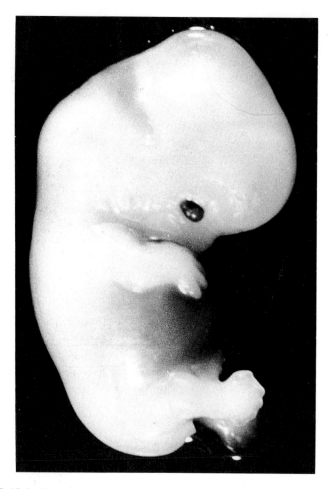

FIGURE 18.6 Later stage in limb development. (From the Anatomy Museum, St Andrews University, by permission.)

(1) If the AER (and *only* the AER) is removed at sequential stages in development, the limb is truncated at more and more distal levels (Figure 18.7). The elements present are normal in size and form but the limb looks as if it has been cleanly amputated. This shows that it develops by sequential distalization.

(2) If an AER is removed cleanly from a limb bud and grafted to the flank of another embryo at a place where no limb forms it induces a complete new limb. This ability is restricted to host embryos in the early embryonic stages.

(3) If an AER from an early limb bud is replaced by that from a late limb bud, the limb develops as normal. This shows that the AER influence does not change during development and does not specify the elements formed in detail.

(4) An early AER grafted to a late limb bud also produces a normal limb.

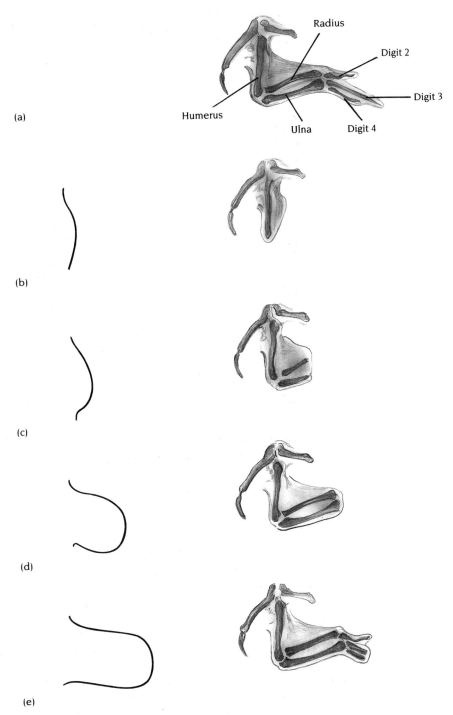

FIGURE 18.7 (a) A normal embryonic chick limb. Note that the wing shown here has three digits, conventionally numbered 2, 3 and 4; (b)–(e) removal of apical ectodermal ridge at progressive stages through development leads to limb truncations at more and more distal levels.

The progress zone theory

To explain these observations, the progress zone theory was devised by Wolpert, Lewis and Summerbell.

This theory proposes that the AER releases a factor that diffuses proximally for a distance of about 300 μm. Cells within this distance of the AER are said to lie in the progress zone.

Initially, when the limb bud is small, all of the cells lie in the progress zone and at this point they have the most proximal value – that of upper limb (Figure 18.8). Each time a cell divides in the progress zone it acquires a more distal character (distal value). However, cell division also leads the limb to grow, and as it elongates, some cells leave the progress zone. When they do so, they commence differentiating with whatever value they have at that time.

Removing the AER removes the progress zone and the cells behave as if they have all left the progress zone. They differentiate with their last value, but no further distalization will occur.

Although this theory is in accord with the observations, it needs to be tested. A critical test has been developed that relies on the fact that radiation

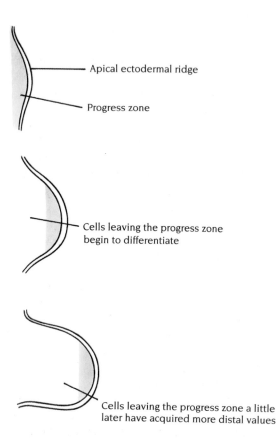

FIGURE 18.8 The progress zone model.

kills cells at random. If the developing limb is exposed to a burst of radiation the progress zone will be partially depopulated. The next cell divisions will repopulate the zone, but few or no cells will be pushed outside the zone's influence. Thereafter the limb will distalize as normal.

This implies that the limb should lack intermediate structures; that, for example, the wrist might be attached to the elbow, depending on the exact circumstances of the experiment. This has been observed experimentally and was seen in some of the children whose mothers were given thalidomide during pregnancy (see Special Topic 9, pp. 369–74).

We have seen that the AER controls distalization – the pattern from shoulder to fingertip. However, differentiation also occurs *across* the limb – from thumb to little finger. In the sense in which the limb buds first appear this is the craniocaudal axis.

The craniocaudal axis

Although the early limb bud lacks any apparent organization other than that of the AER one particular region has very special properties. If cells from this region on the caudal margin are grafted to the opposite, cranial, margin a complete duplication of the craniocaudal axis results (Figures 18.9, 18.10). This special region is consequently known as the **zone of polarizing activity** or ZPA.

The grafted tissue need not contribute to the 'extra' limb structures formed; it can induce the host limb to form the extra structures without itself contributing to any part.

A possible explanation of these observations is that the ZPA is the source of a diffusible substance (a 'morphogen'), which establishes a gradient across the limb bud. Somehow the cells of the limb bud interpret this gradient and give rise to the craniocaudal morphologies in order of increasing distance from the ZPA. In the developing chick embryo the three normal digits of the hand (numbered 2, 3 and 4 craniocaudally) form in accordance with their distance from the ZPA (Figure 18.11(a)).

Grafting an additional ZPA to the cranial limb margin in this model would create a U-shaped distribution of morphogen. The cells of the limb would interpret this as instructions to form digits in the pattern 4 3 2 2 3 4 (Figure 18.11(b)). Bringing the graft more caudal will make the morphogen distribution deeper in the midline, inducing digits 4 3 3 4 only. If made more caudal still the gradient would be consistent with the formation of digits 2 3 4 4 3 3 4 (Figure 18.11(c)). Experimentation has confirmed this prediction of the theory.

Implicit in the theory is the notion that the ZPA signal is quantitative in nature: that is the morphologies arise from the interpretation of the *strength* of the signal. If it could be weakened before grafting the gradient should be correspondingly reduced in slope and height in a predictable manner (Figure 18.11(d)). Experiments were undertaken to expose the ZPA to increasing doses of radiation, and a dose–response curve of signal weakening was indeed observed. In a different approach to the same problem the number of grafted ZPA cells was decreased, until eventually the graft failed to induce first an extra digit 4, then an extra digit 3, and finally an extra digit 2. The startling thing

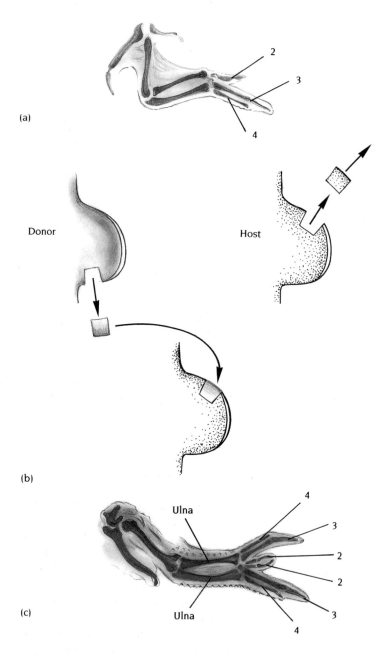

(a)

Donor

Host

(b)

Ulna

4

3

2

2

Ulna

3

(c)

4

FIGURE 18.9 The caudal margin of the limb bud has the special property that it can bring about reduplications of the limb axis when grafted to the cranial margin. (a) Normal limb; (b) grafting method; (c) limb reduplication resulting from such a graft.

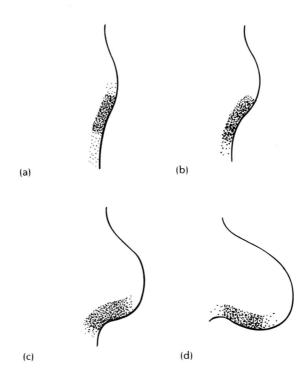

(a)   (b)

(c)   (d)

FIGURE 18.10 (a–d) Distribution of ZPA activity at various stages of limb development. The density of shading is proportional to the activity. Data from Honig and Summerbell (1985).

about this experiment was the small number of cells required: anything over 100 cells gave a complete pattern reduplication, and as few as six cells gave an extra digit 2 on one occasion. The morphogen is extremely potent in its action.

It should be noted that these experiments employed an additional ZPA, rather than trying to weaken the original one. This is because the limb cells 'remember' their highest value when exposed to the ZPA. This value can be pushed upwards by exposing cells to an additional ZPA but if the original ZPA is removed the limb cells remember their last morphogen value and differentiate accordingly. In other words the limb is essentially normal, since the ZPA is present from the earliest appearance of the limb.

The ZPA signal is similar in very different species: if the ZPA from a mouse embryo is grafted to a chick limb bud cranial margin, then it induces a reduplication. (Because the graft itself merely signals to the tissue, the reduplicated digits are chick in nature.) The same happens if ZPAs from human, tortoise and guinea pig embryos, among others, are used.

The observation that the ZPA effect may be progressively attenuated supports the idea of a quantitative gradient of a morphogen but does not of itself indicate what the morphogen might be.

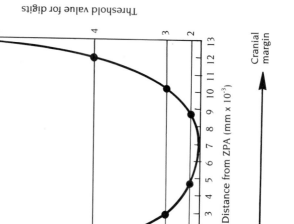

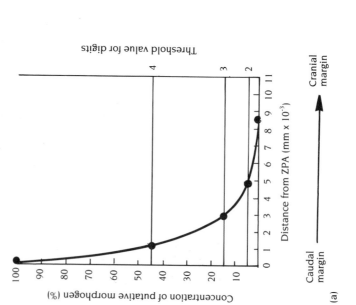

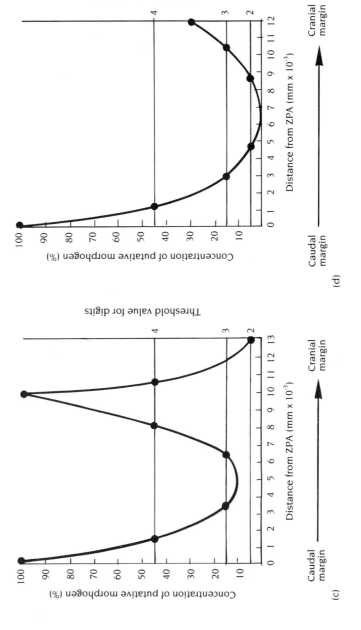

FIGURE 18.11 (a) Gradient of putative morphogen in the normal limb bud; (b) distribution of morphogen after ZPA graft to the cranial margin; (c) distribution of morphogen after graft to midpoint of limb; (d) distribution of morphogen after graft of attenuated ZPA to cranial margin.

The molecular basis of ZPA signalling

The signalling molecule associated with the ZPA was ardently sought but with no success until, for rather indirect reasons, retinoic acid (vitamin A) was applied to the cranial margin of the limb. Not only did this unexpectedly induce reduplications, but it also did so in a dose-dependent manner. High levels produced complete reduplications, successively lower values sequentially induced fewer extra elements. This does not of itself prove that retinoic acid is the genuine limb morphogen, but the case was strengthened by the discovery that it was present naturally in the developing limb bud, and in a graded manner, so that the concentration was highest at the caudal edge. This gradient was found to be rather shallower than expected, and its exact role remains to be established. While it cannot be said beyond doubt that retinoic acid is the natural morphogen, it remains a strong candidate.

This is supported by evidence from two different sources.

Expression of homoeobox genes The first relates to the expression of homoeobox-containing genes in the limb (see Special Topic 6, pp. 174–7). For a number of genes in the *Hox*-4 cluster there is a distinct pattern of expression across the limb (Figure 18.12). At the caudal edge, *Hox* genes 4.4–4.8 are all switched on in the normal developing limb bud; moving more cranially 4.8 is switched off, then 4.7, and so on across the limb, establishing a series of 'nested' regions of gene expression. This fits very well with the action of retinoic acid on homoeobox genes: genes are sequentially activated along a cluster at increasing concentrations. When retinoic acid levels are high, all the genes in a cluster are switched on: at progressively lower levels, the genes in the cluster are switched off in succession. If a ZPA graft or a retinoic acid implant is made to the cranial margin of the limb bud then the pattern of *Hox*-4 expression produces a mirror-image reduplication of thenormal pattern, just as the limb will be a mirror image of the normal morphology.

Elucidation of molecular pathway The second support for the role of retinoic acid in normal development comes from the elucidation of the molecular pathway by which it acts. A number of retinoic acid receptors are present in the limb; one class is found in the cytoplasm. However, these may bind retinoic acid merely in order to inactivate it. A gradient of these receptors is observed, high at the cranial margin and low at the caudal margin: it is therefore the inverse of the retinoic acid gradient. These receptors may steepen the free retinoic acid gradient across the limb. Very different retinoic acid receptors are found in the nucleus. When they bind retinoic acid they become active as transcription factors and specifically initiate the expression of particular genes.

A plausible model is that:

(1) an initially shallow gradient of retinoic acid is amplified by the reverse gradient of the cytoplasmic binding factor;

(2) the remaining free retinoic acid then binds to its nuclear receptor and in a dose-dependent manner initiates the expression of other genes, including the homoeobox-containing genes;

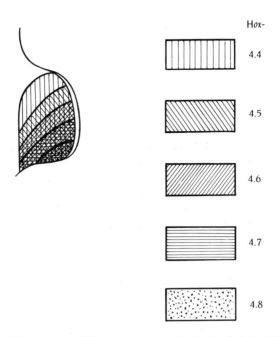

FIGURE 18.12   Distribution of *Hox*-4 gene expression in the limb bud. This is a speculative diagram based on the data of Izpisua-Belmonte *et al.* (1991) and Morgan *et al* (1992).

(3) these 'master' genes in turn initiate the cascade of events, involving many genes, that gives rise to particular morphologies at particular values of the gradient.

The origin of the ZPA

While it is plausible that the origin of limb pattern can be traced to signals produced by the ZPA, this leads inevitably to the question of how the ZPA appears on the caudal margin of the limb. A hint seems to lie in the observation that the primitive node (see Chapter 3) is able to induce reduplications when grafted to the limb cranial margin. It could be that as the primitive streak extends it leaves behind 'ZPA activity' in the regions where the caudal limb margins will develop. This in turn raises further questions, but it would be satisfying to be able to relate limb development to the mechanism of axis formation in the embryo.

Homoeobox gene expression in the proximodistal axis

Homoeobox genes also seem to be involved in the proximodistal axis. *Hox*-7.1 and *Hox*-8.1 have differential patterns of expression from proximal to distal levels, expression being greatest in the distal portions of the limb bud, possibly in response to a signal from the AER. It is not yet known what the inducer is in this case, although a growth-factor-like molecule found to be produced by the AER is a plausible candidate.

Limb defects

In the light of the above discussion many of the common limb defects result from abnormalities of pattern formation in the limb.

Polydactyly Polydactyly is the presence of extra digits. The incidence of this condition varies widely: it is approximately one per 3000 among Caucasian Americans, and one per 200 among African Americans. The extra digit or digits may lie either side of the hand: on the thumb side it may result from the abnormal expression of ZPA activity on the part of cranial limb cells; on the little finger side it may result from the presence of cells sensitive to the ZPA lying caudal to the ZPA itself. Polydactyly has a genetic component, and often runs in families. The extra digit may be removed shortly after birth.

Syndactyly In this condition a degree of 'webbing' persists between the fingers or toes. In severe cases this may result in fusion between digits. The incidence is estimated at one per 3000, but may be greater, because many cases are dealt with by minor surgery without further report. There appears to be a genetic component for this condition; it, too, commonly runs in families.

Transverse defects In this conditions, the limb at birth looks as if it has been amputated at a particular level. This perhaps results from a general failure of the AER at the corresponding stage of development. Complete absence of the limb is known as **amelia**.

Ectrodactyly ('lobster claw') In this condition, midline positional values in the limb are missing, so that digits three and four, for instance, may be missing. This may arise from local failure of the AER to survive.

This last condition introduces the (rather distasteful) habit of naming limb defects from fanciful resemblances to animal limbs. For example, the condition was described on p. 251 in which intermediate proximodistal values are missing. This may result in fingers being attached directly to shoulder elements. On rare occasions this condition may arise spontaneously: more familiarly, it was one of the consequences of maternal ingestion of the drug thalidomide during pregnancy. This condition is known as **phocomelia** (from seal limb), despite the fact that true seal limbs are nothing like this. Fusion of the lower limbs is referred to as **sirenomelia**, in an even more bizarre reference to mermaids.

Amniotic bands Strands of the amniotic membrane may entangle or constrict the embryo and bring about abnormalities. An entangled limb may suffer distortion or vascular damage in consequence. The disrupted vasculature may cause a

haematoma: a collection of blood that may occupy much of the volume of the limb and that results in the destruction of all the tissues in the affected area.

Club foot In club foot, or talipes equinovarus, the foot is abnormally flexed medially, so that the sufferer walks on its outer edge. The cause of this is not certain, but it could arise from mechanical pressures in utero, such as compression of the limbs by the embryonic sac.

Congenital hip dysplasia In this condition the hip is prone to dislocation because of a shallow acetabulum or poorly developed joint capsule. However, these may be consequences of an unknown underlying cause. It is possible that hip dysplasia represents a failure of limb rotation in some way. Because bone can remodel in response to mechanical forces, stress may be applied to the joint to bring about a gradual improvement of the joint shape.

Special Topic 7 Regeneration

As indicated in Chapter 1, the pre-embryo has marked abilities to compensate for tissue removal (and addition). In the embryo, however, complex tissue interactions are taking place, and the consequences of tissue damage are more likely to be harmful. None the less, the embryo is capable of extensive repair of damage. Even the fetus is able to repair wounds with greater speed and neatness than the adult, although in general, this ability decreases with developmental age.

There are exceptions to this general trend, and these present fascinating possibilities for understanding the underlying mechanisms of regeneration and repair.

Limb regeneration

One exception concerns newts and salamanders, which possess the ability to regenerate lost limbs. A blood clot forms at the wound surface and epidermal cells from the stump migrate over the wound. These cells then proliferate to form a layer several cells thick. The tissues underlying the wound epidermis begin to de-differentiate, and give rise to a cap of apparently homogeneous proliferating cells known as the **regeneration blastema**. As cell division proceeds the missing structures are sequentially reformed by the blastemal cells until the end of the limb is reached. At this point the blastema disappears.

Without the formation of a blastema only very limited regeneration will occur. Blastema formation appears to be the key feature determining whether a particular species can regenerate limbs, and mammals do not appear capable of doing so. The degree of regeneration that mammals can show is best described as 'slight'. Mammalian embryos and neonates, for example, may be able to regrow the tips of their digits. Even humans possess a limited capacity to replace missing distal finger structures: if a child who has lost the tip of a finger is treated conservatively by protecting the wound from infection rather than by sewing up the stump the missing section will regenerate as long as it does not extend beyond the first joint. It would be very desirable to enhance this natural ability to the point of real clinical use.

This may be possible if we can gain a better understanding of limb development (Chapter 18). Analogies may be drawn between limb development and regeneration. Formation of the wound epidermis and the undifferentiated blastema during regeneration may be similar to the formation of the AER and the undifferentiated progress zone during development.

A number of empirical procedures have been used to increase the regeneration capacity in poorly regenerating species. These include increasing the supply of nerves and neural factors, electrical stimulation of the limb and manipulation of the process of skin overgrowth of the wound. The degree of success obtained is, however, not striking, and better success may arise from an understanding of the relationship between retinoic acid and the homoeobox genes on which it acts. Specific activation of homoeobox-containing genes may lead directly to further distalization. However, it should be borne in mind that even if complete regeneration can be achieved, the timescale would be long: after all, humans take some 20 years to grow their limbs to the full adult size. It might be most useful to encourage amputated digits to regrow, particularly the thumb and big toe because their loss is severely disabling.

Liver regeneration

A second class of exceptions to the general loss of regenerative capacity in adult vertebrates concerns particular tissues: the liver, for example, preserves considerable regenerative ability. In experimental mammals, 70% of the liver may be removed and yet the liver will then regenerate to almost its full size within a period of weeks. Within 24 h of the removal, the surviving tissue initiates massive cell division.

How this is initiated remains unclear. It could be that the liver cells produce growth factors after wounding to induce cell division; it could be that the liver normally produces an inhibitor that suppresses cell division and that loss of massive amounts of tissue decreases the level of inhibitor to the point where division can begin; it could be that the liver somehow monitors its own function, and responds to a decrease in activity by stimulating cell division. In any case, the controlling factor or factors can be transmitted via the blood: if the circulatory systems of two rats are connected and the liver of one is reduced in size, the liver of the other shows a burst of cell division.

Given the liver's marked powers of regeneration, it may seem puzzling that it should ever suffer severe damage. However, if repeatedly challenged, as in chronic alcoholism, the connective tissue component grows back more strongly than the functional liver cells, leading to a gradual decline in liver function.

Further reading

Bardeen C.R. (1906). Development and variation of the nerves and the musculature of the inferior extremity and of the neighbouring regions of the trunk in man. *Am. J. Anat.*, **6**, 259–391

Bennet M.R., Davey D. and Uebel K. (1980). The growth of segmental nerves from the brachial myotomes into the proximal muscles of the chick forelimb during development. *J. Comp. Neurol.*, **189**, 335–57

Davidson D.R., Crawley A., Hill R.E. and Tickle C. (1991). Position dependent expression of two related homeobox genes in developing vertebrate limbs. *Nature*, **352**, 429–31

Dolle P., Izpisua-Belmonte J-C., Falkenstein H., Renucci A. and Duboule D. (1989). Coordinate expression of the murine Hox-5 complex homeobox-containing genes during limb pattern formation. *Nature*, **342**, 767–72

Gasser R.F. (1982). *Atlas of Human Embryos*. Hagerstown, MD: Harper & Row

Giguere V., Ong E.S., Segui P. and Evans R.M. (1987). Identification of a receptor for the morphogen retinoic acid. *Nature*, 33, 624–9

Honig L.S. and Summerbell D. (1985). Maps of strength of positional signalling activity in the developing chick wing bud. *J. Embryol. Exp. Morph.*, **87**, 167–74

Hornbruch A. and Wolpert L. (1986). Positional signalling by Hensen's Node when grafted to the chick wing bud. *J. Embryol. Exp. Morph.*, **94**, 257–65.

Izpisua-Belmonte J-C., Tickle C., Dolle P., Wolpert L. and Duboule D. (1991). Expression of the homeobox Hox-4 genes and the specification of position in chick wing development. *Nature*, **350**, 585–9

Lewis J.H., Slack J.M.W. and Wolpert L. (1977). Thresholds in development. *J. Theoret. Biol*,. **65**, 579–90

Maden M., Ong D., Summerbell D. and Chytil F. (1989). The role of retinoid-binding proteins in the generation of pattern in the developing limb, the regenerating limb and the nervous system. *Development*, **107** (suppl), 109–19.

Morgan B.A., Izpisua-Belmonte J-C., Duboule D. and Tabin C. (1992). Targeted misexpression of Hox-4.6 in the avian limb bud causes apparent homeotic transformations. *Nature*, **358**, 236–9

Smith J.C. (1979). Evidence for a positional memory in the development of the chick wing. *J. Embryol. Exp. Morph.*, **52**, 105–13

Summerbell D. (1979). The zone of polarising activity: evidence for a role in normal chick limb morphogenesis. *J. Embryol. Exp. Morph.*, **50**, 217–33.

Thaller C. and Eichele G. (1987). Identification of spatial distribution of retinoids in the developing chick limb bud. *Nature*, **327**, 625–8

Tickle C. (1981). The number of polarising cells required to specify additional digits in the developing chick wing bud. *Nature*, **289**, 295–8

Tickle C. Summerbell D. and Wolpert L. (1975). Positional signalling and specification of digits in chick limb morphogenesis. *Nature*, **254**, 199–202

Tickle C., Shellswell G.B., Crawley A. and Wolpert L. (1976). Positional signalling by mouse limb polarising region in the chick wing bud. *Nature*, **259**, 396–7

Tickle C., Alberts B., Wolpert L. and Lee J. (1982). Local application of retinoic acid to the limb bud mimics the action of the polarizing region. *Nature*, **296**, 564–5

Wanek N., Gardiner D.M., Muneoko K. and Bryant S.V. (1991). Conversion by retinoic acid of anterior cells into ZPA cells in the chick wing bud. *Nature*, **350**, 81–3

Wolpert L. (1981) Positional information and pattern formation. *Phil. Trans. R. Soc. Lond. (Biol)*, **295**, 441–50

Special Topic 7

Borgens R.B. (1982). Mice regrow the tips of their foretoes. *Science,* **217**, 747–50

Farrell R.G., Disher W.A., Nsland R.S., Palmatier T.H. and Truhler T.D. (1977). Conservative management of fingertip amputations. *J. Am. Coll. Emerg. Phys.,* **6**, 243–6.

Goss R.J. (1978). *The Physiology of Growth.* New York: Academic Press,

Holder N. (1981). Regeneration and compensatory growth. *Br Med. Bull.,* **37**, 227-32

Illingworth C.M. (1974). Trapped fingers and amputated fingers in children. *J. Paed. Surg.,* **9**, 853–8

Illingworth C.M. and Barker A.T. (1980). Measurement of electrical currents during the regeneration of amputated fingertips in children. *Clin. Phys. Physiol. Meas.,* **1**, 87–9

Sicard, R.E., ed. (1985). *Regulation of Vertebrate Limb Regeneration.* Oxford: Oxford University Press

Wanek N., Muneoka K. and Bryant S.V. (1989). Evidence for regulation following amputation and tissue grafting in the developing mouse limb. *J. Exp. Zool.,* **249**, 55–61

THE BODY CAVITIES AND THE THORAX

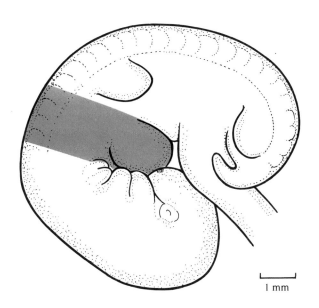

1 mm

19

Body cavities and mesenteries

The body cavities and their mesenteries are complex and clinically important in the adult. Their development is the key to understanding their adult disposition. It is convenient to consider the three main body cavities – the **pleural cavity**, the **pericardial cavity**, and the **peritoneal cavity** – together, and for this it is necessary to review briefly material introduced in Chapter 3.

The intraembryonic coelom develops as a horseshoe-shaped cavity in the embryonic mesoderm, lying on either side of the main body axis and forward from the developing forebrain. This cavity communicates with the chorionic cavity about halfway down the length of the embryo. The embryo, with its amniotic cavity and yolk sac, is attached to the uterine wall via the yolk stalk, which carries the blood vessels running to the placenta.

Figure 19.1 shows the early embryo and its membranes in sagittal section. At about 4 weeks after fertilization the heart is forming inside the forward part of the intraembryonic coelom. Into this space the lungs will also project, as they develop from the gut lying dorsal to the cavity (Chapter 20).

Linings

The primitive pericardial cavity is lined with mesoderm, as is the extraembryonic coelom. The mesodermal cells exposed to the cavity are flattened and can

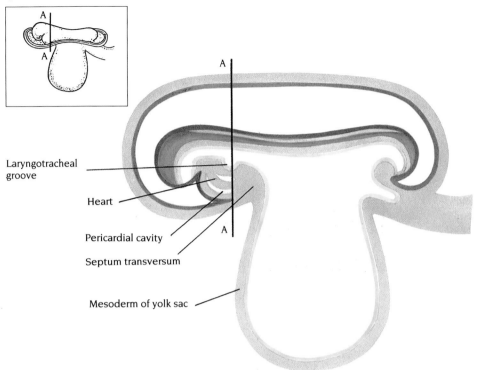

FIGURE 19.1   Diagrammatic sagittal section of embryo early in the embryonic period.

be described as a **mesothelium**, although they are not like a true epithelium in nature. This mesothelium is continuous with the mesoderm lining the chorionic cavity. When the peritoneal cavity appears, it will also be lined with mesothelium.

Mesoderm lying near the gut is described as **splanchnic**; further away it is known as **somatic**. Both somatic and splanchnic mesoderm may be embryonic or extraembryonic. These names all describe differences in position, rather than profound differences in nature, at early stages. However, because the splanchnic and somatic mesoderm will come to lie next to a variety of different neighbouring tissues they will differentiate in different ways (see Chapter 5).

During the course of this differentiation the splanchnic and somatic mesodermal components become known as the **visceral** and **parietal layers**, respectively, of the **serous membranes** or **peritoneum**. Visceral mesoderm will produce the smooth muscle and connective tissue of the gut; parietal mesoderm will form connective tissue and adipose tissue and will be innervated by somatic efferent nerves growing out from the neural tube. Because the visceral layers are not innervated they are not directly sensitive to pain; abscesses in the visceral layers may be experienced as referred pain in the innervated parietal layers.

The mesodermal nature of mesothelium has certain implications for its future behaviour. Unlike true epithelium, it will readily fuse to other layers of mesothelium (a process known as **zygosis**), which influences the deployment of the tissues lying within it. For example, when the gut coils within the peritoneal cavity (see Chapter 23) its visceral mesodermal covering will fuse against the parietal lining of the cavity wherever it comes in contact (**fixation** of the gut). In postnatal life, fusions or **adhesions** may form after surgery. Mesothelium also heals well and, although surgeons routinely suture the peritoneal layers after an operation, it may not be necessary: if left alone the peritoneal layers will heal in 7–8 days, with lower risk of adhesions forming than after suturing.

Perhaps as a result of these extensive healing (i.e. cell division) capabilities tumours of the mesothelium – mesotheliomas – are highly malignant. They may be induced in the lungs by inhaled asbestos or other fibres, which penetrate the endodermal lining layer to interact with the mesodermal tissues.

The pericardioperitoneal canals

The caudal end of the developing pericardial cavity is formed by the floor rising up into a wall (see Chapter 21). This merges with the mesoderm covering the yolk sac to form a mesodermal condensation known as the **septum transversum** (Figure 19.1). The sinus venosi of the heart emerge from this wall (Figure 19.2). The wall continues to rise until it meets the gut with its covering of splanchnopleural mesoderm but there will still be a 'tunnel' of coelom lying on either side of the gut: the **pericardioperitoneal canals**, which represent the legs of the horseshoe-shaped intraembryonic coelom. These continue caudally to open out into the chorionic cavity (Figure 19.2).

The pleural cavity

Within the primitive pericardial cavity, horizontal mesodermal folds begin to grow in from either side, above the level of the heart tube (Figure 19.3). These will meet the dorsal mesocardium, thus separating the definitive pericardial cavity from the pleural cavity (Chapter 20). The linings of the pleural cavity may be described as **visceral peritoneum** around the (endoderm derived) lungs and **parietal peritoneum** over the rest of the cavity. The pleural cavity remains as a patent space throughout adult life, which means that these mesodermal layers do not fuse. This may be due to the fluid content of the pleural cavity, or to the continual movement resulting from breathing. During embryonic and fetal life the pleural cavity expands into the body wall mesoderm to reach its adult disposition (see Chapter 20).

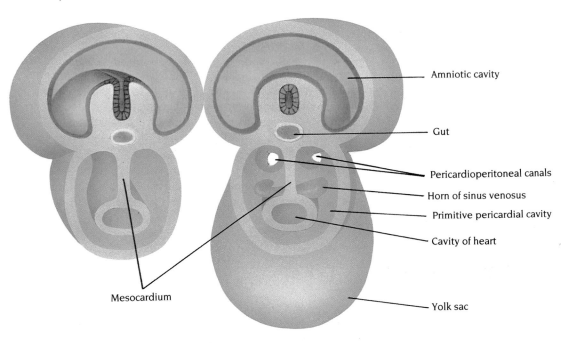

FIGURE 19.2   Section through A–A on Figure 19.1, hinged apart. Looking towards the tail, the pericardioperitoneal canals can be seen opening into the chorionic cavity.

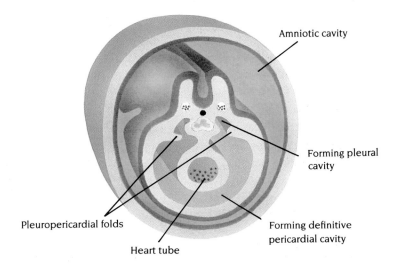

FIGURE 19.3   Similar view to left-hand part of Figure 19.2, at a slightly later stage. The figure shows the beginning of division of the original primitive pericardial cavity into the pleural cavity and the true pericardial cavity by the pleuropericardial folds.

The peritoneal cavity

The primitive pericardial cavity of the fetus thus gives rise to the definitive pleural and pericardial cavities. It is less obvious how the peritoneal cavity develops from the early embryonic arrangement. The key to understanding is the process of folding of the embryo, which can also be viewed as the amniotic cavity expanding to encompass the embryo. Figure 19.4 shows a view of the amnion and yolk sac from the chorionic cavity. (See also Figure 3.13 for transverse sections in the region of the gut.) The amnion will sweep round the embryonic axis as the embryo folds. In the meantime, the yolk sac diminishes in relative size. The yolk stalk, connecting the embryo to the chorionic wall, becomes enclosed in a column of amnion (consisting, of course, of ectoderm and mesoderm). This column encloses the yolk sac remnant and the connecting stalk. Because these last are covered in mesoderm they will eventually fuse with the mesoderm lining the amniotic column, giving the umbilical cord, but in the embryo it remains open to the chorionic cavity.

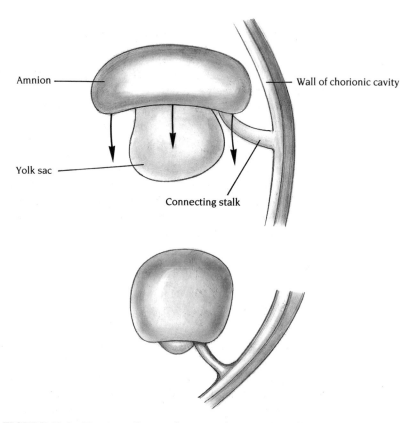

FIGURE 19.4   The expanding amnion, sweeping over the yolk sac.

The sweeping round of the amnion gradually encloses what will become the peritoneal cavity on either side of the gut (Figure 19.4). The peritoneal cavity at the level of the forming umbilical cord is in communication with the chorionic cavity and cranially with the pleural cavity as it forms from the primitive pericardial cavity via the pericardioperitoneal canals. These canals will therefore have to be closed off during lung development (see Chapter 20). The changes in the body cavities are summarized in Figure 19.5.

The gut initially runs in the mesoderm ventral to the neural tube. As development proceeds this mesodermal attachment is sculpted out by the expanding peritoneal coelom (Figure 3.13), so that the gut becomes suspended in a mesodermal sheath (the **dorsal mesentery**, considered in more detail below and in Chapter 23). Ventrally the gut mesoderm is in contact with the anterior abdominal wall at the septum transversum. By analogy with the dorsal mesentery, this brief region of attachment is often called the ventral mesentery but it is not as distinct a band of tissue as the dorsal mesentery becomes. The mesoderm suspending the gut is defined as splanchnopleural or visceral and will differentiate into smooth muscle, connective tissue and adipose tissue.

The dorsal and ventral mesenteries

The gut is surrounded by mesoderm all down its length except at the oral and cloacal membranes. As the body cavities develop during the fourth week the gut from the level of the trachea to the hindgut becomes 'suspended' from the dorsal body wall by its mesodermal covering (Figure 19.6) dividing the body cavities into right and left compartments between the trachea and the yolk sac, since it forms a continuous dorsoventral wall. In the region of the hindgut, the suspending mesoderm is incomplete ventrally and the left and right sides of the peritoneal cavity communicate with each other, except at the hindmost end. This arrangement is usually described by saying that the gut is suspended from a dorsal mesentery and in the fore- and hindgut region is attached to the anterior body structures by a ventral mesentery.

Gut mesenteries and arteries

The dorsal mesentery runs along the entire length of the gut below the diaphragm. Regional names are used locally to describe various parts of the dorsal mesentery as appropriate: **dorsal mesogastrium, dorsal mesoduodenum, mesentery proper**, and the **dorsal mesocolon**. The **lienorenal ligament** (see pp. 308–9) lies between the spleen and the urogenital ridge. The ventral mesentery gives rise to the **lesser omentum** and the **falciform ligament**.

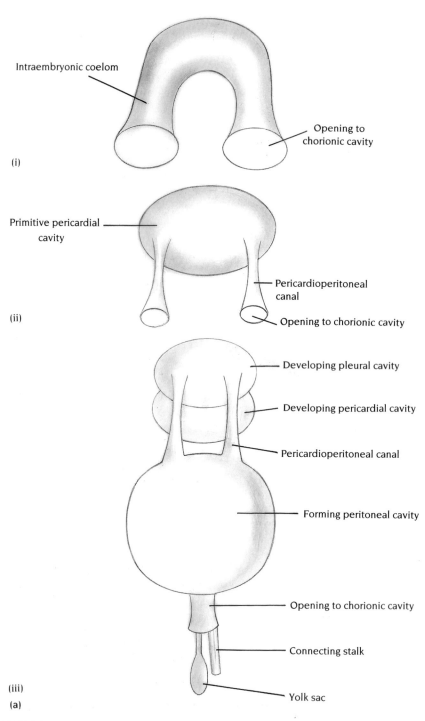

Intraembryonic coelom

Opening to
chorionic cavity

(i)

Primitive pericardial
cavity

Pericardioperitoneal
canal

Opening to chorionic cavity

(ii)

Developing pleural cavity

Developing pericardial cavity

Pericardioperitoneal canal

Forming peritoneal cavity

Opening to chorionic cavity

Connecting stalk

(iii)

Yolk sac

(a)

FIGURE 19.5 (a) Changes undergone by cavities, seen looking forward from above
the tail.

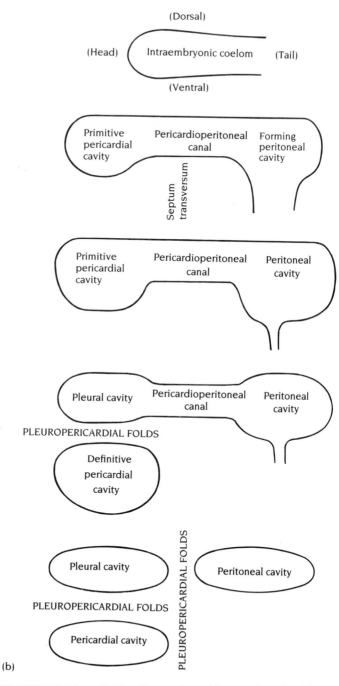

FIGURE 19.5 *(contd)* **(b)**   Changes in cavities seen from the side.

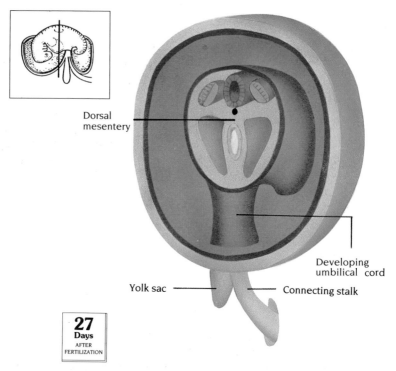

FIGURE 19.6 Section through a 27-day embryo, as shown on inset. The ventral attachment of the embryo, covered by ectoderm, represents the early stages of umbilical cord formation.

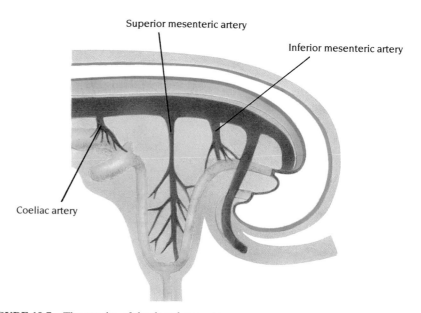

FIGURE 19.7 The arteries of the dorsal mesentery.

Blood supply

Blood vessels run from the dorsal aorta through the dorsal mesentery to the gut (Figure 19.7). The branch supplying the region of the stomach is known as the **coeliac artery**: it also supplies the liver, duodenum, pancreas and spleen. The **vitelline arteries** run to the yolk sac and are substantial in the embryo.

Eventually the vitelline artery continuance ceases as the yolk sac decreases in relative size. The paired arteries fuse, and will supply the midgut loop as the **superior mesenteric artery**. The **inferior mesenteric artery** supplies the hindgut. Caudal to this, the **umbilical arteries** run into the connecting stalk. When the hind limbs form a branch runs to each limb from the corresponding umbilical artery.

Further reading

Callaghan P. (1986). Hands off the peritoneum. *Lancet*, **i**, 849–50

Corliss C.E. (1976). *Patten's Human Embryology. Elements of Clinical Development.* New York: McGraw Hill

Skandalkis J.E., Gray S.W, and Rowe J.S. (1983). *Anatomical complications in general surgery.* New York: McGraw-Hill

Slater N.J., Raftery A.T. and Cope G.H. (1989). The ultrastructure of human abdominal mesothelium. *J. Anat.*, **167**, 47-56

Thomas N.W. (1987). Embryology and structure of the mesothelium. In *Pathology of the mesothelium* (Jones, J.S.P., ed.). Berlin: Springer-Verlag

20

The lungs

EVOLUTION

As indicated in Chapter 14 our ancient fish ancestors obtained oxygen by taking water into their mouths and expelling it through the gill slits.

Shallow water tends to be warm and is therefore worse at retaining oxygen than deep, cold water. As a result, fish living in shallow water near coasts evolved air 'gulping'. This process is aided if the bubbles can be retained, so paired pockets began to develop in the foregut for this purpose. Oxygen absorption is made more effective if these pouches are vascularized, and if their surface area is increased by elongation and branching. Shallow-water fish like this gave rise to the terrestrial vertebrates and to modern bony fish.

The paired condition of the adult lungs has been retained through evolutionary time. However, the embryology of this process has become simplified in higher vertebrates, so that the two lung pockets now arise from a single primordium in the midline of the gut floor. (The primitive condition can still be seen in some amphibian embryos.)

The emergence of vertebrates from the water, and the subsequent evolution of warm-bloodedness, led to continually increasing demands for oxygen. The process of branching and vascularization therefore developed further to give the highly complex lungs of modern mammals. As gills are no longer required their embryonic rudiments may be modified by evolutionary selection to contribute to a variety of different tissues in the head and neck (see Chapter 14).

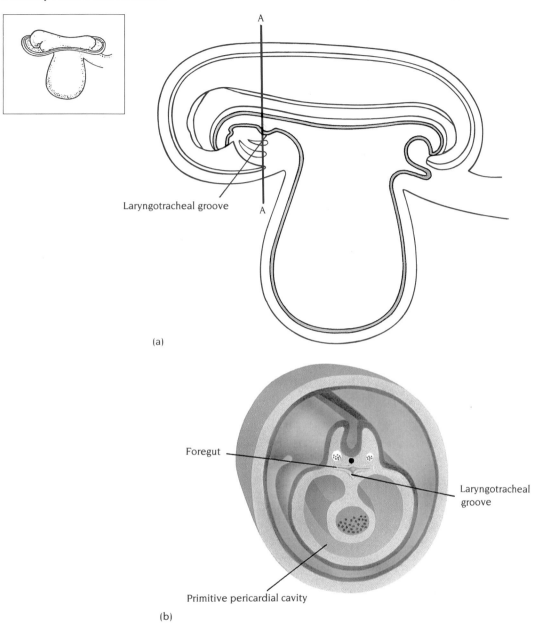

FIGURE 20.1 (a) Sagittal view of fourth week embryo showing position and relations of the laryngotracheal groove; (b) transverse view, through line A–A on part (a).

Development of the lungs

Lung buds

The foregut of the human embryo during the fourth week after fertilization represents a tunnel several times as wide as it is high. The walls are made of ectoderm at the mouth with the frontier with endoderm shifting with developmental age. The endodermal gut tunnel is surrounded by mesoderm (Figure 20.1). Above the mesoderm overlying the roof of the tunnel runs the notochord and developing brain; beneath the mesoderm underlying the floor lies the developing heart in the pericardial cavity.

The formation of the pharyngeal pouches and tongue in the foregut region has already been described. Further down the gut tunnel, as it begins to narrow markedly, a trench or depression develops in the floor (Figures 20.1, 20.2). This marks out the first sign of the development of the lungs. The trench is almost as deep as the tunnel is high and is known as the **laryngotracheal groove** or **laryngotracheal diverticulum**.

At about 28 days after fertilization, **tracheo-oesophageal folds** start to close off the laryngotracheal diverticulum at the caudal end (Figure 20.2(b)). Gradually they will approach each other until, at the caudal end of the depression, they meet in the midline (Figures 20.2(c)). In later development this will represent the point at which the trachea leaves the oesophagus.

The embryo is continuing to enlarge markedly throughout this period. The diverticulum elongates and becomes wider as it grows into underlying mesoderm. At about 35 days the initial diverticulum divides into two further buds, which represent the primary **bronchi** (Figure 20.3(a,b)). These are about the same size as the original lung bud – it appears that there may be a critical size

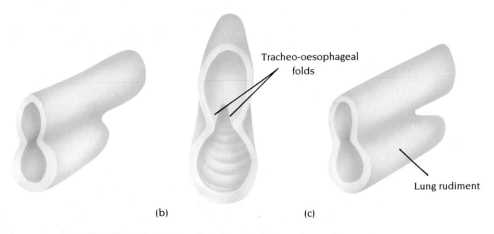

(a) (b) (c)

Tracheo-oesophageal folds

Lung rudiment

FIGURE 20.2 Isolated section of gut showing development of lung rudiment.

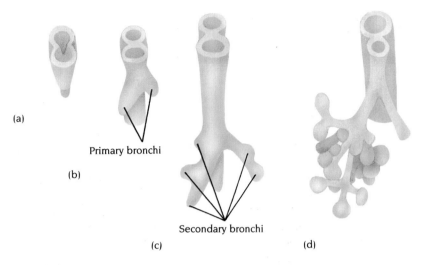

(a)

Primary bronchi

(b)

Secondary bronchi

(c)   (d)

FIGURE 20.3   Ventral view of developing lung rudiment.

for lung outgrowths and as soon as a bud reaches approximately this size, it branches (see Box 20.1). The right-hand bud generally lies pointing more towards the tail than the left. This condition persists to adulthood, and inhaled objects tend to fall into the right bronchus.

During the following week, more buds form as growth continues, until there are three buds on the right and two on the left (Figure 20.3(c)). On the right these buds represent the beginnings of the superior, middle and inferior lobes of the adult lung: on the left they will give rise to the superior and inferior lobes. The lumen of these buds represents the secondary bronchi. Slight variations in bud formation are always possible, which may prove confusing when bronchoscopy is being conducted in adults.

Branching of the lung buds by binary splitting now proceeds continuously (Figure 20.3(d)). At birth there will have been something like 17 or 18 splitting divisions ($2^{17}/2^{18}$ sacs). Branching will continue to occur for perhaps eight years. The size of each terminal sac in the adult is about the same as the initial lung bud in the embryo.

As the lungs grow in size and complexity they require more space: we therefore now need to look at the development of the pleural cavity.

Pleural cavity

The intraembryonic coelom initially forms as a U-shaped space in the intraembryonic mesoderm, with the legs of the U pointing towards the tail of the embryo: these legs open out into the chorionic cavity (see Chapter 19).

The curved base of the U will become the primitive pericardial cavity (see Chapter 22). This will give rise to the pleural cavity and to the definitive pericar-

Box 20.1 Experimental analysis of lung development

In experiments on animal embryos the developing lung buds may be removed and maintained in culture. If the mesoderm normally associated with the bronchus is replaced on one side with mesoderm from the level of the trachea no branching will occur on that side, while on the other side the primary bronchi branch luxuriantly. If tracheal mesoderm is replaced by bronchial mesoderm the normally unbranched trachea begins to bud: this does not happen if the tracheal mesoderm is removed and replaced. Together these findings imply that bronchial mesoderm controls the branching of the endoderm buds – its presence is both a necessary and sufficient condition for branching to occur.

Lung endoderm seems very malleable: associated with mesoderm from the stomach it forms gastric glands, with intestinal mesoderm it generates intestinal villi. Plainly, the mesoderm is playing a key instructive role in influencing the endodermal morphology, as we have seen it do for the ectoderm.

The cellular basis for this mesodermal control in lungs, mammary glands, salivary glands etc. is complex, but as far as branching is concerned it appears to involve the basal lamina – a coat of extracellular molecules including collagen and glycosaminoglycans secreted by and surrounding existing buds. The mesoderm may degrade this at the bud tip and therefore allow this region of the bud to respond to growth factors produced by the mesoderm (Figure 1). Regions between actively budding areas may be stabilized by collagen secreted by the mesoderm.

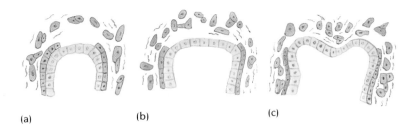

(a) (b) (c)

FIGURE 1 Possible mechanism of branching. The extracellular basal lamina and collagen fibrils are absent at the tip of the bud (a), exposing the endodermal cells to factors stimulating cell division. The resulting enlarged bud (b) buckles and the cleft is gradually stabilized by renewed extracellular matrix production (c).

dial cavity. The legs of the coelom connect the primitive pericardial cavity with what will become the peritoneal cavity (see Chapter 19), and are therefore described as the pericardioperitoneal canals.

The primitive pericardial cavity represents an extensive chamber made of mesoderm, largely filled by the heart hanging from the midline of the roof by its dorsal mesocardium (see Figure 20.1 and Chapter 21). Above the roof mesoderm is the foregut. As the developing laryngotracheal diverticulum grows down from the ventral aspect of the gut it and its mesodermal covering will bulge into the pericardial cavity. This becomes even more marked when the left and right lung buds expand into the primitive pericardial cavity and the pericardioperitoneal canals. Meanwhile, horizontal folds of mesoderm are growing into the pericardial cavity from the sides, starting at about day 35 (Figure 20.4). These are known as the **pleuropericardial folds** because they will divide the primitive pericardial cavity into the pleural cavity dorsally and the pericardial cavity ventrally (i.e. anteriorly in the adult).

The pleural cavity is thus formed from the primitive pericardial cavity and from the pericardioperitoneal canals. As the embryo grows so the pleural cavities expand into the mesoderm of the body wall until they almost encompass the heart (Figure 20.5). Caudally the pericardioperitoneal canals are eventually closed off by mesoderm during development of the diaphragm (see Chapter 22). The pleural cavities also expand into this mesoderm, at what will be the inferior border of the lungs.

The pleuropericardial folds give rise to the fibrous pericardium. The developing lung buds are endodermal in origin, because they are derived from the gut, but they are covered with mesoderm, which becomes increasingly important.

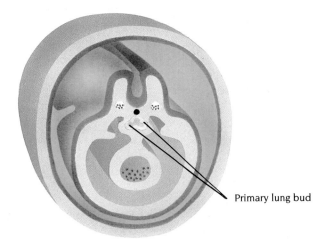

Primary lung bud

FIGURE 20.4   The primary lung buds project into the primitive pericardial cavity.

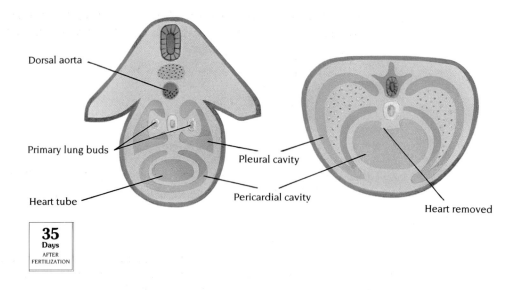

Dorsal aorta

Primary lung buds

Pleural cavity

Heart tube

Pericardial cavity

Heart removed

35
Days
AFTER
FERTILIZATION

FIGURE 20.5 The pleural cavity expands into the mesoderm of the body wall, so that from originally lying dorsal to the pericardial cavity it comes to almost surround it.

Pleural coverings

The lung buds remain covered with mesoderm as they expand. This mesoderm will give rise to bronchial cartilage, smooth muscle and lung connective tissue, including the connective tissue that marks out the lobes of the lung. Round the trachea cartilage rings will form from the mesoderm. An initial network of blood vessels forms in the mesoderm around the lung buds. Eventually branches arise from the nearby branchial arch arteries (see Figure 14.7), perhaps accelerated by production of angiogenic growth factors by the lung buds, to join up with this network.

The pleural cavity is completely lined with mesoderm. Mesoderm associated with gut is described as splanchnic or visceral, and that covering the lungs is later described as the visceral pleura. The mesoderm not covering the lung buds (not associated with endoderm) is described as somatic or parietal and the remainder of the pleural cavity is described as being lined with parietal pleura.

Histology

During the development of the lungs the endodermal lining thins, so that the barrier between the blood vessels in the splanchnic mesoderm and the air that will fill the lungs at birth is as slight as possible. This continuous process is conventionally divided up into four general periods that overlap because differentiation is always more advanced in the cranial part of the lungs than caudally. These periods are:

- Weeks 5–17   Pseudoglandular period
- Weeks 16–25   Canalicular period
- Weeks 24–birth Terminal sac period
- Birth–8 years   Alveolar period

Pseudoglandular period

In the pseudoglandular period, the major lobes and divisions all form. The endoderm cells remain cuboidal.

Canalicular period

In the canalicular stage vascularization begins, and at the end of this period a few terminal sacs develop so the fetus may become just capable of supporting independent life: gestation dates are not exact, of course, and fetuses show individual variation, so survival remains unlikely at this time.

Terminal sac period

As the fetus moves fully into the terminal sac period the lungs begin secreting **surfactant**, a non-wettable phospholipid that keeps the terminal sac endings from touching each other, avoiding lung collapse. This continues through to the alveolar period.

Alveolar period

Before birth the lungs are filled with fluid and will sink if removed and placed in water. This fluid is expelled through the nose and mouth at the first breath, and the lungs will then float. This has been used as a diagnostic test to indicate whether a dead baby was alive at birth or still-born and may be taken as evidence in suspected cases of infanticide.

When the lungs are stretched at the first breath changes occur in circulating levels of bradykinin and prostaglandins, which lead to the gradual shut down of the ductus arteriosus and umbilical arteries.

Defects of the lungs

Lung agenesis In this condition the lung buds fail to form. This failure may be unilateral or bilateral. In unilateral lung agenesis survival is likely after birth, because the remaining lung will increase in size to compensate but bilateral lung agenesis is fatal. Fortunately, lung agenesis is a rare condition.

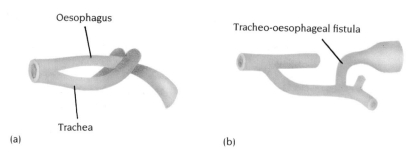

FIGURE 20.6 (a) Positions of the developing lungs relative to the gut; (b) tracheo-oesophageal fistula with oesophageal atresia.

Respiratory distress syndrome In premature babies production of surfactant may be inadequate. The lungs may therefore collapse and the endoderm cell surfaces may be damaged. They then release a glassy protein material (the hyaline membrane, hence the name hyaline membrane disease) that inhibits lung function. About 6000 very premature babies per year in the UK suffer from respiratory distress, and about one third of these die. Surfactant can be obtained from animal and human sources but may be contaminated or evoke an immune response. Recently, however, a pure artificial surfactant has been produced. In clinical trials it was administered immediately after birth to 164 matched pairs of premature babies: 59 babies (36%) in the control group died, compared with 35 (21%) of the treated babies.

Tracheo-oesophageal fistula with oesophageal atresia As the trachea elongates in the embryo the oesophagus comes to lie in between the developing lung buds (Figure 20.6(a)). If the trachea and gut were to come into contact they could fuse, forming a fistula between oesophagus and trachea in the adult. On its own this condition is rare (about one per 100 000 live births), but it is commonly associated with oesphageal atresia – blind ending of the gut – and the incidence is about one per 3000 for the combined condition (Figure 20.6(b)). The newborn baby will gag as its saliva enters its lungs and shows signs of respiratory distress. Milk may be regurgitated on feeding. When the child cries its abdomen may become distended as air is drawn into the stomach.

The prognosis is usually good after surgical repair, especially if this is conducted early, before the child develops pneumonia from inhaling milk and saliva.

Further reading

Balinsky B.I. (1981). *An Introduction to Embryology* 5th edn. New York: Holt Saunders,
Bergsma D. (1979). *Birth Defects Compendium* 2nd edn. London: Macmillan
Emery J. (1969). *The Anatomy of the Developing Lung*. London: Heinemann

Gasser R.F. (1982). *Atlas of Human Embryos*. London: Harper & Row

Hamilton W.J., Boyd J.D. and Mossman H.W. (1962). *Human Embryology* 3rd edn. Cambridge: Heffer

Hildebrand M. (1982). *Analysis of Vertebrate Structure* 2nd edn. New York: John Wiley & Sons

Oliver R.E. (1977). Fetal lung liquids. *Fed. Proc.*, **36**, 2669

Parkinson C.E. and Harvey D. (1981). Amniotic fluid and fetal pulmonary maturity. In *Amniotic Fluid and its Clinical Significance* (Sandler M. ed.), pp. 229–52. New York: Marcel Dekker

O'Rahilly R. and Muller F. (1984). Respiratory and alimentary relations in staged human embryos. *Ann. Otol. Rhinol. Laryngol.*, **93**, 421–9

O'Rahilly R. and Muller F. (1987). *Developmental Stages in Human Embryos*. Carnegie Institution of Washington Publication 637

O'Rahilly R. and Tucker J.A. (1973). The early development of the larynx in staged human embryos. *Ann. Otol. Rhinol. Laryngol.*, **82** (suppl), 1–27

Smith E.I. (1957). The early development of the trachea and oesophagus in relation to atresia of the œsophagus and tracheosphageal fistula. *Contr. Embryol. Carnegie Inst.*, **245**, 36

Stocker J.T., Madewell J.E. and Drake R.M. (1978). Cystic and congenital lung disease in the newborn. *Perspec. Pediatr. Pathol.*, **4**, 93–154

Symchych P. (1978). Developmental anomalies of the lung. In *Pulmonary Physiology of the Fetus, Newborn and Child* (Scarpelli E. *et al.*, eds), pp. 982–98. Philadelphia: Lea & Febiger

Wells L.J. (1954). Development of the human diaphragm and pleural sacs. *Contrib. Embryol. Carnegie Inst.*, **35**, 107–34

Wells L.J. and Boyden E.A. (1954). The development of the bronchopulmonary segments in human embryos of Horizons XVII to XIX. *Am. J. Anat.*, **95**, 163–201

Wigglesworth J.S. and Desai R. (1982). Is fetal respiratory function a major determinant of perinatal survival? *Lancet*, **i**, 264–7

Box 20.1

Alescio T. and Cassini A. (1962). Induction *in vitro* of tracheal buds by pulmonary mesenchyme grafted on tracheal epithelium. *J. Exp. Zool.*, **150**, 83–94

Bernfield M. and Bannerjee S.D. (1982). The turnover of basal lamina glycosaminoglycan correlates with epithelial morphogenesis. *Dev. Biol.*, **90**, 291–305

Deuchar E.M. (1975). *Cellular Interaction in Early Development*. London: Chapman & Hall

Spooner B.S. and Faubion J.M. (1980). Collagen involvement in branching morphogenesis of embryonic lung and salivary gland. *Dev. Biol.*, **77**, 84–102

Wessels N.K. (1970). Mammalian lung development: interactions in formation and morphogenesis of tracheal buds. *J. Exp. Zool.*, **175**, 455–66

Wessels N.K. (1978). *Tissue Interactions and Development*. Menlo Park, CA: W.A. Benjamin

21

The heart

EVOLUTION

In fish, blood is pumped dorsally through the gills from a ventral heart, into blood vessels running dorsally down the axis, then back to the heart. The heart operates as a simple tube pump with valves (Figure 21.1(a)).

The evolution of lungs (see Chapter 20) necessitates the development of a separate blood circulation. Gradually the primitive heart tube became partitioned down the midline (Figure 21.1(b)). This partial separation stage of the two halves in evolution is highly functional in that blood can be readily directed to one side rather than another; for instance when an amphibian dives under the water, it can shut down the blood supply to its lungs and instead divert blood to the skin through which respiration can take place.

Separation of the two sides is usually complete in mammals, although incomplete separation can occur as an anomaly.

Development of the heart

As described earlier, the intraembryonic coelom is horseshoe shaped. Blood islands will form in the floor of the parallel legs of the coelom, differentiating

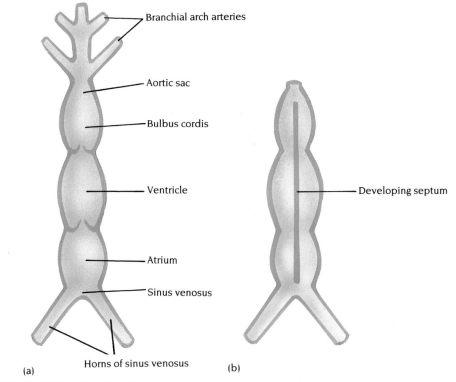

(a)   Horns of sinus venosus   (b)

FIGURE 21.1   Primitive fish heart tube.

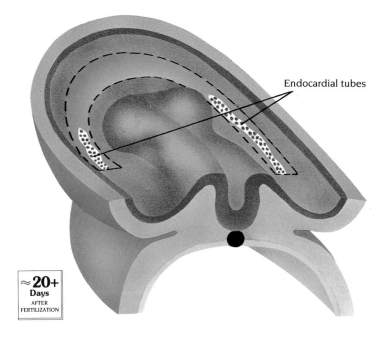

FIGURE 21.2   Blood islands forming in the floor of the intraembryonic coelom.

from splanchnic mesoderm. These islands will gradually become continuous on each side, forming two **endocardial tubes**, one on each side of the midline, by about day 20 (Figure 21.2).

Initially, cardiogenic mesoderm lies on either side, and in front of, the developing forebrain. As a result of the folding of the embryo the most cranial part of the intraembryonic coelom is twisted in such a way that the heart tubes come to lie in the roof rather than the floor (Figure 21.3). Simultaneously the heart tubes will come closer together and will fuse at their cranial ends (Figure 21.4). A single tube is formed, in which constrictions are visible, and these are named in the same way as in those in the fish heart (see Figure 21.5).

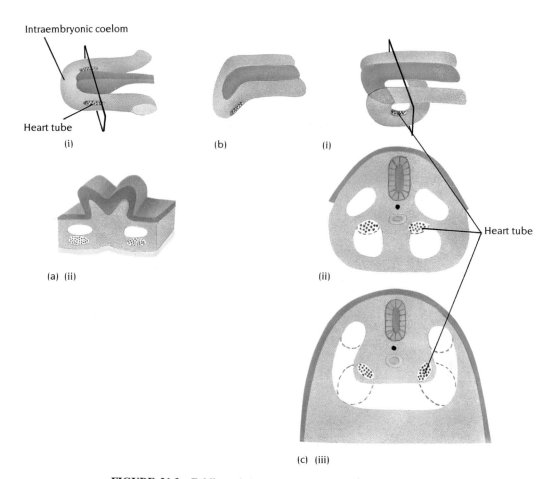

FIGURE 21.3 Folding of the embryo and heart tubes. The intraembryonic coelom is shown as a transparent blue structure. (a) The endocardial tubes form in the floor of the intraembryonic coelom. As the embryo folds (b) these come to lie dorsally to the local coelom (c(i)). A section through the level indicated on the diagram would resemble c(ii); however, the coelom is actually expanding at the same time so in reality it resembles c(iii).

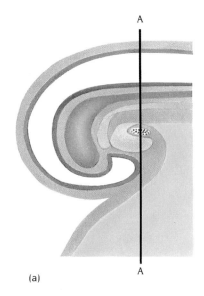

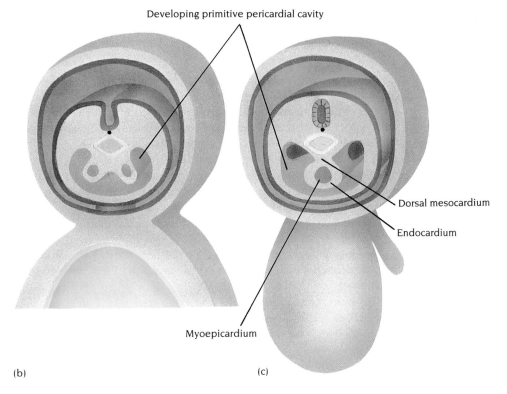

FIGURE 21.4 Fusion of the heart tubes in the midline. A lateral view (a) shows the heart tube in the developing pericardial cavity. A section through line A–A (b) shows how the heart tubes fuse to form a single tube (c).

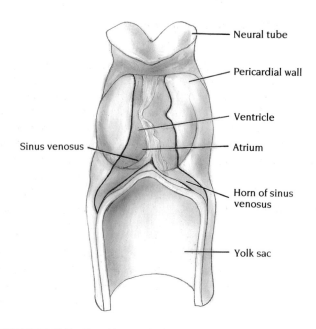

Neural tube

Pericardial wall

Ventricle

Atrium

Sinus venosus

Horn of sinus venosus

Yolk sac

FIGURE 21.5   Fused heart tube in ventral view showing regionalization.

The heart now lies in the primitive pericardial cavity – the descendant of the intraembryonic coelom (Figures 21.3, 21.4). Its walls are made of mesoderm, as is the heart itself. The heart is suspended from the ceiling of the pericardial cavity by the **dorsal mesocardium**, which may be incomplete. The outer covering of the heart is known as the **myoepicardium** because it is in this mesodermal sheath surrounding the endothelial heart tube that cardiac myoblasts will develop. The endothelial heart tube is the **endocardium**. Between the outer myoepicardium and the endocardium the mesodermal cells in section often appear reticulated, although this may be an artefact.

The unfused portions of the primitive endocardial tubes, visible at the caudal end of the heart, become known as the left and right horns of the sinus venosus, by which blood enters the heart (Figure 21.5). They emerge from the mesoderm of the caudal wall of the pericardial cavity, which is a component of the septum transversum (see Chapter 19).

The heart begins to beat during the fourth week after fertilization. The heart is the earliest organ to become functional because it is needed to pump blood through the embryonic and extraembryonic circulations.

Blood flow through the heart

In the early embryo venous blood on each side flows into the left and right horns of the sinus venosus from the placenta via the umbilical vein, from the yolk sac via the vitelline vein, and from the body via the common cardinal vein (see Chapter 7). The horns of the sinus venosus communicate with a small transverse part that leads directly into the primitive **atrium**. This leads in turn into the primitive **ventricle** via the **atrioventricular foramen**. Blood is pumped through the heart by simple sequential contractions of the atrium and the ventricle. The blood flows through the **primary interventricular foramen** to the **bulbus cordis**. This will give rise to part of the definitive right ventricle (hence the name of the foramen) and to the **conus cordis** and the **truncus arteriosus**, which may form a slight expansion at its cranial end, known as the **aortic sac**. From the aortic sac blood enters the **aortic arches** and then the paired dorsal aortae, supplying the head and neck region via branches from the arches and the dorsal aortae. The main blood flow continues caudally down the body in the dorsal aortae, which fuse at the level of the seventh somite during the fourth week. The paired vitelline arteries supply the yolk sac and the paired umbilical arteries supply blood to the placental circulation.

Heart looping

The heart is more or less straight when it is formed by the fusion of the endocardial tubes but during the early embryonic period it begins to bend in two planes (Figure 21.6). As the heart becomes longer it forms an S-shaped loop in the craniocaudal axis. At the same time, the ventral part – the ventricle – of the forming S becomes displaced to the left.

As a result of this looping, the atrium now lies dorsal to the ventricle. As it presses down on the ventricle a left and right division is formed.

The bulbus cordis now curves round to the right to reach the midline once more. The walls of the ventricle gradually become trabeculated during this period.

Entry of blood to the heart

Towards the middle of the embryonic period the systemic venous entry shifts from being bilateral to unilateral (on the right: see Chapter 7). Anastomoses develop across the midline and the blood flow gradually switches over to the right. The right horn of the sinus venosus will become incorporated into the right atrium and the left horn becomes the coronary sinus.

Septation of the heart

The process of septation, which divides the heart into two halves down the midline, is complete by week 5. The process is simple in principle, although it

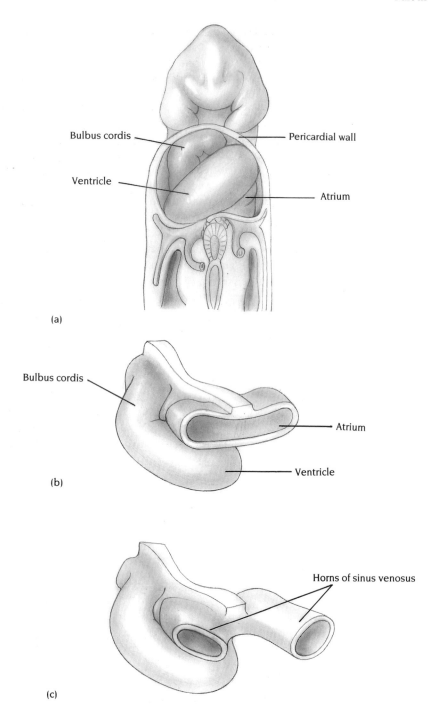

FIGURE 21.6 Heart looping. (a) Ventral view; (b) lateral view, looking forward; (c) similar view from a little more caudally.

appears complex as a result of the looping of the heart. Essentially, partitions grow in the extended heart tube from the ceiling and from the floor (Figure 21.7). This does not happen at the same time in all parts of the heart, and the local names given to the various parts of the partitions and to various other events in heart development tend to conceal the simple nature of the process.

At the atrial end of the heart the roof and floor processes are continuous, forming a crescent-shaped structure known as the **septum primum** (Figure 21.8). It continues to grow cranially towards the atrioventricular foramen; while it is still incomplete the remaining gap connecting the left and right parts of the atrium is called the **ostium primum**. In time the ostium primum will close over as the septum primum reaches the atrioventricular foramen but as it does so another opening begins to form in the septum primum near the roof. This is the **ostium secundum**.

A second septum (the **septum secundum**) begins to grow down on the right hand side of the septum primum (Figure 21.8). It does not reach the atrioventricular foramen, so blood is able to pass from the right atrium through the ostium secundum into the gap between the septae and through the ostium secundum into the left atrium. This is the **foramen ovale**. The blood pressure in the left atrium is low during development, because the blood supply to the lungs is short-circuited by the ductus arteriosus (see Chapter 7) and because the pressure in the lungs is high. The foramen ovale therefore remains open until birth. After birth, the blood pressure on the left side of the heart rises as fluid drains from the lungs and the ductus arteriosus closes. This increased pressure forces the septum primum against the septum secundum, and closes the communication between the left and right atria. In 80% of individuals the septae then fuse permanently; in the remainder they do not fuse but are merely held shut by the blood pressure. This is known as 'probe patency of the foramen ovale'.

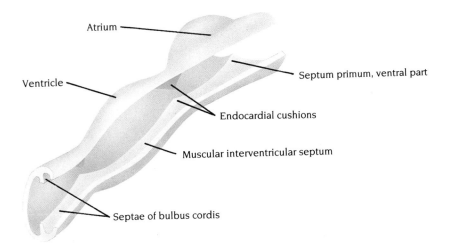

Atrium

Septum primum, ventral part

Ventricle

Endocardial cushions

Muscular interventricular septum

Septae of bulbus cordis

FIGURE 21.7   Notional view of a straightened heart tube, showing septation.

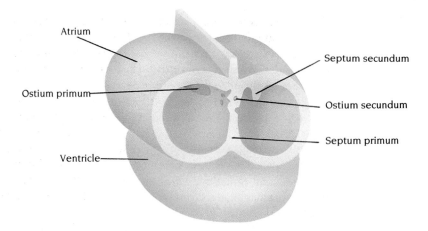

Atrium

Septum secundum

Ostium primum

Ostium secundum

Septum primum

Ventricle

FIGURE 21.8 Septum primum and septum secundum.

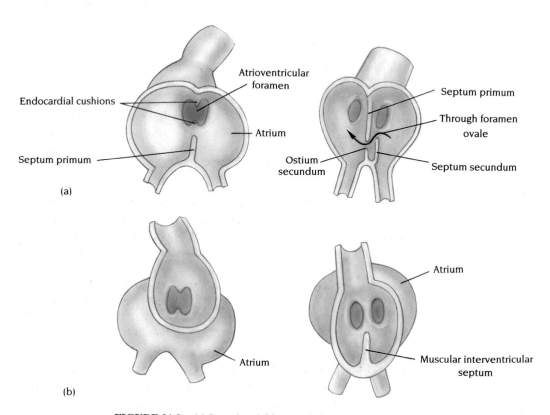

Atrioventricular foramen

Septum primum

Endocardial cushions

Through foramen ovale

Atrium

Ostium secundum

Septum secundum

Septum primum

(a)

Atrium

Atrium

Muscular interventricular septum

(b)

FIGURE 21.9 (a) Dorsal and (b) ventral views of heart.

At the atrioventricular foramen the midline septae are described as the superior and inferior **endocardial cushions** (Figure 21.9(a)). These are the continuations of the septum primum as it passes through the atrioventricular foramen. The cushions grow towards each other and fuse, dividing the atrioventricular foramen into left and right channels (Figure 21.9(b)).

It was indicated above that the primitive ventricle forms much of the right ventricle, while the bulbus cordis will contribute to the left ventricle. Because these structures are initially in 'series' significant changes must be undergone before they are present in 'parallel' and the two channels at the atrioventricular foramen are able to supply the appropriate ventricle. The mechanisms underlying this are not at all clear but a relative shift to the right of the original atrioventricular foramen appears to be coordinated with a widening of the original bulbus cordis (Figure 21.9).

Meanwhile, the ventricle is being divided in two by the **interventricular septum** (Figure 21.9). The bulbus cordis also septates and because this region contributes to the right ventricle the **conotruncal septae** will meet the muscular interventricular septum. The components of the definitive interventricular septum are continuous with the endocardial cushions. In the bulbus region the conotruncal septae form the **aorticopulmonary septum**, which adopts a spiral path as a result of the looping of the heart, and is possibly also influenced by blood flow.

Defects of the heart

Presumably because of this complex series of fusions, heart defects are comparatively common, representing between one-quarter and one-fifth of all abnormalities (41 per 10 000 live births in the Eurocat report). Many heart defects are now detectable by ultrasonography during development (see Special Topic 4, pp. 80–4).

Atrial septal defect Incomplete separation of the left and right atria is described as an atrial septal defect. As described above, 20% of apparently normal adults have probe patency of the foramen ovale, which does not usually cause a problem. However, those few healthy young adults who suffer a cardiac event have an increased incidence of this condition.

True communication between the atria represents 10% of heart defects. Heart murmurs are present as a result of blood flow between the atria. This condition is generally detected not at birth but usually in the second half of the first year. The defect is often corrected surgically when the child is several years old but it is possible to survive into adulthood without treatment.

Ventricular septal defect This is the commonest heart abnormality, representing 25–50% of all heart defects. A small defect results in a characteristic heart murmur. Larger defects create the risk of early congestive heart failure. Surgery has a good chance of correcting these larger defects.

Patent ductus arteriosus The ductus arteriosus normally closes within hours or days of birth. The consequences of failure of closure are related to the degree of patency. In severe cases shortness of breath, respiratory infections, retarded growth and heart failure may result in the first year of life. In minor cases, a characteristic heart murmur is heard but the child may appear otherwise normal. This category represents not quite one-quarter of all heart defects.

Tetralogy of Fallot This represents some 10% of heart defects. Displacement of the conus swellings during development leads to a characteristic set of defects in which there is a ventricular septal defect, stenosis of the outflow of the right ventricle, enlargement of the right ventricle and abnormalities of the right aortic arch. In severe cases cyanosis may be present from soon after birth and becomes progressively more severe. There is a characteristic pattern of heart murmurs. The condition can be resolved by surgery.

Box 21.1 Experimental analysis of heart development

Heart formation

The paired endocardial tubes can be prevented from fusing during development by inserting a thin sheet of material between them. The result is that each forms a complete heart. Fusion is not, therefore, essential to heart development. This ability could be intended as a developmental back-up system, given the importance of heart development.

Development of beating

Perhaps the most remarkable single property of heart tissue is its ability to beat. This is in fact a property of individual cells: if a heart is dissociated into single cells and these are placed in culture conditions, each cell will beat rhythmically at its own rate. When two cells come into contact the slower will entrain on the faster. As the cells continue to divide they will gradually form a large mass in the culture dish in which all the cells are beating in synchrony.

Heart looping

Although the looping of the heart is associated with an increase in length this increase within the confines of the pericardial cavity is not the cause of looping as is sometimes suggested. If the heart is removed from the pericardial cavity at a time when it is still straight, and placed in culture, it will loop on schedule. This appears to be due to differential expansion of the cells in the heart walls.

Special Topic 8 Left and right

Superficially the right side of the body appears very similar to the left but they are far from identical. A composite face made using one half and its mirror image is detectably different from the original. The breasts and testicles also may vary markedly from one side to the other and deep to the surface the differences are even more profound. The heart lies more on the left than the right; the aortic arch lies to the left; the duodenum is thrown in a loop over to the right; there are three lung lobes on the right and two on the left. These differences are derived from handedness in embryological processes. The subtle underlying neural basis for being right- or left-handed also derives its origin early in development.

Sometimes these differences are covert, but they may be revealed in response to particular agents: for instance some teratogens cause defects in one limb rather than the other, and true hermaphrodites are more often male on the right and female on the left.

Although handedness is of considerable medical significance to the embryo in that abnormalities such as heart or gut looping to the wrong side may be life threatening, its underlying basis is still a mystery. However, recent experiments seem to offer clues. These make use of a mouse mutant known as *situs inversus viscerum*. This is a recessive mutation, which in the homozygous condition appears to have no predetermined sense of which ought to be its left or right. Instead, it almost seems as if it tosses a coin: half of the homozygous embryos are normal, and half are mirror images of normal (so that the heart, for example, loops over to the right).

Using this mutant, it is possible to show that the maternal environment does not play a role in influencing left/right decisions. Newly fertilized mutant embryos implanted in normal mothers (see Special Topic 2, pp. 45–6) develop according to their genotype, not according to the mother's genotype, as do normal embryos carried by mutant mothers. Chimaeras may be created between normal and mutant mice: even quite a large proportion of normal cells are not enough to rescue a mutant mouse. Most puzzling of all, drugs that usually affect only one side of the embryo consistently affect only the other side in these mutant mice.

One speculative model to explain these results relies on the fact that some molecules exist as optical isomers: mutual mirror image versions of the molecule identical in chemical constitution but with different chemical properties. If such a 'handed' molecule is present in only one of its optical isomers, and if this molecule were aligned along the axis, then it could generate a 'bias' to one side. A second step would establish a gradient of molecular activity from one side of the embryo to another. This second step is random in principle: the gradient can run from left to right or right to left, but the 'bias' constrains it to run in one consistent direction. A third step would involve the interpretation of this gradient in terms of the physical structures of the body.

If the first step fails to occur correctly – if, for instance, the handed molecule is missing – then the second step would reveal its underlying randomness. This could explain how *situs inversus* mice come to show 50:50 distribution of normal:reversed phenotype.

A chance finding seems likely to shed further light on this process. Research workers carrying out gene injections for an unrelated purpose created a strain of mice which, in the homozygous condition, were completely left/right reversed in all cases. This proved to be because the injected gene had affected the function of a normal gene, which they named *inv*. The nature of this gene awaits elucidation, but it may hold the answer to the riddle of 'handed' development.

Further reading

Allwork S.P. and Anderson R.H. (1979). Developmental anatomy of the membranous part of the ventricular septum in the human heart. *Br. Heart J.*, **41**, 275–80

Anderson R.H., Wilkinson J.L. and Becker A.E. (1978). The bulbus cordis – a misunderstood region of the developing human heart: its significance to the classification of congenital cardiac malformations. *Birth Defects*, **14**, 1–28

Cooper M.H. and O'Rahilly R. (1971). The human heart at seven postovulatory weeks. *Acta Anat.*, **79**, 280–99

Davis C.L. (1927). Development of the human heart from its first appearance to the stage found in embryos of 20 paired somites. *Carnegie Inst. Contrib. Embryol.*, **19**, 245–84

De Vries P.A. and Saunders J. B. De C. M. (1962). Development of the ventricles and spiral outflow tract in the human heart. A contribution to the development of the human heart from age group IX to age group XV. *Carnegie Inst. Contrib. Embryol.*, **37**, 87–114

Fananapazir K. and Kaufman M.H. (1988). Observations on the development of the aorticopulmonary spiral septum in the mouse. *J. Anat.*, **158**, 157–72

Jaffee O.C. (1978). Hemodynamics and cardiogenesis: the effects of physiologic factors on cardiac development. *Birth Defects*, **14**, 393–404

Lomonico M.P., Moore G.W. and Hutchins G.M. (1986). Rotation of the junction of the outflow tract and great arteries in the embryonic human heart. *Anat. Rec.*, **216**, 544–9

Los J.A. (1978). Cardiac septation and development of the aorta, pulmonary tract and pulmonary veins: previous work in the light of recent findings. *Birth Defects*, **14**, 109–38

McBride R.E., Moore G.W. and Hutchins G.M. (1981). Development of the outflow tract and closure of the interventricular septum in the normal human heart. *Am. J. Anat.*, **160**, 309–31

Pexedier T. (1978). Development of the outflow tract of the embryonic heart. *Birth Defects*, **14**, 29–68

Teal S.I., Moore G.W. and Hutchins G.M.(1986). Development of aortic and mitral valve continuity in the human embryonic heart. *Am. J. Anat.*, **176**, 447–60

Walmsley R. (1958). The orientation of the heart and the appearance of its chambers in the adult cadaver. *Br. Heart J.*, **20**, 441–58

Walmsley R. and Monkhouse W.S. (1988). The heart of the newborn child: an anatomical study based upon serial transverse sections. *J. Anat.*, **159**, 93–111

Box 21.1

DeHaan R.L. (1959). Cardiac bifida and the development of pacemaker function in the early chick embryo. *Dev. Biol.*, **1**, 586–602

Goss, C.M. (1935). Double hearts produced experimentally in rat embryos. *J. Exp. Zool.*, **72**, 33–48

Manning A. and McLachlan J.C. (1990). Looping of chick embryo hearts in vitro *J. Anat.*, **168**, 257–63

Special Topic 8

Brown N.A. and Wolpert L. (1980). The development of handedness in left/right asymmetry. *Development*, **109**, 1–9

Yokoyama T., Copeland N.G., Jenkins N.A. *et al.* (1993). Reversal of left–right asymmetry: a *situs inversus* mutation. *Science*, **260**, 679–82

ABDOMEN AND PELVIS

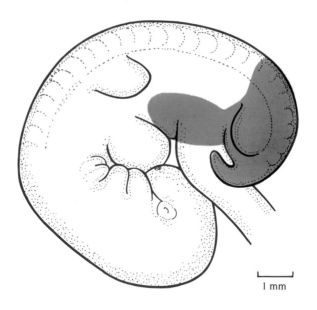

1 mm

22

The diaphragm

The diaphragm in the adult separates the thoracic cavities – the pleural and peri-cardial cavities – from the peritoneal cavity. However, at the time of formation these cavities are connected by the pericardioperitoneal canals between which runs the gut with its surrounding mesoderm. The pericardial cavity is bounded at its caudal end by a wall of mesoderm, which is continuous with the mesoderm cover-ing the yolk sac, and with the mesoderm of the body wall. The formation of the diaphragm must therefore be described in terms of these structures and spaces.

Components of the diaphragm

The diaphragm is conventionally described as having four major components:

- the **dorsal mesentery** at the level of the oesophagus;
- the **septum transversum**;
- the **pleuroperitoneal folds**;
- the **mesoderm of the body wall** (Figure 22.1).

The exact nature of the contribution of each to the adult diaphragm, however, is not definitively established.

The diaphragm is invaded by skeletal myoblasts, ultimately derived from the somites. These include the somites at the level at which the diaphragm origi-

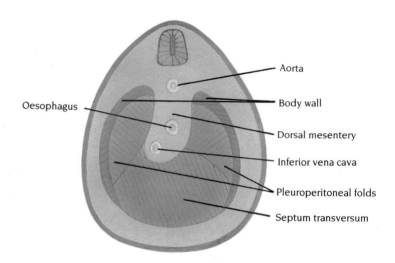

FIGURE 22.1 Components of the diaphragm at about the beginning of the fetal period. The diaphragm is pierced by the aorta, the oesophagus and the inferior vena cava.

nates and the somites at the level at which it will eventually lie, as it undergoes a considerable shift in relative position.

Dorsal mesentery

Because the gut runs through the region where the diaphragm will form, its mesodermal covering (including the dorsal mesentery – see Chapter 21) necessarily contribute. The region formed by the mesentery is invaded by myoblasts, and in the adult, will form the **crura** of the diaphragm. The dorsal mesentery is, of course, mesothelial where it is exposed to the body cavities: here, the pericardioperitoneal canals are running on either side of the body.

The septum transversum

As we have seen, the pericardial cavity is closed off by a wall of mesoderm at its caudal end. From this emerge the horns of the sinus venosus. Dorsal to the wall the pericardioperitoneal canals leave the primitive pericardial cavity for the developing peritoneal cavity. This wall of mesoderm is continuous with the mesoderm covering the yolk sac (see Figure 22.2(a)) and with the ventral mesentery of the gut. The mesodermal structure formed by the caudal end of the pericardium and the cranial mesodermal wall of the yolk sac is known as the septum transversum. It lies at the level of the third, fourth and fifth cervical somites. In an oblique transverse section through the embryo it has the appearance of a wall of mesoderm running across the axis (Figure 22.2(b)). The septum transversum forms a major component of the adult diaphragm, giving rise to

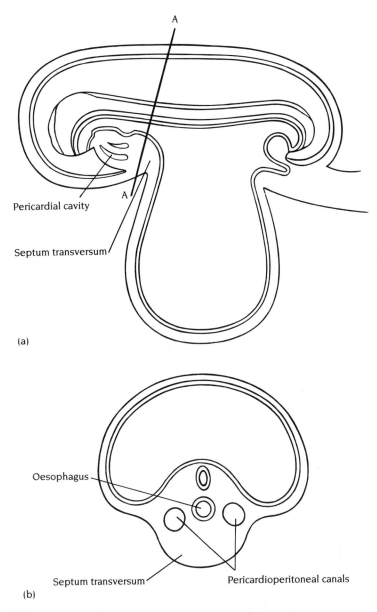

FIGURE 22.2 (a) Midline sagittal section showing the mesoderm of the septum transversum; (b) oblique transverse section (through line A–A in (a)), showing the septum
transversum.

the tendinous part known as the central tendon. It is also of significance in liver
development, as we will see in Chapter 23.

The pleuroperitoneal folds

The pericardioperitoneal canals run through the region where the diaphragm is to develop, and must be closed off during the separation of the primitive pericardial/pleural cavity and the peritoneal cavity. This is achieved by the pleuroperitoneal folds, which grow medially from the mesodermal walls of the pericardioperitoneal canals during the mid-embryonic period, closing off the canals altogether (Figure 22.3). Although the illustration seems to imply that they grow transversely across the canals they actually have an oblique course across the canals. However, for our purposes, we merely need to know that complete occlusion of the tunnels has normally occurred by the end of the sixth week after fertilization. The right-hand canal is generally closed off before the left. The pleuroperitoneal folds thus separate the pleural cavity (see Chapter 20) from the developing peritoneal cavity.

The body wall

The somatic (parietal) mesoderm underlying the ectoderm all the way round the body also contributes to the rim of the diaphragm. Muscle cells from the somites, and associated innervation from the neural tube, will later invade this mesodermal component. However, as discussed below, this represents only part of the innervation of the diaphragm.

Innervation and descent

The mesoderm of the septum transversum is innervated by nerves from cervical roots 3, 4 and 5, because these are the nearest nerve roots when it forms. They run to the septum transversum via the pleuropericardial folds. Subsequently, however, rapid growth of the dorsal cervical part of the embryo leads to a major shift in relative position of the diaphragm. This is known as the 'descent' of the diaphragm. The nerves from C3, 4 and 5, collectively known as the **phrenic nerve**, continue to run in the pleuropericardial folds, as these form what will be the **fibrous pericardium**. These nerves exert motor and sensory control over a major part of the central tendon. The musculature of the rim of the diaphragm is apparently derived from the thoracic segments opposite which it lies after its descent, and these are innervated appropriately.

As can be seen from Figure 22.2(a), the septum transversum lies obliquely across the body axis. After the descent of the diaphragm it will lie much more transversely across the axis.

Defects of the diaphragm

Diaphragmatic hernia The incidence of this condition is approximately 5 per 10 000 live births. It is more common on the left side than on the right and may

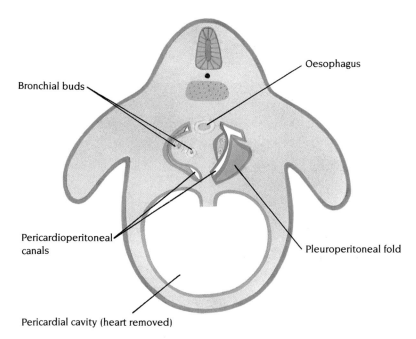

FIGURE 22.3 The angled growth of the pleuroperitoneal folds across the pericardioperitoneal canals.

result from the failure of the pleuroperitoneal folds to occlude completely the pericardioperitoneal canals.

As a result of this failure there is an opening in the diaphragm, and the abdominal viscera may be found in the thorax (Figure 22.4). After birth, the newborn child often experiences difficulty in breathing, with resulting cyanosis. The thoracic organs, the lungs and heart, are often displaced to the side opposite the hernia. The symptoms may increase with time, as the child swallows air which distends the stomach. The diagnosis may be confirmed by radiography of the thorax and abdomen. Fortunately, this defect may be surgically repaired, and the prognosis is good if the condition is spotted before respiratory fatigue and pneumonia develop.

Eventration of the diaphragm This may present with symptoms similar to those of diaphragmatic hernia, but there is no opening present in the diaphragm. Instead an area of muscle weakness or deficiency permits the abdominal contents to 'balloon up' into the thoracic cavity, although they do not penetrate the diaphragm. This condition can result from damage to the phrenic nerve during delivery: because the roots of the phrenic nerve are cervical in origin they are vulnerable to crushing or other damage by obstetric forceps, if these are used to assist the birth. Once the nerves are damaged they fail to maintain the survival of the muscle cells they supply in the normal way (see Special Topic 5, pp. 153–7), and the muscle cells die in consequence.

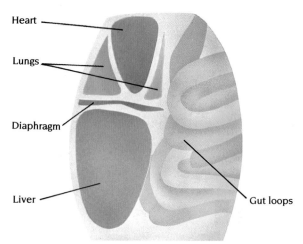

Heart

Lungs

Diaphragm

Liver

Gut loops

FIGURE 22.4   Congenital diaphragmatic hernia: the abdominal contents have displaced the heart and constricted the growth of the lung on the side of the defect.

Congenital hiatus hernia If the crura fail to develop properly the stomach may partially enter the thoracic cavity in the midline. Reflux of the stomach contents may result, especially when lying down. As a consequence the child may show weakness and failure to thrive.

Hiatus hernia may develop during adult life, often as a result of aging. It may be that certain individuals are be predisposed towards this hazard as a result of embryological events, requiring only an appropriate incident to trigger it.

Further reading

Barbin J.Y., Armstrong O., Barbin J.G. and Collin C.L. (1985). Essai de systematisation fonctionnelle du diaphragme. *Bull. Soc. Anat. Paris*, 130–1

Bourdelat D., Barbet J.P., Labbe F. and Hidden G. (1989). The arterial blood supply of the human fetal diaphragm. *Surg. Radiol. Anat.*, **11**, 265–70

Hamilton W.J., Boyd J.D. and Mossman H.W. (1959). *Human Embryology*. Cambridge: Heffer

Pages R. (1966). Sur les hernies diaphragmatiques congenitales de l'enfant, considerations anatomiques, embryologiques, et therapeutiques. *Ann. Chir. Infant*, **7**, 195–207

Wells L.J. (1954). Development of the human diaphragm and pleural sacs. *Carnegie. Contrib. Embryol.*, **35**, 107–43

23

The gut

The gut forms from the endoderm that originally lines the yolk sac. As the embryo folds, so the endoderm is rolled into a simple tube at the cranial and caudal ends, representing the developing foregut and hindgut. The yolk sac is still suspended from the region that will become midgut but will decrease in relative size throughout the embryonic period. More and more of the gut adopts a simple tube shape as the yolk sac diminishes.

This tube will undergo a number of changes throughout embryonic and fetal development. At various locations the gut will alter its width; it will bend; it will twist; it will produce buds; it will elongate considerably. Initially the gut is the same length as the embryo from mouth to anus but in the adult it is several times this length and must therefore be coiled inside the abdominal cavity.

Through these changes the gut will acquire its final deployment and contribute to a number of associated structures. As described in Chapter 19, it is suspended dorsally from a mesodermal mesentery, with a 'ventral mesentery' in the foregut region. These mesenteries will also be thrown into complex arrangements as development proceeds.

Occlusion and recanalization of the gut

During the sixth week the endoderm cells lining the gut rapidly proliferate and occlude the gut lumen; in the late embryonic and early fetal periods the gut recanalizes. The reasons for this are not clear, although it has been suggested that it is to provide enough endoderm to cover the gut as it elongates. Failure of this process is associated with a number of abnormalities (p. 318).

As the diaphragm descends the oesophagus elongates. On the caudal side of the diaphragm the abdominal gut commences, conventionally divided into foregut, midgut and hindgut, on the basis of the arterial blood supply (see Chapter 19). The coeliac artery supplies the foregut, the superior mesenteric artery the midgut and the inferior mesenteric artery the hindgut.

Foregut

Stomach

The stomach forms on the caudal side of the diaphragm. At about 28 days after fertilization the initially simple gut tube begins to dilate (Figure 23.1). By 35 days it is clear that this dilation is asymmetric, with a greater degree of curvature (perhaps due to extra cell division) on the dorsal aspect (Figure 23.2). This represents the **greater curvature of the stomach**. At about 40 days the stomach starts to rotate about its long axis, turning through 90° clockwise as viewed from cranial to caudal (Figure 23.3), which may be associated with an asymmetric thinning of the dorsal mesentery.

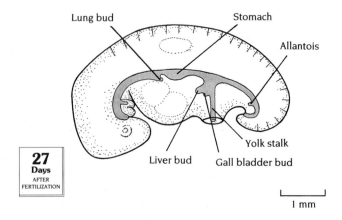

FIGURE 23.1 Early stomach development.

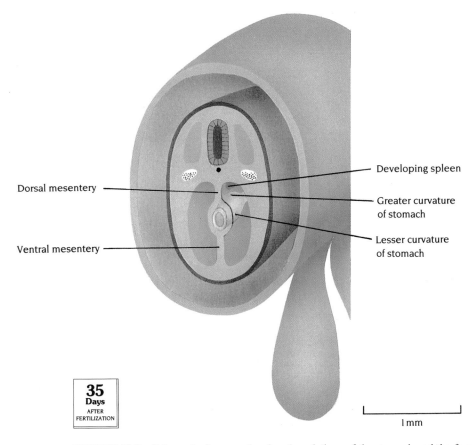

Dorsal mesentery

Ventral mesentery

Developing spleen

Greater curvature of stomach

Lesser curvature of stomach

35 Days AFTER FERTILIZATION

1 mm

FIGURE 23.2 Schematic diagram showing the relations of the stomach and the formation of the greater curvature.

Before the rotation begins, the **vagus nerves** arrive from the spinal cord and so after the rotation the left vagus nerve will innervate the anterior aspect of the stomach, and the right the posterior aspect.

The stomach then shifts to lie more transversely across the abdominal cavity (Figure 23.4) and the duodenum is carried across to the right-hand side of the abdominal cavity.

Formation of omental bursa and lesser sac of the peritoneum

As the stomach rotates the dorsal mesentery moves to the left (Figure 23.3) to form a purse-shaped structure (Latin: *bursa*) which is described as four-layered (there are two layers of mesentery, each of which is bounded by twin outer layers of mesothelium: Figure 23.3, inset). The space within the bursa is the **lesser sac of the peritoneum** and the opening the **epiploic foramen**. When the stom-

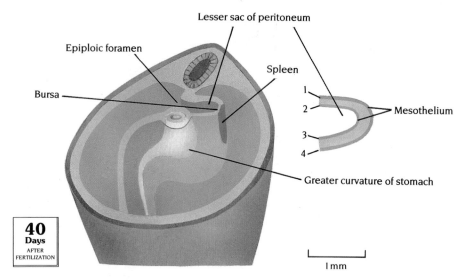

Lesser sac of peritoneum

Epiploic foramen

Spleen

Bursa

Mesothelium

1
2
3
4

Greater curvature of stomach

40 Days
AFTER
FERTILIZATION

1 mm

FIGURE 23.3   Stomach rotation.

ach shifts to a more transverse position the bursa hangs from it over the coiled gut and is hence known as the **omental bursa** or **greater omentum** (from Latin for apron) (Figure 23.4). Its size may vary considerably between individuals.

The stomach is supplied by the coeliac artery, as discussed below.

Spleen

The spleen is entirely mesodermal in origin but it is convenient to consider it with the gut at this point because of its relationship to the stomach. The spleen forms during weeks 4–5 within the dorsal mesentery, just dorsal to the greater curvature of the stomach (Figure 23.2). At this time the stomach still lies in the midline of the body. The spleen develops between the mesothelial layers covering the dorsal mesentery. It forms initially as isolated spleen islands, which then coalesce (in some animals, for example ungulates, the spleen remains as islands).

The spleen makes lymphocytes and produces, stores and destroys red blood cells both in the fetus and after birth. Note that blood-forming tissue develops in a region where the endoderm and splanchnic mesoderm are in close proximity, though they are not in contact.

Adult position of the spleen

As the stomach rotates the spleen is carried to the left with the dorsal mesentery (Figures 23.3, 23.4). The mesentery fuses to the dorsal wall of the coelom where the left urogenital ridge is developing (see Chapter 24). A short stretch of mesentery joins the spleen to the ridge, and is known as the **lienorenal**

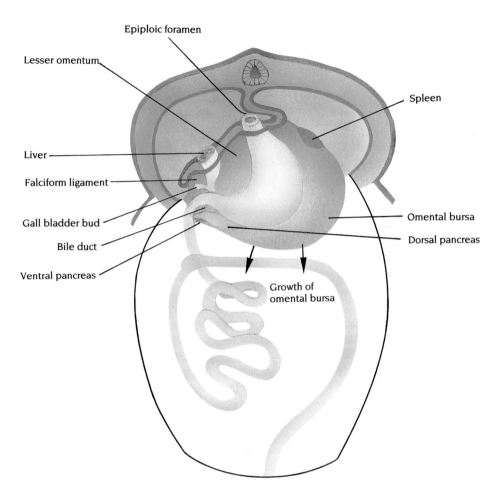

Epiploic foramen

Lesser omentum

Spleen

Liver

Falciform ligament

Gall bladder bud

Bile duct

Ventral pancreas

Omental bursa

Dorsal pancreas

Growth of
omental bursa

FIGURE 23.4   The stomach comes to lie rather more transversely across the long axis
of the body, with corresponding changes to its mesenteries and the neighbouring gut
structures.

ligament. The artery to the spleen is a branch of the coeliac artery and runs in
the mesentery in a tortuous way.

Accessory spleen tissue arises (sometimes even in the pancreas) in as many
as 10% of the population; this anomalous situation in humans therefore corresponds to that found normally in some animals.

Fixation of the duodenum

The rotation of the stomach swings the duodenum round to the right, pressing it
against the dorsal aspect of the peritoneal cavity. Visceral and parietal mesothelium therefore come in contact. The mesoderms fuse ('retroperitoneally' –

against the back of the abdominal cavity) because the space between them is excluded. This fusion is described as fixation of the duodenum and is the local version of a general phenomenon that occurs wherever circumstances allow.

The duodenum occludes at weeks 5–7 and recanalizes by the end of week 8.

Liver

At the fourth week after fertilization, before the stomach and duodenum have begun to rotate, the liver bud or **hepatic diverticulum** starts to grow ventrally from the caudal part of the foregut (Figure 23.1). This bud will also give rise to the primordium of the gall bladder. The bud pushes ventrally and cranially into the mesoderm ventral to the gut. This is often called the ventral mesentery: it represents the attachment of the gut to the ventral body wall, and is continuous with the septum transversum. The region of dorsal mesentery above the bud is known as the **lesser omentum**. The mesentery between the bud and the anterior body wall will develop into the falciform ligament (Figure 23.5).

The liver bud divides into two lobes, left and right, and these continue to invade the mesoderm cranially, ventral to the duodenum and stomach, towards the septum transversum (Figure 23.5). Growth proceeds by outpushing of 'cords' or fingers of endoderm into the septum transversum. Mesothelium (visceral peritoneum) lies on either side of the developing liver, but there is none at the cranial growth points as these are entirely within the mesoderm. Hence, when the septum transversum begins to form the central tendon of the diaphragm, there is no mesothelium between the liver and the diaphragm, producing what will be known as the bare area of the liver.

The right liver lobe becomes bigger than the left. The endodermal liver cords intermingle with blood-filled spaces or sinusoids in the septum transver-

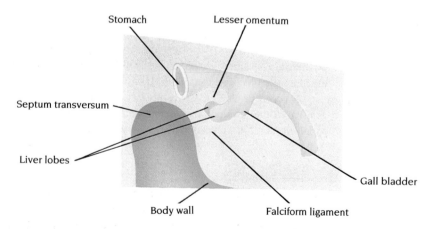

FIGURE 23.5 Formation of the gall bladder primordium.

sum (see Chapter 7), and give rise to parenchymal plates of tissue (the epithelial lining of the intrahepatic part of the biliary apparatus): a substantial part of the liver is therefore endodermal. The mesoderm is believed to give rise to the fibrous, haemopoietic and Kupffer cells of the liver.

At about 6 weeks after fertilization haematopoiesis commences. The liver is a major site of blood formation in the embryo, and this is probably the reason why the liver is relatively larger in the embryo than the adult. By 9 weeks, it represents 10% of fetal weight, compared with 5% of body weight of the adult.

A major part of the liver's haematopoietic role in the embryo is the production of erythrocytes. The fetal liver has been used as a source of haematopoietic cells between weeks 8 and 14 after fertilization as the numbers of post-thymic T lymphocytes are small, which reduces the risk of an immune reaction (often described in this instance as graft versus host disease – GVHD). Such cells might provide stem cells to replace those lost in immunodeficiency syndromes or following chemotherapy for leukaemias.

Gall bladder

During the early embryonic period another bud representing the primordium of the gall bladder appears as an offshoot of the liver bud (Figures 23.1, 23.5), growing caudally and ventrally.

The biliary apparatus makes bile pigments from about 12 weeks after fertilization onwards. These are dark green and colour the contents of the duodenum below the bile duct, which accounts for the dark green appearance of the first bowel movements – known as meconium – in newborn babies. Atresia or stenosis further down the duodenum from the bile duct opening leads to the vomiting of green-stained milk (see p. 319). This may be contrasted with the symptoms of pyloric stenosis (see below). The duct of the gall bladder shifts position in accordance with the movements of the pancreas.

Pancreas

This appears as a **dorsal pancreatic bud** opposite the hepatic diverticulum at 26–27 days after fertilization (Figure 23.6(a)). A **ventral pancreatic bud** develops a few days later from the region of the liver bud/bile duct.

The ventral bud and the opening of the bile duct will migrate round the gut, perhaps due to differential relative growth of the gut wall, and the pancreatic buds will fuse (Figure 23.6(b)). The dorsal portion becomes the **main body** and **tail** of the pancreas, the ventral the **uncinate process** and the **inferior head**. The main pancreatic duct is usually derived from the ventral bud, though there is a degree of variability in this, and two ducts may be present (Figure 23.6(c)). The pancreatic duct and the bile duct normally join to form the **major duodenal papilla** which passes their secretions to the duodenum.

The endocrine cells of the **islets of Langerhans** are believed to come from the endodermal component of the pancreas, as do the exocrine cells that produce

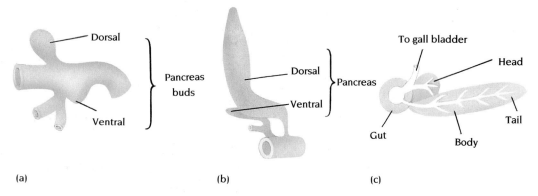

(a)   (b)   (c)

FIGURE 23.6 Formation of the pancreas.

the digestive enzymes. The **septae** and the covering arise from the surrounding splanchnic mesoderm.

Midgut

At about week 5 a loop of gut, attached to the remnant of the yolk sac by the yolk stalk, begins to extend into the chorionic cavity (or extraembryonic coelom) via the forming umbilical cord (Figure 23.7). What makes this happen is unclear, although it has been suggested that it is related to the growth of the liver and mesonephros (see Chapter 24), which reduce the available space in the developing peritoneal cavity. As the gut loop extends, the dorsal mesentery extends with it.

The midgut loop can be considered as having a cranial and a caudal limb (Figure 23.7). The yolk stalk continues to connect the loop to the yolk sac, which diminishes in relative size, at the transition between the cranial and caudal limbs. As described in Chapter 19, the artery of the midgut loop is the superior mesenteric artery, which originally supplied the yolk sac as the paired vitelline arteries.

The midgut loop is then displaced 90° counterclockwise (as seen from the ventral aspect) so that the cranial limb lies to the right and the caudal limb to the left (Figure 23.8). Again, it is not entirely clear how this happens, although it may be related to the rotation of the stomach. If a length of tube incorporating a loop is twisted just above that loop, then the loop is thrown over to one side in exactly this way, as can readily be verified.

Over the next few weeks the cranial and caudal limbs differentiate. The cranial limb elongates rapidly, which necessitates it coiling up to form what is known as the **jejunoileal mass**. This will become the **small intestine** (Figure

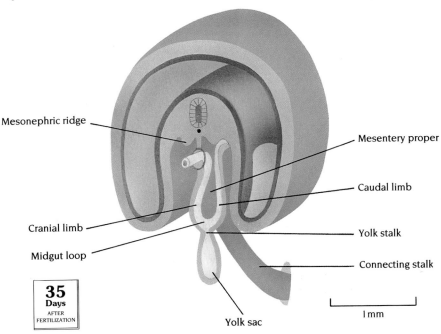

FIGURE 23.7 The extending midgut loop.

23.9). The caudal limb, which does not elongate to anything like the same extent, develops a small protrusion known as the **caecal diverticulum** from which the **appendix** will develop. As a result of the much less extensive growth of the caudal limb and the mesentery the superior mesenteric artery comes to lie rather closer to the caudal limb than to the cranial. The caudal limb will eventually give rise to the transverse and descending **colon**.

At about 10 weeks the liver and kidneys occupy proportionally less of the abdominal cavity and, perhaps as a result, the midgut loop begins to return from

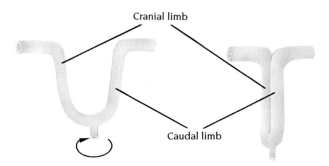

FIGURE 23.8 A lateral view shows how the midgut loop rotates through 90° clockwise as seen from a ventral position.

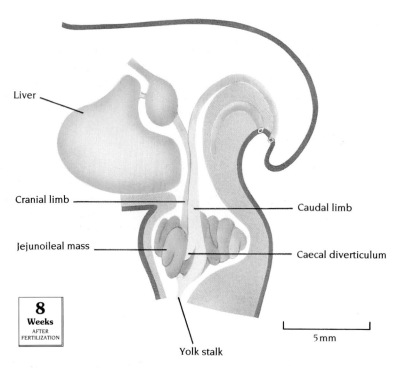

Liver

Cranial limb

Jejunoileal mass

Caudal limb

Caecal diverticulum

8
Weeks
AFTER
FERTILIZATION

5 mm

Yolk stalk

FIGURE 23.9 The jejunoileal mass lies behind the caudal limb.

its position in the umbilical cord and chorionic cavity. The cranial limb forming the jejunoileal mass returns first, slipping gradually through the comparatively narrow entry to the abdominal cavity. Once inside, it lies generally to the right, but is so massive that it spills over the midline to occupy most of the abdominal cavity at this level. The caudal limb (with the superior mesenteric artery) returns to lie on top of the jejunoileal mass. The caecal diverticulum is found under the liver on the right-hand side (see Figure 23.4).

During late fetal development the caecum tends to move down the right side of the abdominal cavity to lie in a more caudal position. This process is not essential to gut function, and in 6% of neonates it has not occurred, so that their caecum remains under the liver. Not infrequently it remains in this position throughout adult life and need present no great problem: it may, however, puzzle a novice surgeon looking for the appendix in the usual place.

These various shifts in relative position are sometimes described as a 180° rotation, which is then added to the original 90° to make 270°. While it is just possible to interpret events in this way, it is not necessary: an initial 90° rotation followed by the return of the elongated cranial limb before the caudal limb is sufficient description.

Fixation

When the gut returns to the abdominal cavity its mesoderm covering is generally pressed against the dorsal aspect of the cavity itself and tends to fuse against the body wall. The mesentery of the midgut is not pressed against the cavity wall in this way, however, so it persists, although its line of attachment alters.

Maturation of the gut

At first, in the fourth week after fertilization, the gut is a simple tube. Villi start to appear in the duodenum in week 8 and villus formation proceeds down the gut until by week 16 the whole intestine possesses villi. The splanchnic mesoderm begins to form circular muscle during week 5, while longitudinal muscle appears early in the fetal period. Peyer's patches develop in week 20. Functional maturation of the digestive capacities of the gut continue up to and after birth.

Hindgut

This is supplied by the inferior mesenteric artery. It includes the last third of the transverse colon and the remaining caudal part of gut down to the point at which it contacts the tail ectoderm. This most caudal part of the gut is known as the **cloaca**, from the Latin word for a sewer. At first it is sealed off by a membrane composed of ectoderm and endoderm – the **cloacal membrane** (compare this with the oral membrane: see Chapter 16).

EVOLUTION OF THE ALLANTOIS

*The evolution of tough, semipermeable eggs enabled the vertebrates to colonize the land. However, this posed the problem for their embryos of how to deal with the poisonous waste products that had previously diffused away in water. A special impermeable sac evolved from the hindgut in which the waste could be stored until hatching. This sac is known as the **allantois**. In mammals the mother removes fetal waste products via the placenta, so there is no real need for the allantois but it still develops in human embryos (just as the yolk sac still develops even in the absence of yolk), and has been modified to fulfil other purposes.*

The allantois develops as an outgrowth from the caudal end of the yolk sac even before the hindgut is fully formed (see Figures 4.3, 23.1). Once the gut has formed, the allantois is seen as a short blind tube running from the gut into the connecting stalk. The umbilical arteries pass the allantois on either side (see Figure 19.6 and p. 108).

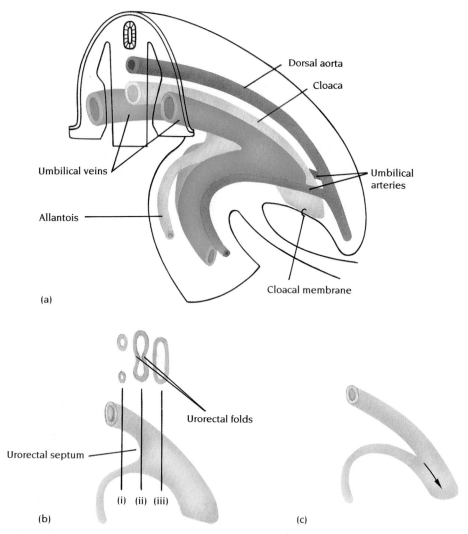

FIGURE 23.10 (a) Hindgut in relation to body wall and the umbilical arteries and veins; (b) sections through the hindgut as described in text; (c) progress of 'urorectal septum' towards the cloacal membrane.

The main part of the hindgut is formed by the cloaca (Figure 23.10(a)).

Figure 23.10(b) shows several transverse sections through the cloaca. At level (i) a transverse section cuts through the gut and allantois, while at level (iii) only the cloaca appears. The intermediate level (ii) shows a transverse section close to the junction of the gut and allantois. The folds apparent at this level are known as the **urorectal folds**; these will come together so that the point of fusion becomes more and more caudal (Figure 23.10(c)). At about 7 weeks fusion has reached the cloacal membrane. The cloaca then divides into the **anorectal canal** and the **primitive urogenital sinus**, closed off by the **anal**

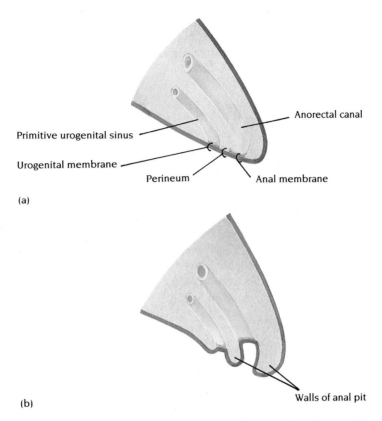

Primitive urogenital sinus

Urogenital membrane

Perineum

Anorectal canal

Anal membrane

(a)

(b)

Walls of anal pit

FIGURE. 23.11   (a) Division of cloacal membrane into anal and urogenital components; (b) formation of the anal pit.

membrane and **urogenital membrane** respectively (Figure 23.11). The region
between the anal and urogenital membranes gives rise to the **perineal body** or
perineum, which derives from the caudal ends of the fused urorectal folds. The
barrier of mesoderm between the anorectal canal and the urogenital sinus
formed by the fusion of the urorectal folds is known as the **urorectal septum**.

Amniotic fluid and the gut

The anal membrane will rupture during weeks 8–9 (compared with the oral
membrane which ruptures at about 4 weeks after fertilization) to create a continuous passage for amniotic fluid through the mouth, along the gut (and yolk sac)
and out again into the amniotic cavity via the anal canal. However, when the
fetus swallows amniotic fluid some is absorbed in the gut, and excess fluid is

removed via the placenta. From about the fourth month the output from the fetal kidneys contributes to the production of amniotic fluid. A balance of removal and production is established, disturbance of which can lead to an excess or deficiency of amniotic fluid.

Anal pit

The mesodermal cells round the anal membrane increase in number until a rim is formed at the outlet of the anal canal. The anal canal now lies at the bottom of a pit – the **anal pit** or **proctodeum** (Figure 23.11(b)). When the anal membrane ruptures the upper two-thirds of the anal canal is lined with endoderm and is supplied with blood from the inferior mesenteric artery. By contrast, the lower third is lined with ectoderm and supplied by branches of the internal pudendal artery. The junction between the ectoderm and endoderm remains visible and is known as the **pectinate line**.

Defects of the gut and associated structures

Defects of the urogenital sinus are dealt with in Chapter 27, as it is important to describe them in association with the development of the urogenital system.

Failure of the gut to recanalize after occlusion, or a local accident such as failure of the immediate blood supply will cause a narrowing (stenosis) or blockage (atresia) that can occur at almost any point along the gut. The position may often be deduced from the symptoms, as described below. A variety of forms of atresia may be found (Figure 23.12). There may be a membrane across the gut, a portion of gut may be replaced by a solid cord or a portion may be missing altogether. The part cranial to the obstruction is often dilated and the part caudal to it correspondingly contracted. The general forms of surgical repair are similar: the obstruction and the distorted region are removed and the remaining portions of gut are joined. Where the gut is difficult to stretch, as in the region of the oesophagus, it may be necessary to interpose a section of gut taken from a more extensible level.

Polyhydramnios One symptom of obstruction may develop in utero: because the fetus cannot swallow properly the amniotic fluid is not circulated through the fetus and absorbed. An excess of amniotic fluid (polyhydramnios) may then develop, which may cause premature birth.

Oesophageal atresia Oesophageal atresia is much rarer than oesophageal atresia with tracheo-oesophageal fistula (see Chapter 20). The symptoms include what appears to be excessive salivation, as the child is unable to swallow its

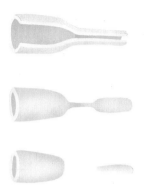

FIGURE 23.12   Various forms of atresia observed in the gut.

saliva. The child will attempt to feed but will regurgitate the meal. If this condition is suspected a catheter should be attempted to be passed down the oesophagus: failure to achieve this indicates that a radiographic examination should be made. Repair may involve replacing the affected section with a length of gut taken from a more caudal level.

Pyloric stenosis   This condition results from hypertrophy of the pyloric muscle at the exit of the stomach. It frequently occurs with an incidence of approximately 40 per 10 000 (or one per 250) live births. It is about four times as common in males as females. The main clinical sign is projectile vomiting after feeding, generally beginning 2–4 weeks after birth. The vomited milk is white or yellow in colour. It is often possible to feel an 'olive-sized' mass in the abdomen where the pylorus muscle lies. The prognosis is very good following surgery but if untreated the child may dehydrate and starve.

Duodenal stenosis/atresia   This is the result of persistent occlusion of the gut. Its incidence is approximately one per 10 000 live births. The symptoms include vomiting of bile-stained fluid. Surgical repair is generally effective, although there is a risk of lung infection if vomit reaches the lungs. Atresias of this kind may be found in association with trisomy 21.

Annular pancreas   This rare defect arises when the pancreatic buds encircle the gut, rather than lying on one side or the other. The symptoms are similar to those of a gut stenosis or atresia at this level.

Accessory pancreatic duct   If the dorsal pancreatic duct persists it forms an accessory pancreatic duct, which empties into the duodenum at a minor duodenal papilla, distinct from the major duodenal papilla.

Intussusception   This occurs when a length of gut slips inside the preceding section and is usually found in young children. It could be due to inadequate fixation. The symptoms can resemble intestinal obstruction and sufferers may pass pieces of sloughed-off gut. An operation is required for repair.

Intestinal duplications Occasionally, when the gut lies closely below the notochord, part of the gut may become attached. As the gut undergoes its various changes in position, this may be pulled into an elongated pouch with the blind end generally deployed cranially. This is an intestinal duplication, and the affected length of gut may be removed or the intervening stretch of gut opened out.

Stenoses and atresias can occur in the midgut in much the same way as in the foregut and oesophagus.

Defects of the midgut loop

A whole series of defects may arise as a result of the curiously cumbersome process of gut herniation and of the presence of the yolk sac.

Meckel's diverticulum The yolk stalk may persist, with a range of degrees of expression. It is found during autopsy or surgery in 2–4% of the population. In about three-quarters of these it is a blind, mobile diverticulum and in most of the rest it is attached by a fibrous cord to the anterior body wall. Rarely, it may persist to the outside as an **omphaloileal fistula**, which exudes faecal material from the umbilicus. Even as a simple diverticulum it may present problems: it may develop ulcerations, become obstructed or develop an appendicitis-like inflammation. There is even a risk that a surgeon pursuing symptoms of appendicitis may fail to identify an inflamed Meckel's diverticulum as the cause.

Omphalocoele This is caused by failure of the midgut loop to return to the abdominal cavity. The protruding gut is covered by peritoneum and an avascular sac of 'amnion'-like material. Its incidence is of the order of one per 6000 live births.

Umbilical hernia A weakness of the musculature of the body wall may lead to an umbilical hernia, in which the umbilical ring is enlarged and the intestines bulge out under a covering of body wall. If the body wall deficiency is lateral to the umbilicus, the condition may be described as gastroschisis. Although in principle this differs from omphalocoele in that the protruding gut is covered by the tissues of the body wall, distinguishing between them may not always be straightforward. Surgical repair is possible, although the abdominal cavity may be too small and there is always a danger of adhesions resulting from the replacement of the gut in the abdomen.

Malrotation of the gut If the gut should rotate in an abnormal manner while in the proximal part of the umbilical cord the return will also be abnormal and could lead to strangulation of the superior mesenteric artery, with consequent adverse effects for the affected segment. Gangrene may develop or the gut may convert into a solid cord and become occluded.

Hindgut Although a number of abnormalities arise during the development of the hindgut, these are best discussed after consideration of the development of the urogenital system.

Box 23.1 Experimental analysis of liver development

How is it possible to establish which germ layer produces particular cell types in the adult liver as described above? An elegant solution to this problem was obtained by Le Douarin, who first mapped the areas of mesoderm and endoderm that contribute to the adult liver then interposed a physical barrier between the liver bud and the mesoderm it normally invaded on one side of the embryo. She found that the presumptive liver mesoderm still gave rise to reticuloendothelial cells and produced characteristic liver enzymes. Prospective liver endoderm from another embryo placed into this mesoderm from which normal liver had been excluded still produced characteristic liver cords despite the disturbance to normal tissue relationships.

Chimaeric embryos, created as described in Box 1.2, have been used to gain further information about the origin of the blood cells in the liver. In mammals the blood stem cells are thought to derive from the blood islands of the yolk sac mesoderm; however, creation of chimaeras in which the cells of the different contributing strains could be recognized indicated that each type of haematopoietic lineage arose from a single cell. This could mean that cells have already specialized before they leave the yolk sac or that they are biased in some way in the liver.

Further reading

Bergsma D. (1979). *Birth Defects Compendium* 2nd edn. London: Macmillan

Corliss C.E. (1976). *Patten's Human Embryology. Elements of Clinical Development.* New York: McGraw Hill

Estrada R.L. (1958). *Anomalies of Intestinal Rotation and Fixation.* Springfield, Il: Thomas

Fitzgerald M.J.T., Nolan J.P. and O'Neill M.N. (1971). The position of the human caecum in fetal life. *J. Anat.*, **109**, 71–4

Frazer J.E. (1931). *A Manual of Embryology.* London: Baillière, Tindall, and Cox

Gasser R.F. (1982). *Atlas of Human Embryos.* Hagerstown MD: Harper & Row

Hamilton W.J., Boyd J.D. and Mossman H.W. (1962). *Human Embryology* 3rd edn. Cambridge: Heffer

Kanagasuntheram R. (1957). Development of the human lesser sac. *J. Anat.*, **91**, 188–206

Lechat M.F. (1989). *Eurocat Report 3.* Surveillance of congenital anomalies. Years 1980–86

Louw H.J. (1959). Congenital intestinal atresia and stenosis in the newborn. *Ann. R. Coll. Surg. Engl.*, **25**, 209–34

Louw J.H. and Barnard C.N. (1955). Congenital intestinal atresia: observations on its origin. *Lancet*, **i**, 1065–7

Odgers P.N.B. (1930). Some observations on the development of the ventral pancreas in man. *J. Anat.*, **65**, 1–7

Potter, G.D. (1990). Intestinal development and regeneration. *Hosp. Pract.*, **25**, 131–44

Salenius P. (1962). On the ontogenesis of the human gastric epithelial cells. *Acta Anat.*, **50** (suppl), 1–76

Severn C.B. (1971). A morphological study of the development of the human liver. I. development of the hepatic diverticulum. *Am. J. Anat.*, **131**, 133–58

Severn, C.B. (1972). A morphological study of the development of the human liver. II. Establishment of liver parenchyma, extrahepatic ducts, and associated venous channels. *Am. J. Anat.*, **133**, 85–7

Skandalkis J.E., Gray S.W., and Rowe J.S. (1983). *Anatomical Complications in General Surgery*. New York: McGraw-Hill

Winter R.M., Knowles S.A.S., Bieber F.R. and Baraitser M. (1988). *The Malformed Fetus and Still Birth*. New York: John Wiley & Sons

Box 23.1

Le Douarin N. (1964). Isolement experimentale du mesenchyme propre du foie et role morphogene de la composante mesodermique dans l'organogenese hepatique. *J. Embryol. Exp. Morph.*, **12**, 141–60

Rossant J. *et al.* (1986). Clonal origin of haematopoietic colonies in the post-natal mouse liver. *Nature,* **319**, 507–11

Wong P.M.C. *et al.* (1986). Properties of the earliest clonogenic hemopoietic precursors to appear in the developing murine yolk sac. *Proc. Natl Acad. Sci. USA*, **83**, 3851–4

24

The urinary system

EVOLUTION

*The evolutionary origin of the excretory and sexual organs not only helps in understanding their form in humans, it also helps explain a variety of defects. It is believed that our early marine ancestors shed waste products directly into their body cavity, and then reclaimed valuable metabolites and fluid via segmentally arranged filtration units, which may have opened individually to the outside (Figure 24.1(a)). However, even if this was once the case, this arrangement soon gave way to one in which the filtrate on each side of the body was passed into an extended tube running tailward to insert into the hindgut for excretion (Figure 24.1(b)). An arrangement of this kind can be seen in modern jawless fish, which retain a number of primitive features. Generally, however, the segmental arrangement of filtration units (described as the **pronephros**) was superseded by the **mesonephros**, in which several filtration units are found in each body segment. Mesonephric kidneys usually begin further down the body axis than the pronephric variety, although they still communicate via lateral paired ducts with the hindgut. Finally the higher vertebrates evolved the **metanephros**, in which the filtration units greatly increased in size and complexity and were confined to discrete paired structures originating near the tail end of the animal.*

To some extent modern mammals recapitulate these events, though it is unlikely that human embryos develop more than a rudimentary pronephros. The

Individual filtration unit

Aorta

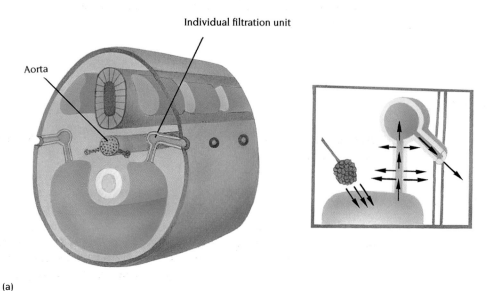

(a)

Common waste duct

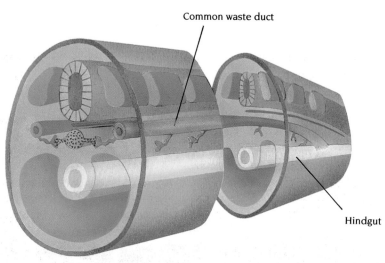

Hindgut

(b)

FIGURE 24.1 Kidney evolution. (a) It may be that the kidneys originated as separate segmental units, each opening to the outside. These may have served to reclaim valuable components from waste secreted to the body cavity (inset: direction of waste flow). (b) A more advanced condition is that in which the segmental units receive waste products directly by diffusion from the blood without passing through the body cavity. The filtrate is then passed in a tube down the body to be excreted via the cloaca. The segmental arrangement of filtration units may be replaced by one in which several units are present per body segment.

evolutionary background is thus a valuable aid to understanding the development of the human urinary system.

Kidney

The kidney develops from the intermediate mesoderm, which lies between the somites and the lateral plate (Figure 24.2).

Pronephros

Human embryos do not possess any substantial structures corresponding to the pronephros. However, transient cell aggregations are observed in the cervical region of the embryo during the first week of the embryonic period and these, although not obviously segmental in nature, may be rudiments of the pronephros.

Mesonephros

A well-formed mesonephros is visible initially at about the level of somite 8 in human embryos during the embryonic period, and is functional during this time.

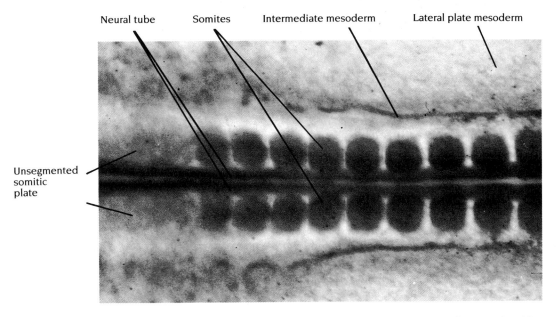

FIGURE 24.2 Dorsal view of 14-somite chick embryo, corresponding to a day 22+ human embryo.

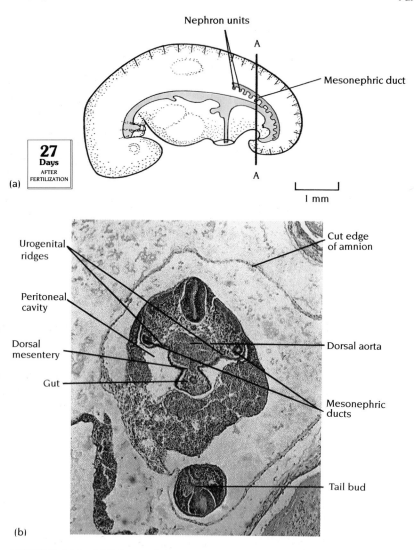

FIGURE 24.3 (a) Mesonephric ducts inserting into cloaca; (b) transverse section through line A–A.

It has two main components: the **mesonephric ducts**, which arise from the dorsolateral part of the intermediate mesoderm, and the **nephron** units, arising medial to the ducts (Figure 24.3: see also Figure 24.9(a)). There are several nephron units per body segment, and these develop communicating links with the mesonephric duct. The duct extends caudally down the embryo until it inserts into the ventral aspect of the cloaca (Figures 24.3(a), 24.4). As the duct extends, corresponding nephron units sequentially differentiate from the caudal intermediate mesoderm. At any one time cranial nephrons are more highly developed than the caudal newcomers.

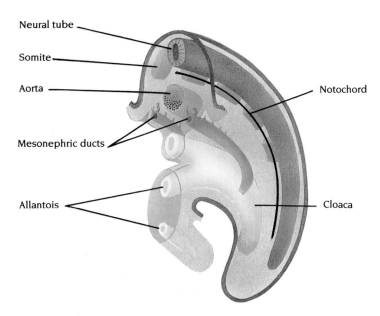

FIGURE 24.4 Diagrammatic view of insertion of mesonephric ducts into the cloaca.

The duct is a substantial structure, and the individual nephron units running into it become more complex and convoluted with time. As a result, distinct **urogenital ridges** develop, projecting down from the dorsal aspect of the peritoneal cavity (Figures 24.3(a), 24.5).

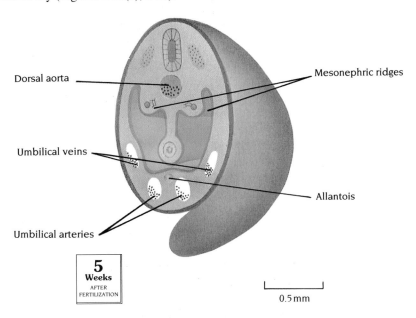

FIGURE 24.5 Diagrammatic view of urogenital ridges.

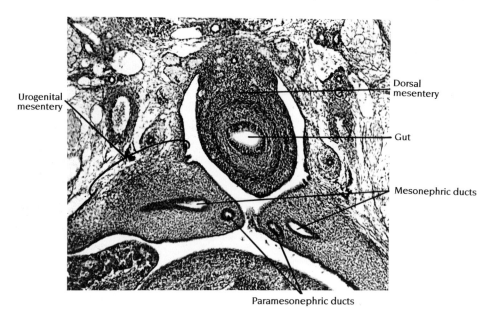

Urogenital mesentery

Dorsal mesentery

Gut

Mesonephric ducts

Paramesonephric ducts

FIGURE 24.6   Urogenital ridges in the midline under the gut.

As described in Chapter 23, the cloaca divides into the hindgut and the urogenital sinus. The mesonephric ducts insert into the ventral part of the cloaca and after this division they insert into the urogenital sinus.

During the embryonic period the urogenital ridges become more distinctly separate from the dorsal body wall, until they are attached only by a narrow band of tissue known as the **urogenital mesentery**. Because the mesonephric ducts run medially to insert into the urogenital sinus, the urogenital ridges approach each other in the midline at caudal levels and eventually meet underneath the gut (Figure 24.6). The ridges are also in contact with the mesodermal covering of the urogenital sinus in the area of the insertion (see Chapter 25). This process is often described as an active one, with the urogenital ridges swinging into the midline to fuse, but in the early embryo the mesonephric ducts run in a continuous mass of mesoderm to join the urogenital sinus, and it may be more accurate to describe the process as resulting from extensions of the coelomic cavity rather than from active movement of bands of tissue.

Whether as a result of the persistence of such tissue or as a result of secondary fusion, the urogenital ridge is attached to the ventral wall of the abdomen by a band of mesoderm that will later form the **gubernaculum**. This will be discussed in Chapter 25.

Although the mesonephric system is functional in human embryos its role is superseded by the **metanephros** (see below). However (as described in the next chapter) in males the mesonephric ducts persist because they are adapted to carry out a new function. In females they remain functionless, and eventually largely degenerate.

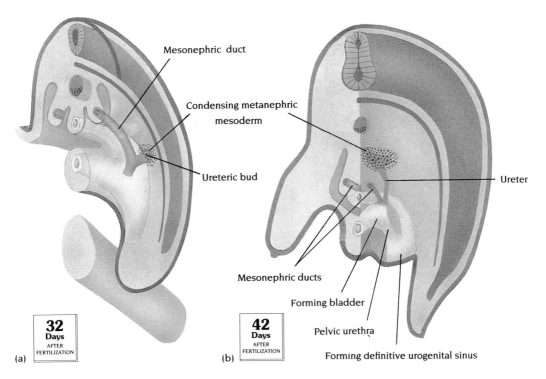

Mesonephric duct

Condensing metanephric
mesoderm

Ureteric bud

Ureter

Mesonephric ducts

Forming bladder

32
Days
AFTER
FERTILIZATION

(a)

42
Days
AFTER
FERTILIZATION

(b)

Pelvic urethra

Forming definitive urogenital sinus

FIGURE 24.7   (a) Formation of the ureteric bud; (b) condensation of metanephric
mesoderm.

Metanephros

This is the definitive kidney and in humans the first sign of its appearance is at
about 32 days after fertilization. It is believed to be functional from as early as
the sixth week onwards, overlapping with the time of activity of the
mesonephros. It appears as the **ureteric bud**, growing out laterally from the caudal part of the mesonephric duct on each side (Figure 24.7(a)), which gradually
becomes surrounded by condensing mesoderm – the **metanephric mesoderm**
(Figures 24.7(b), 24.8). This arises from intermediate mesoderm, as did the
mesonephric duct.

The ureteric bud forms the primitive renal pelvis and continues dividing to
produce the **calyces** (Figure 24.9(c)), which branch to give the collecting
tubules. The metanephric mesoderm develops the Bowman's capsules and the
excretory nephrons or tubules. These consist of the proximal convoluted tubules,
the loops of Henle and the distal convoluted tubules.

The ureteric buds are originally outgrowths from the mesonephric duct but
they will eventually form separate connections to the cloaca – the **ureters**
(Figures 24.7(a,b), 24.9). These develop at the same time as the cloaca is being
divided into the anorectal canal and the urogenital sinus by the urorectal folds

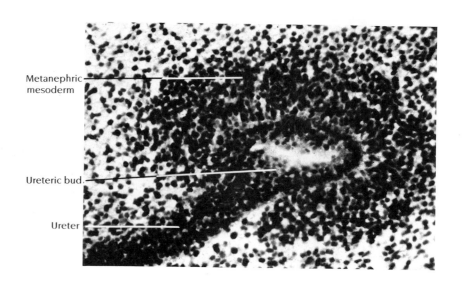

FIGURE 24.8   Condensing metanephric mesoderm. (From the St Andrews' collection, by permission.)

(see Chapter 23). The mesonephric ducts and ureters initially insert into the ventral part of the cloaca, which will become the urogenital sinus. The separate insertions of the ureters may arise as a result of expansion of the urogenital sinus to encompass the region where the bud grew out from the duct. As a result, it is believed that part of the wall of the urogenital sinus has a mesodermal component. This is known as the **trigone of the bladder**. However, it may alternatively be formed by the urogenital sinus endoderm.

Changes in relative position

The metanephric kidneys are at first found at the caudal end of the embryo but differential relative growth in the rest of the body shifts their position sequentially in a cranial direction (Figure 24.9). As this shift proceeds the blood supply of the kidneys continually changes as new branches are induced from the aorta. The 'renal arteries' are merely the last of these induced arterial branches. As a result the blood supply to the kidney displays a wide variety of forms in the adult.

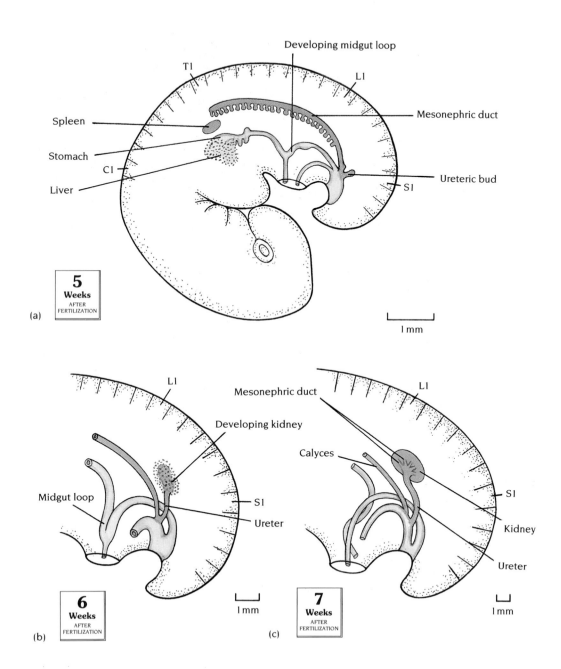

FIGURE 24.9   Relative shift in kidney position with time.

Box 24.1 Experimental analysis of kidney development

In animals with a clearly developed pronephros the pronephric duct normally induces the formation of the mesonephros. If the caudal extension of the pronephric duct is blocked then the mesonephros fails to develop. The mesonephric duct plays a similar role where the pronephros is rudimentary. The backward extension of the duct appears to follow a pre-established adhesion pathway, which is made visible by its expression of cell surface alkaline phosphatase. Neural crest cells placed on this pathway will migrate along it, showing that it is a suitable substrate for general cell migration.

If the bud fails to grow out (as in some mouse mutants) then the metanephric mesoderm cannot form the excretory tubules and if isolated metanephric mesoderm is grown in culture no excretory tubules form. If, however, the bud and the metanephric mesoderm are recombined, even with a filter placed between them, excretory tubules form. This seemed at first to imply that some diffusible influence passed through the filter; however, for this induction to take place it is necessary for very fine cell processes to be able to grow through the filter and contact the metanephric mesoderm directly. Non-kidney structures such as the spinal cord and salivary gland can also induce tubules to form: neurons are in fact the most potent inducer of tubule formation and the early innervation of the ureteric bud might be a key event in bringing about the induction.

If, after tubules have formed, the kidney is disassociated to single cells and then pelleted, the tubules will spontaneously reform. Marking the initial tubule cells before dissociation shows that the same cells reform the secondary tubules. Plainly it is part of their postinduction differentiation programme to develop spontaneously into tubules.

Bladder

As described in Chapter 23, the cloaca is partitioned by the fusion of the urogenital folds so that the urogenital sinus acquires its own separate urogenital membrane. The urogenital sinus continues cranially as the allantois, running in the connecting stalk. The connecting stalk will be incorporated into the umbilical cord. The apical part of the allantois gradually shuts down, forming a cord known initially as the **urachus**, which in turn becomes the **median umbilical ligament**. Cysts or fistulas may form if this closure is incomplete (see below).

The urogenital sinus is divided into three parts: a wide cranial part that will form the presumptive **bladder**, the narrower **pelvic urethra** and the wide presumptive **definitive urogenital sinus**, which is the most caudal part (see Figure 24.7(b)).

In the female the pelvic urethra becomes the **membranous urethra** and its urethral lining gives rise to buds that form the urethral and paraurethral glands. In males the pelvic urethra develops into the **prostatic urethra**, from which the prostate gland arises by budding. The definitive urogenital sinus in females becomes the vestibule of the vagina, and in males the penile urethra (see Chapter 25). The urogenital sinus is an endodermal structure surrounded by mesoderm, and the mesoderm will contribute to the connective tissue of all these structures.

Suprarenal (adrenal) glands

The suprarenal glands are paired ductless glands, secreting their products directly into the bloodstream: the gland is therefore well vascularized.

Tissue types within the suprarenal glands

The glands consist of two different types of tissue. On the outer aspect is **cortical (or interrenal)** tissue, while **medullary** (or chromaffin) tissue lies internally. The cortical tissue is further divided into an outer **zona glomerulosa**, an intermediate **zona fasciculata** and an inner **zona reticularis**.

Suprarenal glands are present in some form in all vertebrates, from jawless fish to humans. In mammals they are discrete encapsulated organs at the anterior pole of the kidneys.

Functions

The cortical tissues secrete steroid hormones and the medulla secretes catecholamines. Catecholamines (such as adrenaline and noradrenaline) are stress hormones that help to regulate heart rate, blood vessel diameter and intestinal movement. High levels are present in the fetus during delivery and birth, to help regulate breathing and to break down stored energy into forms that can nourish cells when the umbilical cord is cut.

Development

Cortex and medulla develop separately, the cortex appearing first as a thickening in the dorsal mesogastrium during weeks 4–5 in humans (Figure 24.10(a)). The medulla cells are derived from the neural crest via an adjacent sympathetic ganglion slightly later. Similar cells may be found scattered throughout the body, but degenerate after birth. Initially cortical and medullary cells are intermingled but later they sort into their respective regions (Figure 24.10(b)). It is suspected that the sorting involves differential mutual adhesiveness between cells: perhaps the medullary cells adhere more strongly to each other than do the

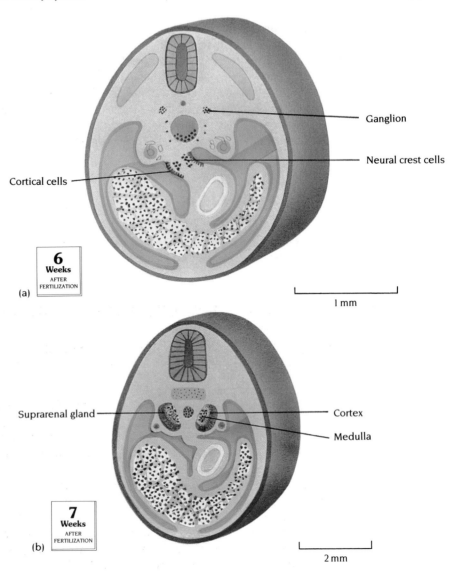

Ganglion

Neural crest cells

Cortical cells

6
Weeks
AFTER
FERTILIZATION
(a)

1 mm

Suprarenal gland

Cortex

Medulla

7
Weeks
AFTER
FERTILIZATION
(b)

2 mm

FIGURE 24.10   (a) Appearance and (b) later development of suprarenal glands.

cortical cells, and as a result an arrangement in which the medullary cells lie internally is favourable in energy terms.

The suprarenal glands are 10–20 times larger in the fetus (as a fraction of body weight) than in the adult; they are even large compared with the kidney (Figure 24.11), but become relatively smaller after birth.

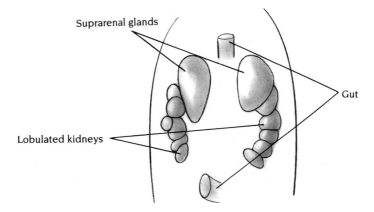

FIGURE 24.11   Position of suprarenal glands during the fetal period. Note their large size, and the lobulated appearance of the kidney.

Defects of the kidney and suprarenal glands

In perhaps 5–10% of all individuals there are asymptomatic deviations from the norm which do not represent abnormalities but which may present surprises for the surgeon in later life.

Renal agenesis This results from failure of the ureteric bud to grow out, probably as a failure of the mesonephric duct to elongate as normal; absence of a kidney is always associated with absence of the ureter on the corresponding side. The much rarer event of double kidney is likewise accompanied by a double ureter.

In the past unilateral agenesis may have gone undetected unless a pelvic examination took place, but it is now recognizable during prenatal ultrasonography. The kidney that *is* present will hypertrophy to compensate and as a result the incidence of this condition is unknown, though it may be 10 per 10 000 pregnancies. The total incidence of bilateral renal agenesis and dysgenesis detected before or around birth in Europe is about 3.5 per 10 000.

Oligohydramnios In bilateral agenesis the amount of amniotic fluid is low (a condition known as oligohydramnios) because the fetus swallows amniotic fluid but does not excrete it via the kidneys. Bilateral agenesis is fatal shortly after birth.

Pelvic kidney In the condition known as pelvic kidney one kidney fails to ascend.

Horseshoe kidney In horseshoe kidney the kidneys fuse at the inferior (medial) pole (Figure 24.12), and both fail to ascend. This occurs in one per 600 live births and is generally symptomless.

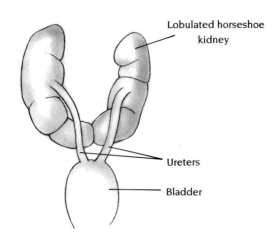

FIGURE 24.12   Horseshoe kidney.

Urachal sinus/cyst/fistula   This arises from persistence of part of the allantois, although there is a range of potential expression. As is often the case, cysts may become infected, leading to a swelling that appears as a moveable midline structure. A patent sinus, developing coincidentally or following this swelling, may leak matter into the bladder or at the umbilical opening. A patent fistula may cause leakage of urine at the umbilical cord.

Polycystic kidney disease   This is a common condition, especially in adults, and its relationship to development is obscure. It is likely that a variety of different conditions are grouped together under this heading. Large urine-filled cysts develop in the kidney, and inhibit normal function in extensive regions. Anything from a few cysts to a mass almost obliterating the kidney may be present. It has been suggested that the congenital version of this condition results from a failure of the collecting and excretory ducts to join up but as it is believed to arise during the fetal period this seems unlikely.

Congenital adrenal hyperplasia   The most common form of this condition is a defect in the enzyme catalysing the conversion of progesterone or 17α-hydroxyprogesterone to deoxycorticosterone and 11-deoxycortisol respectively. The androgen pathway is not blocked, so the fetus is exposed to androgens from approximately 12 weeks on. In females this results in varying degrees of masculinization of the external sexual organs. Males are born apparently normal, but during childhood may show pubertal changes such as voice breaking, growth of pubic and axillary hair and sexual maturation (sometimes known as the 'Infant Hercules' syndrome). Accelerated bone development may result in premature fusion of the epiphysis and hence short stature.

   In some Inuit groups the incidence may be as high as 20 per 10 000 live births. Among the Swiss it is 4 per 10 000, in the USA it is 0.25 per 10 000.

Further reading

Auer J. (1947). Bilateral renal agenesis. *Anat. Rec.*, **97**, 283–92

Bergsma D. (1979). *Birth Defects Compendium*. 2nd edn. London: Macmillan

Bernstein J. (1971). Heritable cystic diseases of the kidney. *Pediatr. Clin. North Am.*, **18**, 395–411

Chester Jones I. (1976). Evolutionary aspects of the adrenal cortex and its homologues. *J. Endocrinol.*, **71**, 3–32

Coupland R.E. (1954). Post-natal fate of the abdominal para-aortic bodies in man. *J. Anat.*, **88**, 455–64

Decker, R.S. (1981). Gap junctions and steroidogenesis in the fetal mammalian adrenal cortex. *Dev. Biol.*, **82**, 20–31

Gardner L.I. (1975). Development of the normal fetal and neonatal suprarenal. In *Endocrine and Genetic Diseases of Childhood and Adolescence* 2nd edn. (Gardner, L.I., ed.), pp. 460–76. Philadelphia: W.B. Saunders

Gasser R.F. (1982). *Atlas of Human Embryos*. Hagerstown MD: Harper & Row

Gruenwald P. (1939). The mechanism of kidney development in human embryos as revealed by an early stage in the agenesis of the ureteric buds. *Anat. Rec.*, **75**, 237–47

Goodrich A.S. (1930). *Studies on the Structure and Development of Embryos*. New York: Macmillan

Hildebrand M. (1981). *Analysis of Vertebrate Structure* 2nd edn. New York: John Wiley & Sons

Lagercrantz H. and Slatkin T.A. (1986). The stress of being born. *Sci. Am.*, **254**, 92–102

Lechat M.F. (1989). *Eurocat Report 3*. Surveillance of congenital anomalies. Years 1980–86

Linnoila L.A., Diagustine R.P., Hervonen A. and Miller R.J. (1980). Distribution of (Met 5)- and (Leu 5)-enkephalin, vasoactive intestinal peptide and substance P-like immunoreactivity in human adrenal gland cells. *Neuroscience*, **5**, 2247–59

O'Rahilly R. and Muller F. (1987). *Developmental Stages in Human Embryos*. Carnegie Institution of Washington Publication 637

Panskey B. (1982). *Review of Medical Embryology*. London: Macmillan

Potter E.L. (1972). *Normal and Abnormal Development of the Kidney*. Chicago: Year Book

Saxen L. (1987). *Organogenesis of the Kidney*. London: Cambridge University Press

Simpoulos A.P. *et al* (1971). Studies on the deficiency of 21 hydroxylation in patients with congenital adrenal hyperplasia. *J. Clin. Endocrinol. Metab.*, **32**, 438–43

Torrey T.W. (1954). The early development of the human nephros. *Contrib. Embryol. Carnegie. Inst*, **35**, 175–97

Wharton L.R. (1949). Double ureters and associated renal anomalies in early human embryos. *Contrib. Embryol. Carnegie. Inst.*, **33**, 103–12

Box 24.1

McLachlan J.C. (1986). Self assembly of structures resembling functional organs by pure populations of cells. *Tissue and Cell*, **18**, 313–20

Sariola H., Ekblom P., and Henke-Fahle S. (1988). Early innervation of the metanephric kidney. *Development*, **104**, 589–90

Sariola H., Ekblom P. and Henke-Fahle S. (1989). Embryonic neurons as in vitro inducers of differentiation of nephrogenic mesenchyme. *Dev. Biol.*, **132**, 271–81

Torrey T.W. (1965). Morphogenesis of the vertebrate kidney. In *Organogenesis* (DeHaan R.L. and Ursprung H., eds), pp. 559–79. New York: Holt, Rinehart & Winston

Zackson S.L. and Steinberg M.S. (1986). Cranial neural crest cells exhibit directed migration on the pronephric duct pathway: further evidence for in vivo adhesion gradient. *Dev. Biol.*, **117**, 342–53

Zackson S.L. and Steinberg M.S. (1988). A molecular marker for cell guidance information in the axolotl. *Dev. Biol.*, **127**, 435–42

25

Internal and external sexual organs

Internal genitalia

EVOLUTION

*In early vertebrate evolution gonads were generally both male and female, with the male component lying deep in the gonad, and the female superficial. Their owners could self fertilize – eggs and sperm were both shed into the body coelom. However, even for hermaphrodites (individuals who are both male and female) it is best to have sexual reproduction, in which genetic information is exchanged between individuals. The gametes must then be kept separate within the individual. The solution evolved was that sperm made use of the increasingly redundant mesonephric duct to travel via the cloaca to the outside world, while eggs were shed into the coelom and passed out through abdominal slits. Even now, female humans still shed their eggs in the body coelom, although this carries the risk that they may implant in the abdominal cavity (see Chapter 2). However, the evolution of a separate tubule to carry the eggs went some way towards alleviating this risk. This new tubule runs along the side of the mesonephric ridge – and is named the **paramesonephric** tubule – to insert into the cloaca. Hermaphrodite animals have both sets of tubules and can control whether eggs or sperm are deposited. When the sexes become completely separate, as in mammals (including humans), one set of tubules must degenerate.*

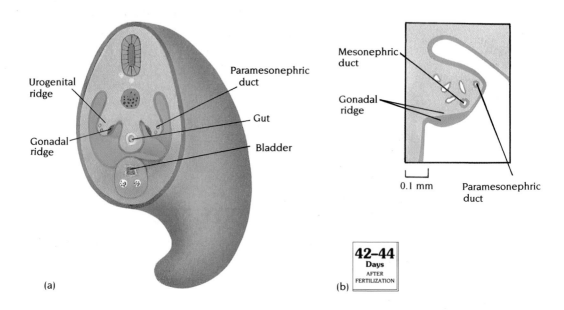

FíGURE 25.1 (a) Section through embryo showing urogenital ridge. (b) Section through urogenital ridge.

Gonads: indifferent stage

During the fifth week after fertilization a swelling appears on the medial and caudal aspect of the urogenital ridge: this is the **gonadal ridge** (Figure 25.1). This is a mesodermal structure, projecting into the coelomic cavity, and its outer layer is mesothelial in nature. This mesothelial layer thickens to form the **coelomic epithelium**, which then begins to invade the underlying mesoderm. This unusual invasive behaviour suggests that a signalling event of some kind has occurred (see below). The invading cells will form the **primitive sex cords** by the sixth week after fertilization (Figure 25.2).

The invasion is caused by the arrival of the **primordial germ cells** (PGCs). As described in Chapter 26, the germ line is kept separate from the somatic cells: the PGCs differentiate outside the body in the yolk sac mesoderm and then migrate by amoeboid movement over the yolk sac and gut into the dorsal mesentery and then on to the gonadal ridge by week 6. If they do not arrive the gonadal ridges develop no further. Normally, however, when they do arrive sexual differentiation commences.

Femaleness is the baseline condition, from which males are diverted during development by the influence of powerful chemicals. If a fully functioning Y chromosome, and the appropriate receptor systems for gene products activated

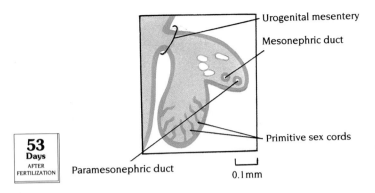

Urogenital mesentery

Mesonephric duct

Primitive sex cords

53 Days AFTER FERTILIZATION

Paramesonephric duct

0.1 mm

FIGURE 25.2 Primitive sex cords.

by the Y chromosome, are present the individual becomes male: otherwise, she remains female.

Ducts: indifferent stage

The paramesonephric ducts form lateral to the mesonephric ducts (Figures 25.1, 25.3) during the sixth week, by the development of a craniocaudal thickening which then sinks to become a duct, in a manner not unlike the formation of the lacrimal glands. The tube thus formed remains open cranially into the peritoneal cavity: caudally, it crosses into the middle to meet its counterpart from the other side and both insert into the dorsal aspect of the urogenital sinus (Figure 25.4).

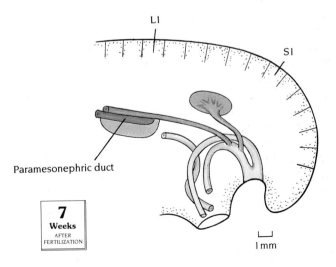

L1

S1

Paramesonephric duct

7 Weeks AFTER FERTILIZATION

1 mm

FIGURE 25.3 The cranial end of the paramesonephric duct.

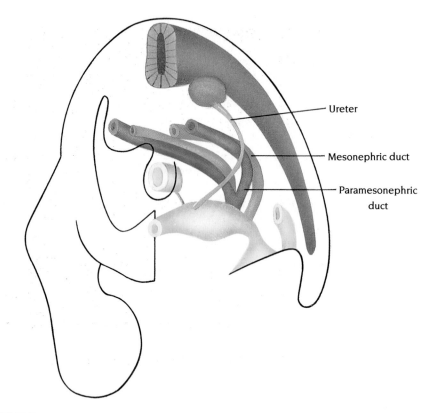

FIGURE 25.4 Insertion of paramesonephric ducts into urogenital sinus.

Ureter

Mesonephric duct

Paramesonephric duct

The supporting band of tissue is known as the urogenital mesentery (see Figures 25.2, 25.6). By the start of the fetal period the gonadal ridges fuse in the midline (Figure 25.5).

A little cranial to this position the gonadal ridges are in contact with the ventral aspect of the peritoneal cavity, although it is unclear whether this represents a persistence of an existing band of tissue or a secondary fusion (Figure 25.6). A line of mesodermal fusion runs down to the caudal end of the peritoneal cavity on each side producing the **plica gubernaculi**, which will contribute to the gubernaculi in both males and females. They continue into the urogenital mesentery, running in the mesoderm until they reach the **labioscrotal** (or **genital**) **swellings** (see below) on either side of the cloacal membrane. There they attach just under the surface.

This means that a band of tissue runs in mesoderm from the gonad to the inner aspect of the ectoderm of the labioscrotal swellings.

With time the gonads will come to lie more caudally in the coelom and it is generally believed that the gubernaculum plays a part in this process as described below.

A pocket, the **processus vaginalis**, develops on each side of the body at the caudal end of the coelomic cavity. The gubernaculum runs just under the lining wall of these pockets. Again, they form in both males and females (Figure 25.7).

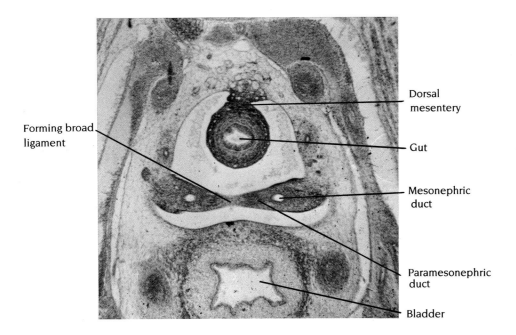

Forming broad ligament

Dorsal mesentery

Gut

Mesonephric duct

Paramesonephric duct

Bladder

FIGURE 25.5 Formation of the broad ligament of the ovary.

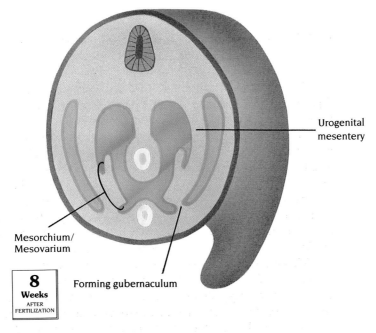

Urogenital mesentery

Mesorchium/ Mesovarium

Forming gubernaculum

8
Weeks
AFTER
FERTILIZATION

FIGURE 25.6 Formation of the plica gubernaculi. The gonad is attached to the urogenital mesentery by a band of tissue known as the mesorchium in males and mesovarium in females.

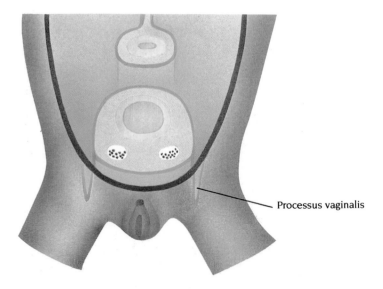

Processus vaginalis

FIGURE 25.7 Formation of the processus vaginalis.

As the basal condition of mankind is female, we will consider the ovaries first.

Development of the ovaries

The tissue lineages during female development are summarized in Figure 25.8.

In females the primary sex cords degenerate and are replaced by **secondary sex cords** (Figure 25.9). These will go on to give rise to the **follicular cells** which, in association with the PGCs, form the **follicles**. The deep mesoderm of the ridge produces the **ovarian medulla**. A thin layer of extracellular matrix fibres, the **tunica albuginea**, develops under the basement membrane during fetal development.

The paramesonephric duct persists to form the **uterine tube**, the **uterus** and

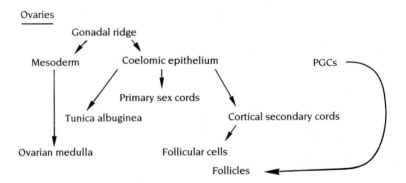

FIGURE 25.8 Tissue lineages during female development.

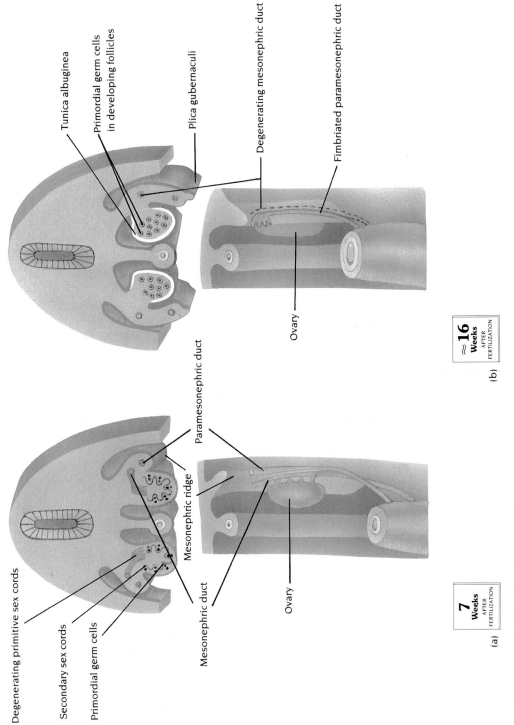

FIGURE 25.9 Later development of the ovary.

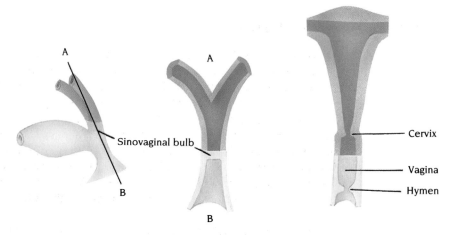

Cervix

Sinovaginal bulb

Vagina

Hymen

FIGURE 25.10 Formation of the vagina and hymen.

the superior part of the **vagina**. The cranial part remains open to the coelom and becomes fimbriated at the upper end. Eggs are shed into the coelom from the gonadal surface and are gathered into the upper end of the uterine tube. At the caudal end the paramesonephric ducts fuse to form the **uterovaginal canal** (Figure 25.10). In females the **mesonephric** ducts degenerate, apart from an occasional minor remnant. When the urogenital ridges come together they form the **broad ligament of the uterus**.

The ovary moves caudally under the influence of the gubernaculum, but does not enter the processus vaginalis. The gubernaculum fuses to the para-mesonephric duct and as these ducts fuse the ovaries are pulled into the gonadal ligament. The gubernaculum in the female becomes the **ovarian ligament** superiorly and the **round ligament of the uterus** inferiorly.

The attachment of the ovary to the urogenital ridge becomes more and more attenuated, forming a band of tissue known as the **mesovarium** (see Figure 25.6).

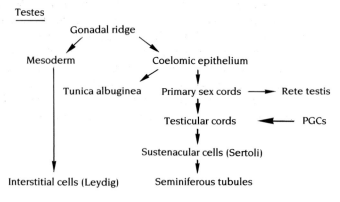

FIGURE 25.11 Tissue lineages during male development.

Development of the testes

The tissue lineages during male development are summarized in Figure 25.11.

The outermost mesothelium will in time form a thick outer layer known as the tunica albuginea (Figure 25.12). This is markedly more developed than the equivalent structure in the female and is the first histological sign of sexual differences in the gonads. It is evident from week 16. The primary sex cords persist as the **testicular cords**, and will form the **sustentacular** or **Sertoli cells** of the **seminiferous tubules**. In addition, they form the **rete testis**, which connects the seminiferous tubules with the mesonephric system. The PGCs make a functional association with the seminiferous tubules where they give rise to sperm. The mesoderm of the testis contributes to the **interstitial** or **Leydig cells**.

In the postpubertal male, sperm will pass from the seminiferous tubules through the rete testis into the mesonephric duct via the remnants of functional renal units known as **efferent ductules**. The cranial mesonephric duct becomes highly convoluted to form the **epididymis**. Its continuation will be the **vas deferens**. The paramesonephric duct degenerates. An outgrowth from the caudal mesonephric duct develops into the **seminal vesicle**. (The **prostate gland** arises from the urethra, as do the bulbourethral glands: see Chapter 24.)

The attachment band of the testis to the original urogenital ridge is known as the **mesorchium** (see Figure 25.6).

Descent of the testes (Figure 25.13)

The descent of the testes is much more marked than that of the ovaries. By the late fetal period each testis lies just outside the processus vaginalis. It then enters the wall of the processus through the inguinal ring to pass down the inguinal canal to lie in the area that will become the **scrotum**, bringing with it the vas deferens. It is believed that this final stage occurs in a rather short period of time. It is mediated by the gubernaculum, which is contractile under the influence of testosterone. The descent process occurs at some point between the 22nd and 23rd week after fertilization.

During this movement the testis remains under the surface of the mesoderm: it does not enter the coelom. After the testes have 'entered' the wall of the processus vaginalis, the gubernaculum largely atrophies.

Subsequently, the processus vaginalis will generally obliterate, although it remains a point of weakness in the body wall. A patent or potential space, the **tunica vaginalis**, remains associated with the testis. It is lined with what is essentially peritoneum – the mesothelial lining of the coelomic cavity. The vas deferens, too, becomes wrapped in mesothelium.

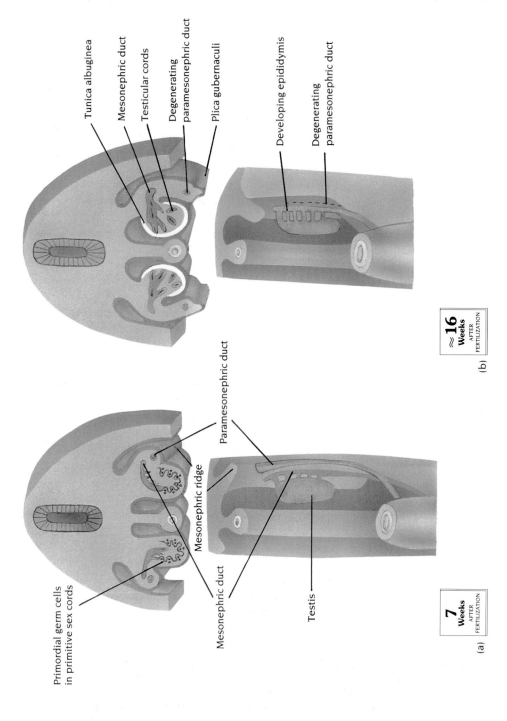

FIGURE 25.12 Later development of the testis.

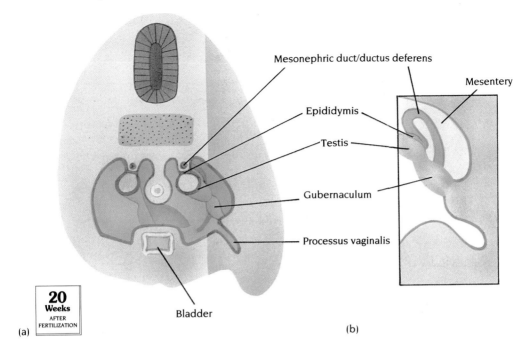

20
Weeks
AFTER
FERTILIZATION

Mesonephric duct/ductus deferens

Mesentery

Epididymis

Testis

Gubernaculum

Processus vaginalis

Bladder

(a)

(b)

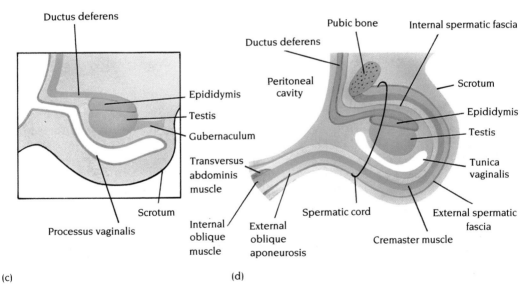

Ductus deferens

Pubic bone

Internal spermatic fascia

Ductus deferens

Peritoneal
cavity

Scrotum

Epididymis

Epididymis

Testis

Testis

Gubernaculum

Tunica
vaginalis

Transversus
abdominis
muscle

Scrotum

Spermatic cord

External spermatic
fascia

Processus vaginalis

Internal
oblique
muscle

External
oblique
aponeurosis

Cremaster muscle

(c)

(d)

FIGURE 25.13   The descent of the testes. (a) The plica gubernaculi, the degenerating mesonephric ridge, and the caudal attachment of the mesonephros, form the gubernaculum testis. The processus vaginalis (see Figure 25.7) develops ventral to the attachment of the gubernaculum to the caudal end of the peritoneal cavity (b). At about 21 weeks after fertilization, the testes descend, probably rather rapidly, to lie dorsal to the processus vaginalis. They now lie on either side of the developing penis, in what will be the scrotum. Subsequently, muscle layers differentiate around the testis, and the processus vaginalis closes to leave a space, the tunica vaginalis, which is lined with peritoneal mesoderm (d).

External genitalia

EVOLUTION

After the evolution of sexual reproduction, both sexes shed their eggs and sperm outside the body for external fertilization. This is a successful strategy for marine animals but is not possible on land. The solution to this problem lay in the development of intromittent organs (also found in some fish), to enable internal fertilization to take place.

For some unknown reason, spermatogenesis fails at mammalian body temperatures, so the testes are placed in an external sac to keep them cool – a solution rather lacking in engineering elegance.

Development of the external genitalia

Like the internal sex organs the external genitalia are initially the same in both sexes (Figure 25.14(a–e)).

Around the cloacal membrane **urogenital folds** and **labioscrotal swellings** develop, as does a mass of tissue at the cranial end: this is the **genital tubercle**. As described in Chapter 23, the urogenital and anal membranes separate and the anus comes to lie at the base of the anal pit. The anal and urogenital membranes rupture at about the seventh week after fertilization. The urogenital opening is the outlet of the bladder.

Female external genitalia

Females change little from this initial condition. The urogenital folds become the **labia minora**, the labioscrotal swellings become the **labia majora** and the genital tubercle the **clitoris** (Figure 25.14(b)).

The paramesonephric ducts insert into the urogenital sinus and induce a solid endodermal swelling to grow from it (see Figure 25.10). Spaces begin to develop in this swelling, which eventually becomes the inferior part of the vagina. A remnant may persist (the **hymen**), which is therefore endodermal in origin. The hymen has been known to be attributed a cultural importance far in excess of its embryological interest.

The urethral orifice will open out, so that the vagina is eventually surrounded by endodermal tissue.

Because the female external genitalia undergo comparatively little change during development major abnormalities are unusual. The same cannot be said for fusion of the paramesonephric ducts, as is described below.

Male external genitalia

In males the urogenital folds 'zip up', beginning from the most caudal end (Figure 25.14(h–j)) during the early fetal period (weeks 9–11). At the same time

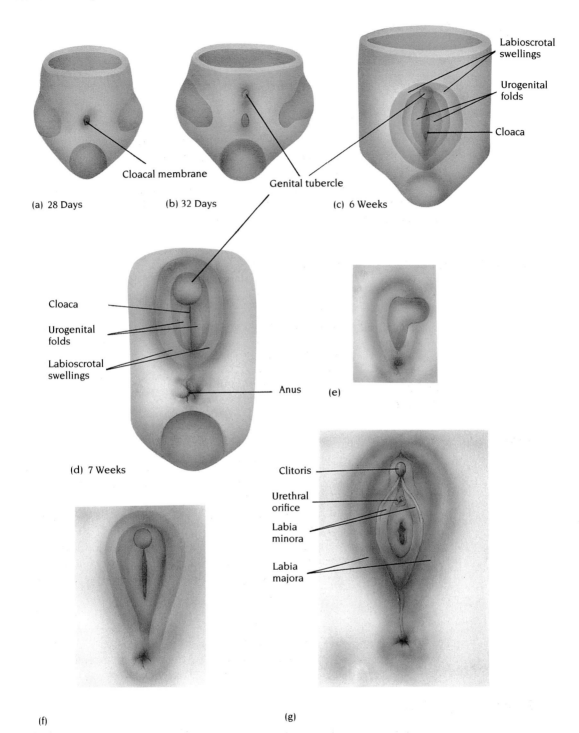

(a) 28 Days

(b) 32 Days

(c) 6 Weeks

Cloacal membrane

Genital tubercle

Labioscrotal swellings

Urogenital folds

Cloaca

Cloaca

Urogenital folds

Labioscrotal swellings

Anus

(e)

(d) 7 Weeks

Clitoris

Urethral orifice

Labia minora

Labia majora

(f)

(g)

FIGURE 25.14 (a–d) Development of the external genitalia to the indifferent during the embryonic period; (e) Lateral view of genital tubucle; (f–g) further development of the female genitalia.

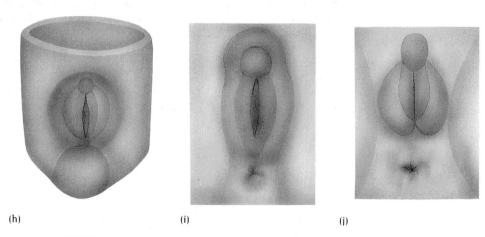

(h)   (i)   (j)

FIGURE 25.14 *(contd)*   (h–j) Further development of the male genitalia.

the genital tubercle begins to extend. This will form the **penis**, which is analogous to the clitoris in females. The urethra will be enclosed within the penis but the orifice at its tip develops separately from the ectoderm. A cord of ectoderm forms from the tip to meet the urethra and then hollows out (Figure 25.15). Ectoderm also invades from the tip to mark out the **foreskin**, and these ectodermal ingrowths undergo programmed cell death to form patent spaces.

This process relies on the coming together of a number of components, and defects are therefore likely.

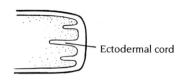

Ectodermal cord

FIGURE 25.15   Ectodermal cord of penis.

Defects of the internal and external sexual structures

Cryptorchidism (undescended testes) This is found in one in three premature male babies, reflecting the lateness of testicular descent. The testes may descend spontaneously thereafter. It is also found in one in 30 full-term males. Sperm are not viable at normal body temperatures; sterility will result if the condition persists. Furthermore, undescended testes may develop tumours. If the testes have not descended by the age at which puberty usually occurs they may be removed surgically.

Congenital inguinal hernia (Figure 25.16) The weakness in the body wall created by the processus vaginalis creates the possibility that a loop of bowel may pass into the tunica vaginalis during adult life, particularly when abdominal pressure is increased by lifting a heavy weight. When the loop is

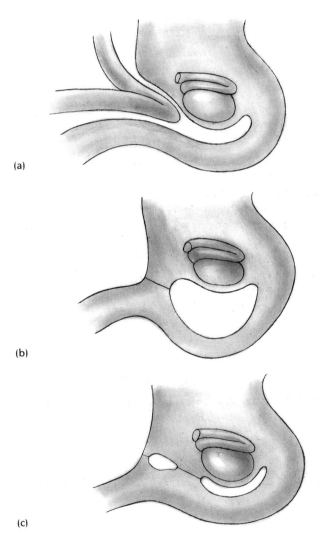

(a)

(b)

(c)

FIGURE 25.16 (a) Indirect congenital inguinal hernia arising from failure of the processus vaginalis to close; (b) hydrocoele, arising from incomplete closure of the cranial portion of the processus vaginalis.

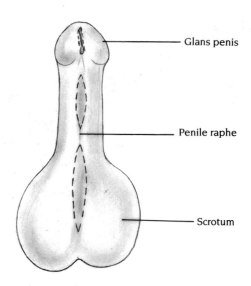

FIGURE 25.17   Hypospadias can occur in almost any position along the penile raphe.

present at birth a mass is observed in the groin, and pain results from straining or crying. Approximately three times as many cases occur on the right as on the left. As the processus vaginalis forms in both sexes this condition is also seen in females, although it is ten times more common in males.

Hydrocoele A patent space of the kind represented by the processus vaginalis could fail to close or re-open pathologically. Large fluid accumulations in the region of the processus and tunica vaginalis are described as hydrocoeles and may arise from a variety of causes.

Hypospadias In this condition the urethra opens on the ventral aspect of the penis (Figure 25.17), causing problems with urination. The opening is in the glans region of the penis in 60% of cases. The penis may be underdeveloped and may curve downwards (a condition known as chordée penis) in 50% of cases. The condition may be due to insufficient androgen production resulting in failure of the urogenital folds to fuse. Incidence may be as high as one per 200 live births, making it an extremely common defect.

Incomplete uterine fusions (Figure 25.18) In females a spectrum of defects involve incorrect fusion of the paramesonephric ducts, with a total incidence of one per 1000 live births. Defects may range from completely separate uteri to a slight additional structure in the uterus. Sufferers may show repeated spontaneous miscarriage.

Anorectal atresias and fistulas (Figure 25.19) This also represents a spectrum of conditions usually classified together. Now that we have described the development of the genital apparatus, it is possible to understand the varieties that may be observed. An underdeveloped anal canal with no communication to

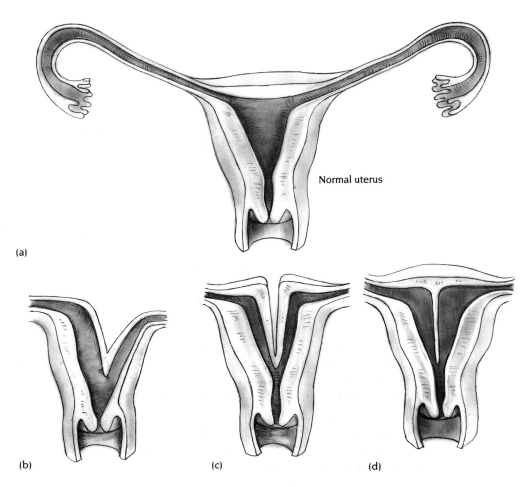

(a)

(b)   (c)   (d)

FIGURE 25.18   (a) Normal uterus. Various forms of abdominal uterine development may give (b) separate uteri; (c) a partitioned uterus; (d) maldevelopment of one uterine horn.

the rectum may be associated with a fistula to the vagina in females or to the urethra in males. The anal canal may also come to a blind end. The incidence of this category of conditions is approximately one per 3000 live births, although it varies markedly with social conditions.

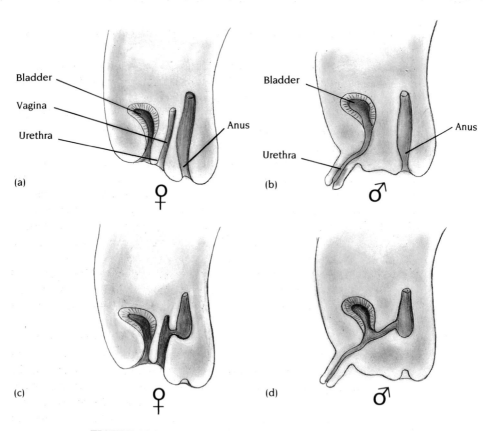

FIGURE 25.19 Anorectal atresias and fistulas in males and females.

Box 25.1 Experimental analysis of sex development

Males and females are physically distinct and this distinction normally correlates with an XY (male) and XX (female) sex chromosome complement. The basal condition is female: the presence of the Y chromosome normally initiates maleness, but there are a considerable variety of morphologies between these conditions.

Given that the Y chromosome is not essential for life, and that one X chromosome is sufficient, there is a greater number of viable monosomies and trisomies of the sex chromosomes than of the autosomes.

The presence of a single X chromosome (usually described as XO) is known as *Turner's syndrome*. Sufferers are female, short in stature with a broad chest and 'webbed' neck. They are infertile and do not mature sexually.

The sex chromosome complement XXY is known as Klinefelter's syndrome: affected males are tall and thin with long limbs. They too may be infertile and may show some signs of breast development.

XXX females occur at the same frequency as XXY males but are generally normal in appearance and fertile; similarly, XYY males are normal in appearance.

The incidence of each of these three trisomies is about one per 1000 live births. This is similar to that of trisomy 21, and offers a hint of the spontaneous incidence of non-disjunction events in human development. If we assume that no chromosome is more likely than another to show disjunction and (less likely) that the sex trisomies have no deleterious effect on developmental survival, then we might expect something like 46 trisomies per 1000 pregnancies. Each trisomy has a corresponding monosomy; this represents 92 non-disjunction abnormalities per 1000 pregnancies, most of which must result in death during development. This rough estimate is likely to understate the true figure but it indicates how common this problem may be.

Possession of the correct complement of sex chromosomes does not, however, guarantee normal sexual morphology. Sexual maturation depends on the correct functioning of the sex hormones and there may be defects in the production of, or response to, the hormones during development and adolescence producing a variety of intermediate forms between male and female. True hermaphrodites also exist, with both male and female internal sexual organs: it is even possible for an individual to be male on the right and female on the left. We will return to this concept below.

It could be said that males are females whose bodies have been distorted by powerful steroid hormones. Some simple experiments further illustrate the interaction between the gonads and the sex hormones during the development of the genital ducts. Normal females retain the paramesonephric ducts and lose the mesonephric ducts, while in males the opposite is true. Addition of antitestosterone to a male fetus causes loss of the mesonephric ducts only: removal of the testes also results in retention of the paramesonephric ducts. From this we can conclude that in males testosterone stabilizes the mesonephric ducts, but another substance is produced by the testis to make the paramesonephric ducts degenerate. This is now known to be a member of the TGF-β family of growth factors (see Special Topic 10, pp. 384–5).

The question remains as to how production of these substances is initiated. Under normal circumstances, possession of a Y chromosome is the determining factor in mammals for maleness.

Occasionally XY females are found; these usually lack a small region from the tip of one of the arms of the Y chromosome. It is now known that the missing region includes a Y-encoded gene known as *Sry* in mice and *SRY* in humans. It is a zinc-finger protein, which means that it can bind to the coils of DNA, leading to specific gene expression (of the paramesonephric duct inhibiting substance and testosterone, for instance). On occasion XX males are found, but many of these possess an *SRY*-containing region translocated to another chromosome. *SRY* thus seems to be the key factor in initiating the cascade of maleness. In the absence of *SRY*, ovary-controlling genes lead to the development of ovaries, giving the female phenotype. In perhaps the definitive test, a female mouse genetically engineered to possess the *Sry* gene developed as a male. *Sry* is expressed in the gonadal ridge at the time of testis determination.

However, this does not explain all the abnormalities, for example those individuals who are male one side and female on the other (oddly, usually male on the right and female on the left). This may require a further explanation involving more than just the genetic constitution. Perhaps it is related to timing: the embryo may have to be at an appropriate stage to respond to sex initiating signals. If male signals are received at this time males develop, otherwise development is female. This idea is supported by the observation that male fetuses are a little bigger than female, even from early stages, while within an embryo the right side is a little bigger than the left. It may be that sex determining genes plays a role in moderating the speed of development.

Further reading

Brewster S.F. (1985). The development and differentiation of human seminal vesicles. *J. Anat.*, **143**, 45–55

Byskov A.G. (1981). Gonadal sex and germ cell differentiation. In *Mechanisms of Sex Differentiation in Animals and Man* (Austin, C.R. and Edwards, R., eds), pp. 145–57. Cambridge: Cambridge University Press

Byskov A.G. (1986). Differentiation of the mammalian embryonic gonad. *Physiol. Rev.*, **66**, 71–7

Frazer B.A. and Sato A.G. (1989). Morphological sex differentiation in the human embryo: a light and scanning electron microscopic study. *J. Anat.*, **165**, 61–74

Heyns C.F. (1987). The gubernaculum during testicular descent in the human fetus. *J. Anat.*, **153**, 93–112

Johnson M. and Everitt B. (1980). *Essential Reproduction*. London: Blackwell

Peters H. and McNatty K.P. (1980). *The Ovary*. London: Paul Elek

Sadow J.I.D. (1980). *Essential Reproduction*. London: Croom Helm

Setchell B.P. (1978). *The Mammalian Testis*. London: Paul Elek

Box 25.1

Behringer R.R. *et al.* (1990). Abnormal sexual development in transgenic mice chronically expressing Mullerian Inhibiting Substance. *Nature,* **345**, 167–70

Jost A. *et al.* (1973). Studies on sex differentiation in mammals. *Rec. Progr. Horm. Res.,* **29**, 1–41

Koopman P. and Gubbay J. (1991). The biology of *Sry. Semin. Dev. Biol.,* **2**, 259–64

Koopman P., Gubbay J., Vivian N., Goodfellow P. and Lovell-Badge R. (1991). Male development of chromosomally female mouse transgenic for Sry. *Nature,* **351**, 117–21

McLaren A. (1990). Of MIS and the mouse. *Nature,* **345**, 111

Mittwoch U. (1988). The race to be male. *New Scientist,* **22 October**, 38–42

Neu R.L. and Gardner L.I. (1975). Abnormalities of the sex chromosomes. In *Endocrine and Genetic Diseases of Childhood and Adolescence* 2nd edn (Gardner L.I., ed.), pp. 793–814. Philadelphia: W.B. Saunders

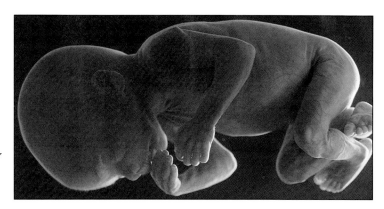

PART IV

The succession of generations

26

Germ cells and inheritance

The fact that characteristics can be transmitted from parents to children must have been evident from early times yet the mechanism of transmission, risky and uncertain as any study of hereditary monarchy proves it to be, remained obscure until it was investigated by scientific methods in the nineteenth century. At this time a popular view, reluctantly espoused by Charles Darwin, was that of **pangenesis**. Particles were assumed to be distributed throughout the body, carrying information on their local environment. Copies of the particles were thrown off from time to time and collected in the germ cells. During embryonic development each particle could direct the reforming of its region of origin. This theory is testable because it implies that characters acquired during life can be inherited: August Weismann accordingly docked the tails of 15 generations of mice but observed no effect on the tails of the offspring, in the same way that circumcision over hundreds of generations in some cultural groups has not affected the development of the human foreskin.

From these (and similar) experiments Weismann suggested that part of the developing embryo – the **germ plasm** – is set aside and the rest of the embryo goes on to form adult structures – the **soma**. Germ plasm will produce the next generation: it therefore continues from generation to generation. The adult is the germ plasm's way of carrying itself forward.

Primordial germ cells

What evidence is there for the existence of this germ plasm? In some animals visible regional specialization of the egg cytoplasm can be seen which, as the egg cleaves, is partitioned into cells that will become sperm or eggs: the **germ cells**. Only in insects has it been possible to prove definitively that this germ plasm actually converts cells into true germ cells that in time will give rise to gametes, but it may also be true in some vertebrates such as frogs. Given that mammalian embryos are highly regulative, however, it is unlikely that germ plasm is set aside in exactly this way, and the mechanism by which germ cells are established in humans remains unknown.

The early precursors of germ cells, known as the **primordial germ cells** (PGCs), in humans are typical of vertebrate germ cells in general. They appear comparatively early in development (about 24 days after fertilization): at this time, like all other cells in the body, they are diploid (that is, they possess a full, double, set of chromosomes) and they bear no resemblance to the definitive germ cells they will later form. They may be slightly larger than the neighbouring cells and can be identified by their positive staining reaction with alkaline phosphatase. They arise in a site remote from their eventual home in the internal sexual organs: in fact they originate outside the body of the embryo, in the wall of the yolk sac (Figure 26.1), and have, as a result, to cover considerable distances to populate the sex organs. This is achieved by amoeboid movement through the gut mesentery. This raises two questions: why they first appear at such a distant site, and how they then find their way to the gonads. No clear answer is available for the first of these: it may be to keep the PGCs away from morphogenetic signals in the body of the embryo (see Chapter 5). The second question is easier to study. It is known that the direction of movement is influenced by the substrate over which they move: if amphibian PGCs are dropped onto a piece of gut mesentery in culture they line up in the direction that they would normally take in vivo, and this seems to reflect an orientation established in the cytoskeleton of the gut cells. In addition, there seems to be a chemical attractant produced by the gonads, as shown by the following experiment.

An agar covered slide is prepared and three wells are cut in it: PGCs are plated in the centre well; in one of the side wells a gonadal ridge is placed and in the other a control organ. After several days the PGCs have migrated towards the side of the well nearest the gonadal ridge.

From time to time a PGC may get lost, and may then give rise to a particular type of cancer (see Special Topic 10, pp. 384–5).

The numbers of PGCs are initially small – perhaps as few as 100 in the yolk sac. However, they multiply during migration and by the time they arrive at the gonad may be several thousand strong. They then continue to multiply mitotically (see p. 366). In the female fetus the PGCs differentiate into **oogonia**; in males they will form **spermatogonia**, but only at puberty. Spermatogonia replace themselves by continued mitotic division, so the number of sperm that

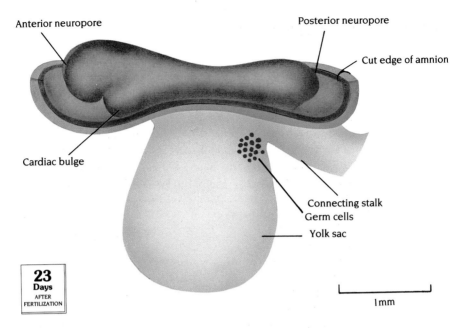

FIGURE 26.1 Site of origin of human primordial germ cells.

can be produced is vast: oogonia, by contrast, are limited in number. Their number rises to perhaps 7 million or so in the 5-month fetus, then many degenerate so that by birth there may be only a million or fewer functional germ cells present. These are generally **oocytes**, oogonia that have commenced meiotic division (see below) and have therefore entered upon the process that will lead to them becoming haploid (possessing only one full set of chromosomes). Spermatogonia, by contrast, remain fully diploid till the onset of puberty, whereupon they re-enter mitotic division: they become haploid only as they enter terminal differentiation.

The reason for this reduction in chromosome complement was identified by Weismann even before chromosomes were discovered. He pointed out that each time male and female germ cells fused the number of 'units of heredity' (whatever those were) would double. Because this cannot continue to occur in every successive generation, Weismann proposed that a 'reduction division' took place at some stage in germ cells, so that the number of heredity units halved compared with a normal body cell. But Weismann also knew that some animal eggs will complete development parthenogenetically, without being fertilized by a sperm, so even the reduced number represents one full set. It followed then that before the reduction division cells have two full sets of heredity units. We now know that these units of heredity are genes, and we can describe the underlying processes in detail.

Mitosis and meiosis

Humans possess 46 chromosomes: 22 (autosome) pairs and two sex chromosomes (Table 26.1).

Mitosis

In mitosis the single chromosomes double, and the double chromosomes then separate to give twice the number of *single* chromosomes. One set of 46 single chromosomes goes to each daughter of the associated cell division. Each chromosome undergoes this process separately: it does not associate with its corresponding pair partner.

Meiosis

It would be possible to generate a reduction division simply by missing out the replication step and giving one chromosome of each pair to each of the daughters. However, this does not happen, for reasons we will examine shortly: there are in fact two divisions.

Before the first division the single chromosomes become double as in mitosis, but then each chromosome pairs up with its corresponding partner. At the first division one of each pair of *double* chromosomes goes to each of the daughters, giving each daughter 23 double chromosomes. This is followed by a second division in which each of the daughter cells acquires a single chromosome from each of the double ones, so it has 23 single ones.

Why is this complex mechanism adopted? While the chromosomes are paired the strands of DNA break and rejoin in such a way that segments of one chromosome transfer to the other and when the pairs separate a unique recombination of the genes provided by the mother and father has been generated. This gene recombination increases the amount of variability in the population, and provides the raw material for evolution.

Although the principles of meiosis are the same in both sperm and eggs the timing of events, and the distribution of cytoplasm to the daughter cells, are very different and must be considered separately.

Oocyte development

In the development of oocytes a pause occurs during the first meiotic division, after the exchange of genetic material but before complete separation of the pairs and hence before the daughter cells separate. Parts of the new genome may be transcribed at this point to make proteins for later use. At birth essentially all the surviving germ cells have reached, and are arrested in, this **primary oocyte** stage. Each primary oocyte is surrounded by flattened cells derived from the

TABLE 26.1   Checklist for mitosis and meiosis.

	Number of cells	Number of chromosomes	Structure	DNA
Mitosis				
Begins with	1	46	single	2n
Replication	1	46	double	4n
Division	2	46	single	2n
Meiosis				
Begins with	1	46	single	2n
Replication	1	46	double	4n
Pairing	1	2×23	double	4n
First meiotic division	2	23	double	2n
Second meiotic division	4	23	single	n

ovarian tissue, as described in more detail in Chapter 27; these ovarian cells and the primary oocyte are together referred to as a **primordial follicle**.

Primordial follicles remain in this state until at least the onset of puberty then in each menstrual cycle a small number of primordial follicles begins to undergo hormonally induced changes (see Figure 27.1). The primary oocyte starts to enlarge and the surrounding ovarian cells become cuboidal. An acellular matrix layer (the **zona pellucida**: see Chapter 2) is deposited round the oocyte and a space opens up between some of the follicular cells. The primordial follicles undergoing these processes are called **primary follicles.** Generally, only one or perhaps two of these will reach full maturity: when they do so the first meiotic division of the oocyte is at last completed. However, the two daughter cells are very unequal in size: one inherits essentially all the cytoplasm and is known as the **secondary oocyte**; the other is the known as the **first polar body** (see Chapter 2). The first stages of the second meiotic division are now completed rapidly, followed by another pause. **Ovulation** – expulsion of the egg and its surrounding cumulus cells from the ovary – now occurs and the egg enters the ampulla of the oviduct. If the egg is fertilized, the second meiotic division will be completed: again, one of the daughters is small, becoming the **second polar body**. The first polar body might divide again.

It is not fully understood why only one primary follicle normally matures: more can be induced to do so under hormonal treatment (see Special Topic 2, pp. 45–6).

Spermatogenesis

By the time migration and initial multiplication of PGCs in the male is complete the germ cells lie in the primary sex cords (Chapter 25). Here they remain until puberty, at which time the sex cords become tubular structures and the germ cells – now known as spermatogonia – come to lie along the inner surface of the tubule. At this stage they may re-enter mitotic division. The events that lead particular spermatogonia to initiate meiotic division are unknown but some – known as spermatocytes – do so, and generate four haploid **spermatids** once their meoitic divisions are complete. The spermatids are at first fairly unremarkable rounded cells, but then undergo dramatic differentiation to form the definitive spermatozoa.

Defects of meiosis

Primary oocytes may wait many years for external signals to complete the separation of the chromosome pairs and to enter the first meiotic division. As a result there is a risk that other chance events – exposure to low-level cosmic radiation or to substances found in the environment, for instance – may deleteriously affect the ability of the chromosome pairs to separate successfully. If this happens for one pair, then one daughter cell will have only 22 double chromosomes and the other will have 24. At the second meiotic division the first daughter can produce two cells with 22 single chromosomes and the second two cells with 24 (of course, in practice three of these four cells will be polar bodies). Fertilization, which adds a full set of 23 chromosomes, means that zygotes are produced which have either only one version (monosomy) or three versions (trisomy) of a particular chromosome. Monosomies are rarely seen, apart from those affecting the sex chromosomes, probably because they are lethal early in development. Trisomies are more common, but usually only children with trisomy of chromosome 21 have reasonable life expectancy (see Table 26.2). A number of other trisomies survive to birth, but it is rare for them to live long (again, sex-chromosome trisomies are the exception).

Trisomy 21 Trisomy 21 (also known as Down's syndrome) has some characteristic physical signs. The face may be broad and flat, the palpebral crease of the eyelid is missing and there may be a single crease running across the palm of the hand. Some degree of mental dysfunction is frequently present: this is often described as 'mental retardation' but this term implies more than is known for sure. Exactly why these signs result from the underlying trisomy is unknown. It is, however, interesting that the gene for β-amyloid protein is present on chromosome 21. This protein accumulates in the brains of patients suffering from Alzheimer's disease and may be associated with the loss of mental function observed in this condition. Perhaps overexpression of β-amyloid arising from the three copies present in trisomy 21 sufferers also affects mental function.

Sex chromosome trisomies and monosomies also have a better chance of survival than most disjunction events, because only one sex chromosome (the X chromosome) is essential to survival. These are dealt with in Chapter 25.

Deletions and translocations Occasionally a complete region of one chromosome may attach to another chromosome during meiosis. On separation one daughter cell will inherit a chromosome with a region missing (a deletion) while the other has an extraneous piece (a translocation). There are too many variations to describe individually, but they may resemble monosomies and trisomies.

TABLE 26.2   Incidence of chromosomal abnormalities.

Abnormality	Per 10 000 pregnancies	Per 10 000 live births (where different)
All autosomal	19.3	15.83
Trisomy 21	13.6	12.1
Trisomy 18 all	2.0	
Trisomy 13 all	0.8	
Klinefelter (XXY)	10	
Turner (XO)	20	1
XXX females	10	10
XYY males	10	10

Maternal age and abnormality

The likelihood of many kinds of abnormality increases with maternal age. This is probably due to the increased time the oocytes have spent arrested in first meiosis, in extreme cases up to 50 years. The relationship between trisomy syndrome and maternal age may serve as an example: it occurs in five or six pregnancies per 10 000 in women under 25 but in women over 40 it may occur in 100 pregnancies per 10 000. Fetal screening and therapeutic abortion is significantly reducing the number of live-born trisomy 21 sufferers.

Special Topic 9 The abnormal fetus

Introduction

The study of developmental abnormality is often described as **teratology** (from the Greek *teratos*, monster). From this root comes **teratogenesis** – the formation of 'monsters' and **teratogen**, an agent with this ability.

In Europe just over 2% of all live born children have a significant abnormality detectable within the first 6 months; others have abnormalities which may not become apparent until much later, but these are not recorded in the same way, so the figures are imprecise. Many more have one or more **anomalies**: slight variations from the normal form that are unlikely to have any negative consequences.

Considerable local variations are recorded even within Europe. Incidences of significant abnormalities range from 1.2% of births in west Flanders to 3.2% in Glasgow. Such variation reflects economic and genetic differences between subpopulations. The social and personal consequences of birth abnormalities are considerable and identifying their causes is a major medical task.

The historical names given to individual conditions were often whimsical rather than informative. No less whimsical were the proposed causes: it has been a popular belief since classical times that experiences of the mother during pregnancy could lead to specific defects in the child. The reality is rather more complex.

There are two main strands in the causation of congenital abnormalities: the genetic and the environmental. These are formally separate but in practice are closely linked. For example, two strains of rat show similar incidences of spontaneous cleft palate development under normal conditions but if pregnant rats of each strain are given the same dose of a teratogen, they show markedly different rates of palatal clefting. The effect of a particular teratogen is therefore dependent on the animal's genetic background. It is likely that there is a complete spectrum ranging from defects that are caused entirely by the genetic background to those entirely caused by some external agent, with the majority of cases lying between these extremes. Although precise figures are hard to come by, it has been suggested that 25% of all abnormalities are assignable to genetic defects, and 10% are associated with known environmental factors. The remaining 65% cannot be ascribed definitely to one of those two causes. Many abnormalities may be caused by currently unknown genetic or environmental factors, but some of the defects not assigned to specific causes could arise from developmental 'accidents'. Development is not deterministic in the sense that events unfold and induce each other in an inflexible manner: rather it is probabilistic and interactive. A number of similar mechanisms may tend to support a particular outcome and there may be variation between embryos as to what exactly is going on at any particular time. The probabilistic nature of each mechanism could imply that, by chance, a proportion of the final outcomes will go wrong.

Genetic sources of abnormality

These may result from point mutations, rearrangements of segments of chromosomes or changes in chromosome number (see Chapter 26 for more information on this last category). When expression of the gene (or set of genes) is initiated the corresponding proteins may be abnormal or abnormally expressed, and as a result the associated functions cannot be carried out properly. Many such defects are not expressed until after birth and some of those that are expressed before birth are concerned with physiological processes that are not strictly developmental, although they may be necessary to normal development. It is likely that a genetic defect in a major pathway of development would lead to massive developmental failure early on. The fascinating world of genetic abnormality is largely outside the scope of this book, with three exceptions:

(1) Non-disjunction of chromosomes (see p. 368).
(2) Abnormalities of sexual development (see Chapter 25).
(3) Genetic imprinting (see Box 1.1). This is of major developmental interest because it reflects differences in genes according to whether they pass through the egg or the sperm.

Environmental sources of abnormality

Environmental factors include chemical agents ingested by the mother, physical agents such as radiation, heat and pressure, and biotic agents (such as bacteria, viruses and fungi). As described above, these exert their effects in different ways against particular genetic backgrounds. The effect of environmental factors is also influenced by the time at which they act and to a lesser extent by their nature.

Timing

As described earlier, there are three main phases of development: the pre-embryonic, the embryonic and the fetal. Each of these stages shows a different response to environmental insult, which is worth reviewing here.

Pre-embryonic period

The pre-embryonic period runs from fertilization to the end of the third week. During this time cell numbers increase rapidly, the pre-embryo implants in the uterine wall and individuality is established at gastrulation. The pre-embryo shows marked regulative behaviour (see Chapter 1). As a result, response to harmful agents is rather unpredictable. If only some of the cells are killed or affected then the unaffected cells may compensate for their absence or altered behaviour. In mouse pre-embryos normal development may continue even after 80% of the cells have been killed; however, a point will eventually be reached at which the pre-embryo cannot survive. A spontaneous abortion will then occur, though at this stage it is unlikely that the mother will even be aware that she has been pregnant.

Embryonic period

The embryonic period extends from the beginning of the third week to the end of the eighth week. The main organ systems form during this phase, though by its end the embryo is still only some 3 cm long.

   The embryonic period is characterized by many delicate and complex tissue interactions, disturbance of which almost inevitably leads to abnormalities. As a result the embryonic phase is sometimes referred to as the **critical period**. The most complex interactions are usually the most frequently affected; palate and lips, eyes, ears, brain and neural tube and heart are all highly susceptible.

   At the beginning of the embryonic phase the mother will have missed one menstrual period, but because these are often erratic in any case or because some bleeding may have occurred at implantation she may still not realize that she is pregnant. Caution must therefore be used in prescribing any medicines for women of child-bearing age.

Fetal period

The fetal period occupies the time remaining until birth. The main events of morphology have been completed by the beginning of this phase but the fetus continues to grow steadily, and the organ systems mature towards a functional state. This is particularly true of the nervous system in which functional connections are being established and the skeletal system as cartilaginous precursor elements are replaced by bone. Extensive cell death also occurs in the nervous system and the reproductive system. Abnormalities induced during this period therefore have less dramatic effects on morphology than those in the embryonic phase but may affect growth, formation of the hard tissues and the ordering of neural connections. This last is of particular importance, because it may result in mental dysfunction.

By looking at the particular defects that have arisen in an affected child it is possible to speculate on the time at which exposure to a teratogenic agent may have occurred. Within the eventful embryonic period it is even possible to identify organ systems at particular risk at particular times, usually the time of their first appearance. This suspected time can be compared with the mother's medical history and possible causative agents may be indicated.

Two key points must be borne in mind during this process. One is that teratogens are in general rather non-specific in their action (see below), so the cause of the defect cannot readily be inferred from the nature of the defect: different teratogens acting at the same developmental stage may have similar effects. The second is that teratogens interact with the genome of the embryo, as indicated above, so simultaneous administration of a teratogen to different embryos will affect each differently.

However, once an agent is suspected of having a teratogenic action, controlled comparisons can be made retrospectively to indicate whether women who have been exposed to this agent are at increased risk and a strong circumstantial case made against that agent.

Nature of teratogens

A distinction must be drawn between agents that affect the developing child and those that affect the DNA of the parental germ cell line: the latter act primarily as **mutagens**. Primary oocytes are established before birth, and do not divide until ovulation; the female germ line is therefore much more susceptible to mutagens than the male. (Sperm are produced anew by mitotic division throughout life. However, there is increasing evidence that exposure of males to a number of environmental influences can affect developmental processes in their children.)

The list of confirmed and suspected teratogens is extensive. Of the three main categories, thalidomide is perhaps the most notorious chemical teratogen, ionizing radiation the best known physical agent and German measles (rubella virus) the most familiar biological agent: these are discussed in more detail below. Others are less easy to assess: alcohol, for instance, has been associated with birth defects (the 'fetal alcohol syndrome') and as a result pregnant women have been advised to abstain from all alcohol. However, while heavy drinkers are at a higher risk of having an abnormal child, this risk may be caused by their lifestyle in general; associated use of tobacco and illegal substances, poor nutritional status, poor attendance at antenatal clinics etc.

A number of medical treatments are known to have teratogenic activity. Tetracycline antibiotics affect hard tissue formation during the fetal period, affecting the long bones and teeth. Anticonvulsant drugs may also have teratogenic effects.

Dietary deficiencies may cause fetal abnormalities. Extensive trials suggest that supplementing the diet of women considering pregnancy with folic acid reduces the incidence of spina bifida. Unfortunately, there is also evidence that excesses of some vitamins – particularly vitamin A (retinoic acid) – can also cause abnormalities. (This might be expected because retinoids are believed to play key morphogenetic roles during development (see Chapter 17).)

The effects of a teratogenic agent can be direct or indirect.

Direct effects

Direct agents exert their primary effect on the embryo or fetus: radiation of various sorts falls into this category. Chemicals and viruses must cross the placental barrier to have a direct effect. Most small molecules can cross the placental barrier by direct diffusion, but some larger molecules are transported across it. Viruses including cytomegalovirus, hepatitis and HIV are able to cross the placenta.

Indirect effects

Indirect agents exert their primary effect on the mother, in such a manner that fetal development is affected. For instance, cigarette smoking causes hypoxia in the mother. This in turn affects the fetus, which is smaller than normal. If the mother's diet is deficient in calcium or iron the fetus will maximize its supply via the placenta, at the expense of the mother.

Type examples

Thalidomide   In the late 1950s, the German company Grunenthal marketed a new drug as a sedative that was subsequently licenced in other countries under a variety of trade names, including thalidomide, although stringent regulations in America prevented its general introduction there. One particular category of patient thalidomide was recommended for was the pregnant mother. No appropriate testing of pregnant animals or controlled human studies had been carried out before such marketing. In countries where it was being used, however, the incidence of rare abnormalities began to increase. Limb abnormalities attracted particular attention. Medical histories of the mothers of children with these defects revealed that most had taken thalidomide during their pregnancy. Animal testing confirmed that thalidomide is an extremely potent teratogen and it was subsequently withdrawn from markets world-wide, amid extreme legal acrimony. (In men, and in women outside child-bearing age, thalidomide is once more prescribed for a variety of conditions.) World-wide, thousands of children are known to have been severely affected. More thorough animal testing of new drugs, greater caution on the part of doctors in prescribing to women of child-bearing age and closer monitoring of population birth abnormality rates make it unlikely that a disaster on this scale will occur again in the developed world.

Radiation   Large doses of radiation have been given to pregnant women on a number of occasions. The dropping of atomic bombs on Japan during World War II is the largest involuntary experiment of this kind, though on an individual basis it may occur when women are being treated for cancer by radiotherapy. Large doses in the range 100–1000 rads are very damaging, and the majority of fetuses are severely damaged in consequence. Doses in the range 25–100 rads are known to be harmful to CNS development and a woman exposed to this level of radiation is usually advised to have the pregnancy terminated.

Direct diagnostic X-rays fall in the range 0.3–2 rads and are unlikely to cause direct harm to the embryo or fetus. However, a whole-body maximum of 0.5 rads is the permitted limit in the UK, and women of child-bearing age should not be given abdominal X-rays unless pregnancy can be ruled out (during menstruation, for instance) or the need is overwhelming. Scattered radiation from non-abdominal X-rays does not appear to pose a significant risk.

Rubella   The rubella virus – the causative agent of German measles – was one of the first infectious agents to established as a teratogen. The virus, like a number of others such as cytomegalovirus and herpes simplex, crosses the placenta to attack the embryo or fetus. It is possible to plot the effect it exerts at different stages of development. In accordance with the organs being formed at that time, the proportion of mothers infected with the rubella virus during the first 12 weeks of pregnancy who have an abnormal child can reach 20%.

Specificity of teratogen action

Despite the impression that is sometimes conveyed teratogens are generally rather non-specific in their effect. Agents that affect basic cell processes such as division, movement, secretion, survival and differentiation are likely to be deleterious to development. For instance, palatal shelf fusion depends on the shelves growing at the proper time and place, on hyaluronic acid being secreted on schedule, on the ectodermal covering breaking down at the right time and on fusion between the mesodermal layers occurring subsequently. If *any* of these processes are altered clefting of the palate may result.

As a result it is often difficult to identify a teratogenic agent from study of the defect. Even in one individual a particular teratogen may affect each side of the body in different ways, perhaps reflecting slight differences in microenvironment.

Despite this, particular defects are often assigned to particular drugs. For example, the effects of thalidomide were often associated with an unusual limb defect (often known as phocomelia, 'seal limbs': see Chapter 18). In fact, thalidomide causes a wide spectrum of defects, and was first identified as a teratogen by its association with bowel atresias. Many women did not recollect that they had been given thalidomide during their pregnancy until they were interviewed with this in mind and their medical records were checked.

Lack of teratogenic specificity can have important medical consequences, in that it may be harder to track down the agent responsible for malformations. It may also have important legal consequences: in a recent court case in America, a judge held that a spermicidal jelly was responsible for defects of a child's left arm, left shoulder and right hand but not for the child's cleft lip and nostril and optic nerve defect. This judicial certainty must have some unique basis rooted outside scientific evidence.

Further reading

Baker T.G. (1963). A quantitative and cytological study of germ cells in human ovaries. *Proc. R. Soc. Lond. (Biol.)*, **158**, 417–33

Eddy E.M., Clark J.M., Gong D. and Fenerson B.A. (1981). Origin and migration of primordial germ cells in mammals. *Gamete Res.*, **4**, 333–62

Fawcett D.W. and Bedford J.M., eds. (1979). *The Spermatozoon*. Baltimore: Urban & Schwarzenberg

Godin I., Wylie C.C. and Heasman J. (1990). Genital ridges exert long range effects on mouse primordial germ cell numbers and direction of migration in culture. *Development*, **108**, 357–63

Neu R.L. and Gardner L.I. (1975). Abnormalities of the sex chromosomes. In *Endocrine and Genetic Disease of Childhood and Adolescence*, pp. 793–814. Philadelphia: W.B. Saunders

Peters H. and McNatty K.P. (1980). *The Ovary*. London: Paul Elek

Simpson J.L. (1977). *Disorders of Sexual Differentiation*. Chicago: Year Book Publishers

Therman E. (1986). *Human Chromosomes: Structure, Behaviour, Effects* 2nd edn. New York: Springer-Verlag

Witschi. E. (1948). Migration of the germ cells of human embryos from the yolk sac to the primitive gonadal folds. *Contrib. Embryol.*, **32**, 67–80

Wylie C.C., Heaysman J., Swan A.P. and Anderton B.H. (1979). Evidence for substrate guidance of primordial germ cells. *Exp. Cell. Res.*, **121**, 315–24

Special Topic 9

Jones K.L. and Smith D.W. (1973). Recognition of the fetal alcohol syndrome in early pregnancy. *Lancet*, **ii**, 999–1001

Kantor A.F., Curnen M.G.M., Meigs J.W. and Flannery J.T. (1979). Occupations of fathers of patients with Wilms' Tumour. *J. Epidemiol. Commun. Health.*, **33**, 253–6

Milunsky A., Jick S.S. Jick S.S. *et al.* (1989). Multivitamin/folic acid supplementation in early pregnancy reduces the prevalence of neural tube defects. *JAMA*, **262**, 2847–52

Savitz D., Whelan E.A. and Kleckner R.C. (1989). Effects of parents' occupational exposures on risk of stillbirth, pre-term delivery and small-for-gestational-age infants. *Am. J. Epidemiol.*, **129**, 1201–18

Seeman P., Sellars E.M. and Roschlan W.H. (1980). *Principles of Medical Pharmacology* 3rd edn. Toronto: University of Toronto Press

Sepkowitz S. (1988). Teratogens and perinatal epidemiology. *Lancet*, **i**, 115

Whittle M.J. and Hanretty K.P. (1986). Identifying abnormalities. *Brit. Med. J.*, **293**, 1485–8

Wilson J.G. (1977). Present status of drugs as teratogens in man. *Teratology*, **7**, 3–16

Zuckerman B.S., Hingson R. (1986). Alcohol consumption during pregnancy: a critical review. *Dev. Med. Child. Neurol.*, **28**, 649–61

27

The menstrual cycle and pregnancy

As described in Chapter 26, in each menstrual cycle a few **primary follicles**, selected by some unknown means, begin to develop. Of these, only one (more rarely two) will usually complete ovulation. On average this occurs once every 28 days, although there is a considerable degree of variability around this mean value. Changes in the follicles are co-ordinated with changes in the uterine lining.

In ovulation, morphological events are under hormonal control. However, this hormonal control involves complex positive and negative feedback events, which may confuse the issue on first reading. In the hope of imparting familiarity with basics, the morphological events will be described separately from, and before, the hormonal events.

Morphological events in the menstrual cycle

In the absence of pregnancy, the menstrual cycle begins with the shedding of the prepared endometrial lining of the uterus. Five or six days after this commences, a small number of primordial follicles begin to enlarge in the ovary (See Figure 27.1) and cells in the uterine endometrium recommence proliferation. The endometrium again begins to grow thicker in consequence (Figure 27.1).

The primordial follicles will undergo further differentiation to become primary follicles. The oocytes inside these enlarge slightly and the zona pellucida is laid down by the follicular cells and the oocyte. Cortical granules also begin to appear. The follicular cells within the growing follicle now begin to proliferate but most of these growing follicles will degenerate, leaving only a few to continue development.

In the meantime vascularization has commenced in the endometrial lining of the uterus.

In those few follicles that develop further a space or **antrum** begins to develop between the follicular cells. The ovarian cells surrounding these **antral follicles** become vascularized. Finally, only one of these follicles will proceed in its development; the others will degenerate. The oocyte in the successful follicle will become surrounded by **cumulus oophorus**, which after ovulation will be known as the corona radiata cells.

By midway through the menstrual cycle, at about day 14, the endothelium is at its maximum thickness.

Shortly after this meiosis recommences in the remaining oocyte and within 24 hours it has completed its first meiotic division and started the second, although it will arrest before this is completed.

The follicle wall thins in preparation for ovulation, which takes place within about 12 hours of the first meiotic division. The oocyte and its accompanying cumulus cells emerge from the follicle and enter the ampulla of the oviduct under the influence of the fimbria, to await fertilization. The follicle now begins to collapse and the remaining follicular cells are invaded by blood vessels. At this stage it is described as the **corpus luteum**.

The corpus luteum will degenerate over a period of approximately 14 days. A new group of oocytes will then proceed with primary follicle formation.

When the corpus luteum forms, the thickened endometrium wall also develops glands that secrete glycogen. Once the corpus luteum has degenerated, however, the endometrium begins to break down and the cycle recommences.

Fertilization

If fertilization occurs a different set of events is initiated. The zygote arrives in the uterus when the uterine wall is at its thickest and when the glands and blood vessels are best developed. This is to aid the survival and nutrition of the embryo as it implants. Once implantation has occurred the uterine wall must not be sloughed off or the conceptus would be lost. Instead the endometrium survives under the influence of signals produced by the corpus luteum and the implanting conceptus. Further ovulation is redundant during the pregnancy, and is inhibited by chemical signals.

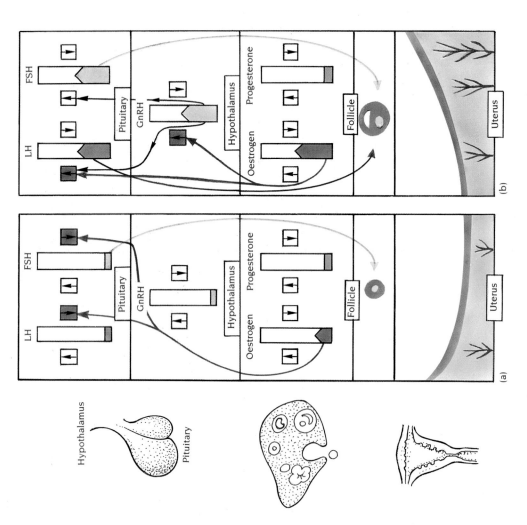

FIGURE 27.1 Changes in the uterus, the follicles in the ovary, the hypothalamus and the pituitary during the menstrual cycle. Hormones are shown with an 'up' button and a 'down' button which can be pressed by a variety of signals. Changes are continuous, as is shown by the associated hormone

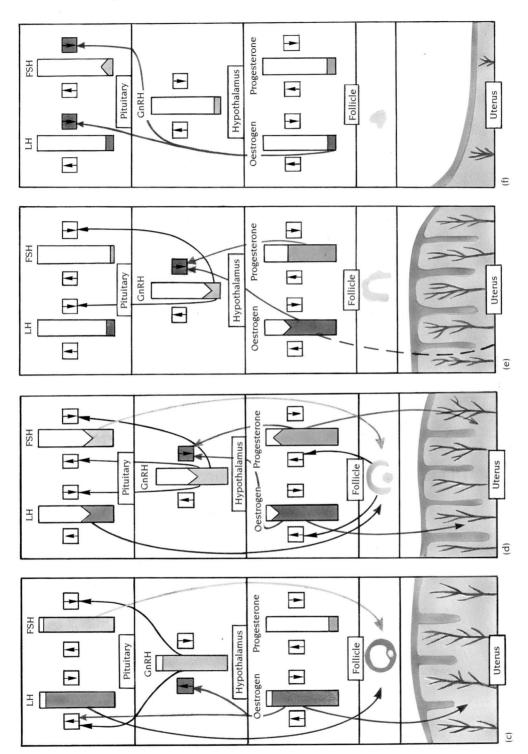

FIGURE 27.1 (continued)

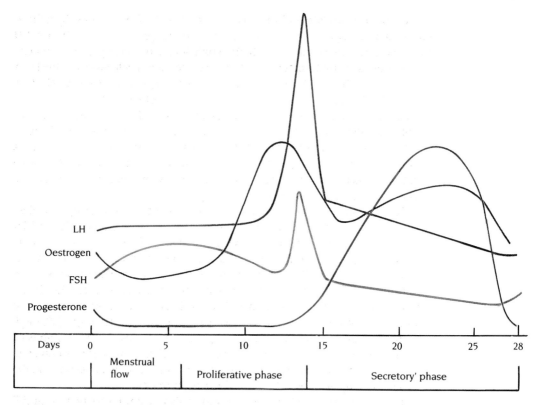

FIGURE 27.2 Hormonal changes, shown in arbitrary units.

Hormonal events in the menstrual cycle

So far this has been a morphological description only. However, the events in
the ovary and the events in the uterus must be closely coordinated. Other behavioural and physical changes occur in the body during the cycle, and these too
must be coordinated with ovarian and uterine events. Coordination is achieved
by means of an interacting series of hormonal signals in which the ovary, the
uterus, the pituitary and hypothalamus all communicate with each other in a
complex manner.

   The description may commence with the primary follicles in the ovary. As
they develop, the follicular and ovarian connective tissue cells secrete levels of
oestrogen that are initially low, but will rise sharply as the follicle matures
(Figure 27.1(a)). While low levels of oestrogen are present production of the
pituitary hormones **follicle stimulating hormone** (FSH) and **luteinizing hormone** (LH) are inhibited. As oestrogen levels rise (Figure 27.1(b)), they stimulate the uterine wall to become thicker and more vascularized. Once levels have
peaked, they fall as quickly as they rose. This **oestrogen surge** stimulates the

production of **gonadotrophin releasing hormone** (GnRH) from the hypothalamus (Figure 27.1(b)). This in turn sharply increases production of FSH and LH from the pituitary (Figure 27.1(b,c)). High levels of oestrogen also directly increase the sensitivity of the pituitary LH releasing mechanism to GnRH. A sharp increase in LH therefore follows the oestrogen surge (Figure 27.1(c)). Levels of FSH also increase under the influence of oestrogen.

Until now, the follicles have been largely insensitive to LH due to lack of specific receptors, but at this point these receptors also begin to increase in number. In response, therefore, to the LH and FSH surges the oocyte recommences meiosis, the follicle cells prepare for ovulation and ovulation itself takes place about a day later. The remaining follicular tissue is stimulated to form the corpus luteum by LH (hence 'luteinizing hormone').

Having initiated these events the levels of LH fall off as sharply as they rose (Figure 27.1(d)). This may be due to 'down regulation'; occupation of LH-stimulating receptors leads to them being internalized in the cell (as is the case for many receptor–ligand complexes), and as a result they are no longer available at the cell surface. The receptors will reappear after internal processing, but for the moment the pituitary cells are insensitive to stimulation and LH levels therefore fall in proportion to the speed at which they rose. In the meantime, the LH has stimulated the cells of the corpus luteum to produce oestrogen (although this does not reach its former levels) and progesterone. Now under the influence of progesterone as well as oestrogen, the endometrium continues to vascularize and develops glands. These secrete fluid that helps sustain the pre-embryo in the uterus before implantation (if fertilization has occurred).

But progesterone and oestrogen together also inhibit production of GnRH in the hypothalamus (Figure 27.1(e)), so rates of FSH and LH production fall even further. The corpus luteum, dependent on LH, will therefore begin to degenerate, decreasing oestrogen and progesterone levels. The endometrium, dependent on these hormones to maintain its thickened vascular state, degenerates as the endometrial arteries go into spasm. This represents the onset of the flow phase of menstruation, when the endometrial lining, some blood and the unfertilized oocyte are lost.

Released from the inhibitory effects of the progesterone produced by the corpus luteum, FSH levels begin to rise once more (Figure 27.1(f)) until enough is present to stimulate new follicles to develop, and the process can recommence.

In addition to the events described above, the sex hormones play a variety of other roles. They bring about behavioural changes and induce contractions of the common musculature that connects the uterine tubes, the uterus and their supportive ligaments.

Of the phases of the menstrual cycle, that involving the development of the follicle and proliferation of the endometrium is the most variable in duration. The luteal phase, in which the endometrium is developing its secretory role, tends to be consistently about 13–15 days. The 'flow' phase of menstruation lasts for 4 or 5 days. Variation in the 'proliferative' phase means that complete menstrual cycles may vary from 20 to 40 days, with considerable variation occurring both between and within individuals.

Pregnancy

Fertilization must somehow interrupt this normal succession of events: this is achieved by the pre-embryo producing its own hormonal signal (**human chorionic gonadotrophin**: hCG, which acts on the corpus luteum to support it even in the absence of LH. As a result, the corpus luteum will continue to produce oestrogen and progesterone. This means in turn that the endometrium is preserved in its thickened state and that menstruation does not occur. Recent findings indicate that the pre-embryo may also produce oestrogen and progesterone.

The urine of newly pregnant women contains hCG; this is the basis for pregnancy tests.

By 12 weeks after fertilization the placenta is producing substantial amounts of progesterone and the corpus luteum, now redundant, finally degenerates.

The uterine contractions that lead to birth are induced by oxytocin, which is produced by the posterior pituitary. Synthetic oxytocin analogues are widely used to induce labour. Prostaglandins also play a role in inducing contractions, and during pregnancy these are inhibited by the production of gravidin, levels of which decrease sharply before labour.

Contraception

Pregnancy can be prevented in a number of ways in addition to abstinence from sexual intercourse, which does not appeal to many people of child-bearing age.

The sperm and the egg may be physically prevented from coming into contact with each other, for example by withdrawal of the penis from the vagina before ejaculation occurs or by avoidance of intercourse during ovulation. Both methods are risky. In the US, out of 100 women and partners using either of these methods 23–24 women will become pregnant each year, compared with 90 taking no precautions at all. Alternatively, the man may wear a rubber condom over his penis or the woman may wear a diaphragm in the upper part of her vagina or a cap over her cervix. Used properly, these can give a conception incidence of 2 per 100 women per year: in practice, the incidence varies between 10 and 20 pregnancies, so we may assume that they are often used suboptimally. A female condom, lining the vagina, has recently been added to this list.

All these methods may be used in association with spermicidal agents, which are in themselves rather ineffective contraceptives.

Alternatively, gamete encounters may be prevented by tying off the vas deferens in men or by removing a portion of the oviduct in women. These methods are comparatively safe and highly effective, but are very difficult to reverse.

A reversible method of achieving the same end is to inhibit ovulation by means of synthetic hormones. A combination of oestrogen and progesterone is generally used to block FSH and LH production, as described above. These hormones are most commonly administered in the form of a daily pill, although longer-lasting injections and dermal patches have also been employed. This is a highly effective method of contraception, with conception incidence of between 0.5 and 2 pregnancies per 100 women per year, and although there are associated risks, these are currently lower than those of pregnancy.

Finally, devices may be placed inside the uterus (hence intra-uterine device or IUD) which usually prevent pregnancy occurring, perhaps by inhibiting implantation, although the method by which they operate is not yet completely clear. These are not quite as effective as the pill, with optimal and actual pregnancy incidences of 1–2 and 5, respectively.

Termination of pregnancy

Termination of pregnancy is legal in a number of countries. While generalizations are difficult, there appears to be a hierarchy of grounds for legal termination. Danger to the life of the mother is more widely accepted than abnormality of the fetus, which in turn is more generally accepted than the desire of the mother not to have a child. However, in some countries abortion is used as a means of contraception, in default of availability of contraceptive advice or devices. As indicated in Special Topic 9 (pp. 369–74), legalized termination can bring about a significant reduction in the incidence of abnormalities among full-term children.

A variety of methods are available.

(1) In early pregnancy, the artificial steroid RU 486 can be used to compete with progesterone for binding to the progesterone receptor. Progesterone is necessary for the continuation of pregnancy, although the exact molecular mechanism involved remains unclear. The presence of RU 486 on the progesterone-binding site prevents this from happening. In association with prostaglandins, RU 486 therefore induces an early abortion. It is too early to say definitively if this method will result in fewer side-effects than the alternatives, although it may be easier to administer.

(2) A common alternative method in early pregnancy is vacuum aspiration to remove the contents of the uterus. Curettage is the physical removal of these contents. Both methods pose minor risks of uterine damage or incomplete removal of the contents.

(3) At later stages, prostaglandins may be administered to the mother to induce uterine contractions to expel the fetus.

(4) Injection of hypertonic saline into the amniotic sac achieves the same effect, although it is not entirely clear how.

Although termination of pregnancy poses physical risks which increase sharply as pregnancy progresses, these are significantly lower than the risks of pregnancy itself, at least where abortion is legal.

Special Topic 10 Embryos and cancer

Cancer cells differ from normal adult cells in that they tend to divide rapidly while remaining comparatively undifferentiated. They are also capable of migration through the body, both as single cells and as invasive sheets, as opposed to most normal cell types which, with a few exceptions, are rather static. Together these properties of rapid growth and of movement (or **metastasis**) through the body represent the clinical dangers posed by cancers.

However, these are also in many ways the properties of embryonic cells: indeed, embryos grow faster than most malignant cancers. Extensive cell movement also occurs, including the invasion of cells as groups (as seen during integument development), the migration of single cells (as seen in neural crest development) and the movement of cells in the blood (as occurs with osteoclasts). There are therefore grounds for viewing the cancerous properties of cells as representing a reversion to embryonic behaviour, with one crucial difference: while these cell behaviours are tightly controlled in the embryo they are quite uncontrolled in malignancy. It may be that cancer cells have lost the ability to respond to environmental signals; however, it is also possible that in at least some instances the environmental signals have ceased to operate normally.

One indication that this is the case has been described in Box 1.2. Teratocarcinoma cells, originally malignant, may be restored to normal behaviour by placing them together with early embryo cells: stable 'bad behaviour' on the part of the tumour cells can be corrected by the environment. The same conclusion can be drawn from the observation that mouse embryos removed from their mother and grafted into an ectopic site in another mouse can give rise to teratocarcinomas in their new site. Here no genetic change has occurred: merely a change in how the cells behave.

Wilms' tumours are tumours of the embryonic kidney that often seem to have a hereditary component. In appearance they appear to represent an aberration of mesenchymal cell differentiation that particularly affects the kidneys and genitalia. A candidate gene has been identified that is missing in Wilms' tumour patients, indicating that it is normally active as a suppressor gene. The pattern of expression of this gene in normal development is, as might be expected, particularly marked in the developing kidneys and internal sexual organs. While the precise function of this gene is as yet unclear, it is plainly important in kidney development in some way, and provides evidence of yet another link between development and cancer.

Growth factors

Other similarities between embryos and tumours can be seen in the role of growth factors. These are extracellular polypeptides, generally acting at the cell membrane, that play key roles in regulating cell division and differentiation. They are usually distinguished from peptide hormones by their local action: in general, they affect cells in the vicinity of the producing cells rather than distant cells via the blood supply.

Many growth factors were originally identified from tumour cells: in fact many tumours appear to be related to abnormal expression of, or responsiveness to, growth factors in some way. As a result they often produce growth factors in large amounts. These growth factors can then be shown to play a variety of roles in vitro, including stimulation of cell division and modulation of differentiation. One class, the transforming growth factors, may serve as an example.

Transforming growth factors

These make normal cells behave like tumour cells in assays in vitro. Normal cells will not divide without the presence of a solid substrate, but tumour cells will. However, normal cells *will* divide in culture conditions in the presence of transforming growth factors. This transformation to tumour behaviour is temporary: when the growth factors are withdrawn the cells revert to normal behaviour.

As might be expected, abnormalities of transforming growth factor action are associated with a number of tumours. Such abnormalities may take the form of excess production of normal growth factors, abnormally high sensitivity to existing factors or production of a hyperactive version of the transforming growth factor.

What, then, are the normal roles of transforming growth factors? One key class of roles is in normal development. When Mullerian inhibiting substance, the agent that induces regression of the paramesonephric ducts (Chapter 00), was finally characterized it turned out to be a member of the transforming growth factor family. Bone morphogenetic protein, an agent that promotes chondrification, likewise proved to be a member of this family. Transforming growth factor family members proved to be active in heart development and the early stages of axis formation in *Xenopus* also involve a molecule in this class. In fact, even within this one family of growth factors instances of their involvement in development are too numerous to recount here. In the adult growth factors also play roles in wound healing and regeneration, which in some ways may be seen as survival of embryonic behaviour.

Other kinds of growth factor are no less interesting or important in development and cancer: endothelial cell growth factors are known to play a role in angiogenesis that is equally vital in both tumour biology and normal development (see Special Topic 5, pp. 153–7); fibroblast growth factors are involved in many developmental processes and in adult wound healing in addition to their role in cancer.

Growth factors can even interact with homoeotic mutations (see Special Topic 6, pp. 174–7). When the main body is being established, growth factors initiate the differential activation of homoeobox genes in the same way that retinoic acid does during limb development.

Together all these discoveries indicate that cellular and developmental biology are undergoing an enormous intellectual simplification in which common molecular controls are being discovered to underlie cell division and differentiation, development and the abnormal behaviour of cancer cells. Understanding the nature of these controls, usually tightly regulated during development, offers the reasonable hope of finding ways of regulating them in cancer also.

Further reading

Austin C.R. and Short, R.V., eds (1984). *Reproduction in Mammals 3. Hormonal Control of Reproduction* 2nd edn. Cambridge: Cambridge University Press

Baulieu E.-E. (1989). Contragestion and other clinical applications of RU 486, an antiprogesterone at the receptor. *Science*, **245**, 1351–7

Hatcher, R. *et al.* (1986). *Contraceptive Technology* 1986–87. New York: Irvington

Hogarth P.J. (1978). *Biology of Reproduction*. Glasgow: Blackie

Liggins G.C. (1989). Initiation of labour. *Biol. Neonate*, **55**, 366–75

Special Topic 10

Akhurst R.J. *et al.* (1990) TGF beta in murine morphogenetic processes: the early embryo and cardiogenesis. *Development*, **108**, 645–56

Burgess A.W. (1989). Epidermal growth factor and transforming growth factor-alpha. *Br. Med. Bull.*, **45**, 401–24

Carrit B., Parrington J.M., Welch H.M. and Povey S. (1982). Diverse origins of multiple ovarian teratomas in a single individual. *Proc. Natl Acad. Sci. USA*, **79**, 7400–4

Heath J.K. and Smith A.G. (1989). Growth factors in embryogenesis. *Br. Med. Bull.*, **45**, 319–36

Hsuan J.J. (1989). Transforming growth factors-beta. *Br. Med. Bull.*, **45**, 425–37

Jakobovits A. (1986). The expression of growth factors and growth factor receptors during mouse embryogenesis. In *Oncogenes and Growth Control* (Kahn, P. and Graf, T., eds), pp. 9–17 Berlin: Springer-Verlag

Kaplan C.G., Askin F.B. and Benirschke K. (1979). Cytogenetics of extragonadal tumours. *Teratology*, **19**, 261–6

Kimmel D.L., Moyer E.K., and Peale A.R. (1950). A cerebral tumour containing five human fetuses. A case of fetus in fetu. *Anat. Rec.*, **106**, 141–65

Pritchard-Jones K. *et al.* (1990). The candidate Wilms' Tumour gene is involved in genitourinary development. *Nature*, **346**, 194–7

Ruiz i Altaba A. and Melton A. (1989). Interaction between peptide growth factors and homeobox genes in the establishment of antero-posterior polarity in frog embryos. *Nature*, **341**, 33–8

Sporn M.B. and Roberts A.B. (1985). Autocrine growth factors in cancer. *Nature*, **313**, 745–7

Waterfield M.D. (1989). Epidermal Growth Factor and related molecules. *Lancet*, **i**, 1243–6

Clinical problem-based learning section

Clinical problems do not present themselves with the neat appearance of an embryology textbook. In particular, their resolution may require the integration of many kinds of knowledge, including that of surgery, immunology, general medicine, statistics and even law, psychology and ethics, among others. No textbook can possibly address all of these issues. In this section, clinical problems are posed of a kind that might be encountered in practice. To answer the questions asked will require not merely integration of material from this book, but also from a range of other sources, and identifying the answers will therefore require that you carry out further reading and research. This need not be done on an individual basis. There are many advantages to working in small groups and sharing the information that each member collects.

Since the resolutions of the problems may be extensive and wide-ranging, and may differ from place to place, no set 'answer' is provided. However, there is another reason for this; embryology is a rapidly developing subject and a set answer might well be out of date in a rather short time as techniques, skills and diagnoses improve. You should therefore aim to find the most up-to-date solutions and be aware that these may have changed by next year!

Naturally, these are only a very small proportion of the embryologically-related clinical situations you could encounter. However, my hope is that the skills you develop in dealing with these questions will be of general applicability throughout your career.

1 An ultrasound scan 16 weeks into a pregnancy shows the developing fetus to have a grossly abnormal brain and skull. Only the basal portions of the frontal, parietal and occipital bones are present. The brain tissue is greatly reduced and is exposed to the amniotic cavity at the back of the head. What is this condition called, how common is it, and what factors may have contributed to bringing it about? Working within your local legal framework, what course of action would you recommend?

2 You are looking after a newly pregnant female who has a history of spontaneous second trimester abortions. What are the possible underlying causes for this? Which of these causes have a developmental origin? What precautions would you take during her pregnancy?

3 You are asked to look after a newborn child with DiGeorge syndrome. In this condition, the embryological derivatives of the 3rd and 4th pharyngeal pouches fail to form properly. Which structures in the head and neck would normally be affected? What clinical consequences would you expect to see in the child, and what measures should you take to deal with them?

4 A pregnant woman shows signs of polyhydramnios (excess of amniotic fluid). What tests would you wish to carry out and why? If an ultrasound scan revealed that only one fetus was present, that it possessed no detectable neural tube defects and that the stomach could not be identified, what embryological condition might you suspect? What action would you take? If oligohydramnios had been observed, what are the appropriate tests to consider and what conditions might be suspected?

5 A 17-year-old male patient is found to have an enlarging mass of tissue in the roof of the nasopharynx. On sampling the mass proves to contain epithelial-lined cysts. What would this suggest to you? How would you explain the origin of the mass to your patient? Would you recommend surgery for this condition? If you did, how would you describe to him the risks and the likelihood of success?

6 Four cases of trisomy 13 from approximately 10 000 live births are reported in a county that contains a nuclear power station. Is this likely to represent a significant variation from normal? Can you conclude that the presence of the nuclear power station is responsible for these abnormalities? What other factors might influence the reported incidence?

7 A child is born with irideal coloboma – a defect of the iris such that there is a gap or notch in the lower quadrant. In this case the notch reaches internally as far as the retina. In addition, the whole of the affected eye is smaller than normal. The mother reports that on a foreign holiday four months into her pregnancy she had a frontal radiograph of the chest. She now wishes to sue the hospital concerned for damages. What advice would you give her concerning the connection between the X-ray and the occurrence of the defect?

8 An adult male patient presents with symptoms typical of appendicitis, and in addition has passed blood clots in his stool. However, during the operation the appendix proves to be healthy in appearance. In addition, the appendix is not obviously kinked or otherwise obstructed. What would you check next?

9 A woman who is breast-feeding her first-born child reports that a mole on her thorax, just above and slightly lateral to her left breast, has become enlarged and painful, and is dribbling a milky fluid. How would you advise her in these circumstances?

10 A newborn infant in your care shows signs of respiratory distress. On feeding, he/she chokes and regurgitates milk. When he/she cries the abdomen

becomes hard and distended. What condition might you suspect? What investigations would you wish to carry out in order to resolve your suspicions?

11 A young woman with severe acne who is being treated with retinoid skin cream discovered that she is in the early stages of pregnancy. What advice would you give her and what action would you take?

12 A helicopter pilot in your care gives birth to a child whose skull is narrow mediolaterally but elongated in the anterior–posterior direction. She asks you whether it could have been influenced by her exposure to crop-spraying chemicals during the first month of her pregnancy, how it can be treated, and how likely it is that this condition will be present in any subsequent children that she has. How would you answer her questions?

13 Two mothers in neighbouring beds in the maternity hospital give birth to children with cleft palate. In one case primary cleft palate is present, while the other child has secondary cleft palate. How would you reply if they asked you how likely it was that a common cause underlay the defects in their children? What treatment would you recommend in each case?

14 A newborn male child in your care has difficulty in breathing and is cyanosed. These signs seem to be getting worse as time passes. An X-ray shows that the heart is displaced to the right and that abdominal viscera are displaced into the chest region on the left hand side. What embryological condition would you suspect here and what action would you recommend?

15 A mother gives birth to a congenitally deaf child. She is concerned that this defect may have been caused by some event during her pregnancy. In investigating this possibility, at which stage of pregnancy would you concentrate your review of her medical history? What factors might you suspect as potential causes?

16 A woman who has difficulty in conceiving following an illegal abortion in her youth consults you on the likelihood of a successful pregnancy arising from in vitro fertilization. How would you advise her?

17 A newborn infant in your care shows a faecal discharge from the umbilicus. How would you explain to the parents the nature of the underlying defect? What course of action would you recommend pursuing?

18 A child is born with a hand defect. The mother reports that, up till the time that her pregnancy was confirmed, she was taking a tranquillizer (Diazepam). What effect (if any) might this have had on the embryo?

19 During the herniation and return of the midgut, a loop of intestine becomes abnormally twisted and the blood supply to a section of ileum is cut off, leading to the formation of a solid gangrenous cord over part of its length. What consequences might result for mother and child during the pregnancy and after the birth?

20 A child is born with an enlarged head. The anterior fontanelle is tense and the scalp veins are distended. What condition would you suspect, and how would you treat it? Why are these symptoms observed?

21 A mother who has previously given birth to a child suffering from spina bifida asks you how likely this condition is to recur in a subsequent pregnancy, and what steps she could take to reduce any risks. How would you advise her?

22 A newborn male child is observed to have the urethral opening on the ventral (inferior) aspect of the penis rather than at the tip. The parents ask you if this condition can be remedied, and if it will affect their son's subsequent sexual functioning. How would you reply?

23 A routine ultrasound scan 18 weeks into a pregnancy reveals the presence of a sac-like malformation in the umbilical region of the fetus. What condition would you suspect here, and what special precautions might you consider during the pregnancy and birth? Would you recommend an operation to correct the malformation immediately after the child is born, or would it be better to wait to allow the child to gain strength before the operation?

24 A baby girl, on learning to walk, shows a pronounced waddle. Her left leg appears slightly shorter than the right, and it cannot be extended as far as the right leg. The buttock skin folds are asymmetric. What condition would you suspect, and how would you treat it?

25 A young male adolescent attends your surgery with a small swelling that has recently developed in the mid-line of his neck. It is not fixed to the underlying structures. You tell him that it may be a thyroglossal cyst. Would you also recommend that it be surgically removed? How would you reply if he asked you if the operation would leave a disfiguring scar and if the cyst was likely to recur? Are the patient's age and sex of any significance in this condition?

26 A male child of 15 months has a persistent hydrocoele, and has a large mass present on the right side of the groin. The mass is more evident on straining or crying. What condition would you suspect, and how would you treat it?

Index

E

ear 229–34
  defects 238
  evolution 230
  external 234
    defects 238
  inner 230–4
  middle 230–4
ectoderm xv
  derivatives 53
  differentiation in birds and mice
    91–2
  embryonic **39**, 132
  interactions with mesoderm 134–5
  primitive (epiblast) 16, **32**
ectomesenchyme 149–50
ectopic pregnancy 44
ectrodactyly 258
efferent ductules **349**
egg(s) 3, *4*
  freezing 46
  maternal influences 6, 8
  organization inherent in 9–11, 37
  see also oocyte(s); zygote
embryo **xiii**, xiv
  and cancer 384–5
  diagnosis in postimplantation 80–4
  diagnosis in pre-implantation 18–21
  folding 59, *60–1*
  freezing 46
  orientation xv
embryonic disc 33
embryonic period **xiii**, xiv
  response to harmful agents 371
enamel **136**, *137*
encephalocoele 188
endocardial cushions *291*, *292*, **293**
endocardial tubes **286**
  fusion 286, *287*
  prevention of fusion 294
endocardium **288**
endochondral bone 125
endocrine cells, neural crest-derived
  150
endoderm xv
  derivatives 53, 74, *75*
  embryonic **39**
  extraembryonic 33
  primitive (hypoblast) 16, **32**
endolymphatic duct *233*, **234**
endometrium 376–7, 381
endothelial cell growth factors 156,
  385
enteric ganglia *147*
epiblast (primitive ectoderm) 16, **32**
epidermis 132–3
epididymis **349**
epidural space **100**
epiglottal cartilages 209
epimere *119*, *121*
epiploic foramen **307–8**
epithalamus *167*, **168**
erector pili muscles 139
erythrocytes (red blood cells) 112,
  311
ethmoid *181*, 182
excesses, regulation of 13–14
external auditory meatus **203**, *233*,
  234

extraembryonic membranes **xiii**, 71–4
  see also amnion; chorion
extraembryonic structures 70–84
  evolution 70–1
eye 224–9
  defects 238
  development 225–9
  evolution 224–5
eyelids 229

F

face 211–23
  bones *181*, 185
  deformities 211, 220–2
facial clefts 214, 220–2
  lateral 221
  median 221
  oblique 221
facial (VII) nerve *196*, 197
facial prominences 211–17
  fusion 213–17
falciform ligament **269**, 310
fallopian tube (uterine tube) *26*, **346**
Fallot's tetralogy 294
feather formation 134–5
female 340–1
  external genitalia 350, *351*
  internal genitalia 344–6
  tissue lineages *344*
fertilization 24, 25–8, 377
  in vitro, *see* in vitro fertilization
fetal alcohol syndrome 372
fetal cells, in maternal blood 84
fetal period **xiii**, xiv
  response to harmful agents 371
fetal surgery 84
fetoscopy 83
fetus **xiii**, xiv
  abnormal, *see* congenital
    abnormalities
  orientation xv
fetus-in-fetu (included fetus) 64
fibroblast growth factor (FGF) 37,
  38–9, 119, 228, 385
fibronectin 151
fingerprints 133
first and second arch syndrome 188
fish
  gills 191, *192*, 274
  heart tube 284, *285*
fixation, gut *266*, 309–10, 315
folic acid 372
follicles **344**
  antral **377**
  primary 367, **376**
  primordial **367**, 376–7
follicle stimulating hormone (FSH)
  380, 381
follicular cells **344**, 377
fontanelles **186**, *187*
foramen caecum **205**
foramen ovale 113, **291**, *292*
  closure 114, 291
  probe patency 291, 293
forebrain (prosencephalon) 164, *165*
  division 166
foregut *75*, 306–12

foreskin **352**
fourth ventricle *169*, *170*, **171**
fragile X syndrome 8
frenulum **236**
frontal bone *181*, 184
frontal sections xv-xvi
frontonasal prominence **211–13**
  fusion 214, *215–16*
fruit fly (*Drosophila*) 174–7
functional structures, formation of
  153–7

G

gall bladder *310*, 311
gamete intrafallopian transfer (GIFT)
  46
ganglia, nerve 98, *99*, *147*, 148
gastroschisis 320
gastrula **xiv**
gastrulation **xiv**, 34–9, 49
  mechanisms 36–9
gene clusters 174–5
genes 365
  in early development 5–9
genetic defects
  correction at gene level 20–1
  prenatal diagnosis 18–21
genetic imprinting **6**, **8**, 370
genitalia
  external 350–2
    defects 352–5
    development 350–2
    evolution 350
  internal 339–49
    defects 352–5
    development 340–9
    evolution 339
genital (labioscrotal) swellings **342**,
  350
genital tubercle 350, *351*
German measles (rubella) 372, 374
germ cells 363–74
  primordial, *see* primordial
    germ cells
germ layers **39**
  derivatives 53–9
  see also ectoderm; endoderm;
    mesoderm
germ plasm **363**
gestation **xiii-xiv**
gills, fish 191, *192*, 274
gingival laminae *135*
glial cells **96**, *97*, 148
glossopharyngeal (IX) nerve *196*, 197,
  236
Goldenhar's syndrome 188
gonadal ridge **340**, 342
gonadotrophin releasing hormone
  (GnRH) **381**
gonads 339
  indifferent stage 340–1, 342
  see also ovaries; testes
gradients, diffusible substances 92–3,
  251–3, *254–5*
gravidin 382
grey crescent 37, 38, 39
grey matter *97*, **98**